The Secret to a Healthy Spine

The Secret to a Healthy Spine

A User's Guide to Overcoming Back Pain

Jason Gilbert

NH
NEW HOLLAND

First published in 2022 by New Holland Publishers
Sydney • Auckland

Level 1, 178 Fox Valley Road, Wahroonga, NSW 2076, Australia
5/39 Woodside Ave, Northcote, Auckland 0627, New Zealand

newhollandpublishers.com

A record of this book is held at the National Library of Australia.

ISBN 9781760794446

Group Managing Director: Fiona Schultz
Project Editor: Duncan Perkinson
Designer: Andrew Davies
Production Director: Arlene Gippert
Printed in Australia by SOS Print + Media Group

10 9 8 7 6 5 4 3 2 1

Keep up with New Holland Publishers:

NewHollandPublishers

@newhollandpublishers

The Secret To a Healthy Spine

By the time most of us think about how important spinal health is, we've already entered into a painful state of dysfunction, or worse still, already have irreversible degenerative changes. If you suffer from back pain, think about all the important aspects of your life that have been negatively impacted. Does it affect your work, your concentration, or possibly even your earning potential? Does it affect your mood and therefore your personal relationships with your loved ones? What about your favourite sport or exercise? How are they affected by your back pain or limitations? Now think about how important these aspects are to your overall happiness and general health. Back pain reduces our quality of life and health on so many levels.

Unfortunately, this is exacerbated by our society's paradigm of worrying about something when it is already bad, when disease has set in or health and function have been lost, instead of focusing on providing our body with what it needs and helping it avoid what it doesn't. Most of us end up in this position not because we lack responsibility, but because we were never taught how to care for our spine in the same way we care for our teeth, in other words, care for instead of treat (when disease has already occurred).

Back pain is not like the flu. It is a normal reflex that our brain activates to advise us that our spine is not functioning correctly, just like hunger is a normal reflex to advise us that we need to nourish ourselves or tiredness when our body needs to rest. If our body is signalling its need for attention via pain and we ignore or turn off that signal via medication or alternative methods, we are regrettably allowing it to stay in its state of dysfunction, and invariably delaying and intensifying the suffering that we will experience in the future. While flu symptoms improve when the body has dealt with the cause, pain symptoms don't. They have an underlying cause and if it is not rectified, the symptoms will return, usually more frequently and more intensely in the future.

Back pain and other associated symptoms need to be unpleasant to motivate us to act and focus on the underlying problem. In this book you will learn about the underlying causes of back pain, enabling your body to return to normal function and consequently allow it to relieve the unpleasant back pain symptoms itself, instead of overriding the reflex and relieving the pain temporarily while the spine continues to function incorrectly and eventually and invariably, degenerate precociously.

You will be empowered with the knowledge necessary to recognize and eliminate the factors in your life that are worsening your spinal health all while learning to introduce factors that your body needs for correct function.

The Secret to a Healthy Spine is the definitive instructional manual, a user's guide, on how to care for, maintain, and rectify problems when they occur. It works. Over 100 000 people all around the world have benefited from this knowledge over the last 25 years. It presents a refreshing, common-sense approach to spinal care, one that I am sure will not only allow your back to be pain-free in no time but one that also promotes the longevity of your spine and quality of your health throughout your life.

ABOUT THE AUTHOR

Wealthy people are experts in making, saving, and managing money and as such are frequently listened to by those who would like to accumulate wealth. Similarly, sportspeople who have refined their sport, elevated their fitness to its optimal level, and mastered the discipline required to exceed in their chosen sport, become great coaches. As a highly qualified individual in the area of spinal health, Jason Gilbert not only has profound experience as a professional in his chosen area but also as a patient who started experiencing back pain early in life. Following his spinal surgery, he has had to join the dots to reach a pain-free but highly functional state of spinal health.

Jason first felt back pain at the age of seven. He didn't know it at the time, but his functional and structural spinal problem would eventually lead him to spinal surgery. Well before this, however, these problems led him to study and complete a 5-year master of Chiropractic program, which allowed him to work with hundreds of thousands of people all around the world and, as a result, develop a profound understanding of why back pain occurs. During his journey he has also accumulated extensive knowledge that contributes to the wealth of understanding that he passes on to you via this book, *The Secret to a Healthy Spine*.

Contents

This book is dedicated to my family in the influence that they directly or indirectly had on my passion for health. Especially to my brother Daniel who supported me financially while I was doing my masters degree. And of course to the amazing people, colleagues, clients and mentors that have enabled me to acquire the knowledge detailed in this book.I will be forever grateful to all of you.

WHY DO YOU NEED TO LEARN HOW TO CARE FOR YOUR SPINE?

Without being aware of the effects that everyday activities like sleeping, sitting, working, or playing sports have on our spine, we use our body and wait until it degenerates or starts to cause obvious symptoms like pain before we start considering its importance. Our spine protects the critical parts of our nervous system, the spinal cord, and nerve roots, which are responsible for transferring all the information from the brain to the body via nerve impulses. If there are blockages in the communication of these nerve impulses, the body simply starts to change from a state of health or 'ease' to a state of 'disease' because its cells, tissues, and organs cannot function correctly without 100% of the electrical nerve information that originates in the brain. This often happens without any obvious signs (especially in the early phases of any disease process). We continue our lives oblivious to the harmful effects that our traumas, bad posture, minor aches, and a variety of other symptoms derived from emotional problems, job responsibilities, and other daily activities, have on our health and vertebral columns.

The reduction in the normal function of the body occurs so gradually that we do not perceive when it happens. Signs of dysfunction like the black smoke, vibrations, and overheating in the case of a faulty machine become a high fever, pins and needles in the arms, sciatic pain, and headaches in the case of our body. A person who suffers from these symptoms must know that they are actually the consequence of some other cause and not a bodily defect or plain old back luck as many would be inclined to think. Some may even recognize that something, be it a certain activity, posture, action, or even a lack of exercise or nutrients could be contributing to the way they feel. However, most of us do not stop to discover the real cause of these symptoms.

Most people know that taking pain killers to relieve pain or anti-inflammatory medication for something like a herniated disc or osteoarthritis only masks the problem; yet most of the time, they genuinely do not know how else to resolve it. They know that they are not treating the real cause of the symptom and it's just a matter of time before the condition returns and

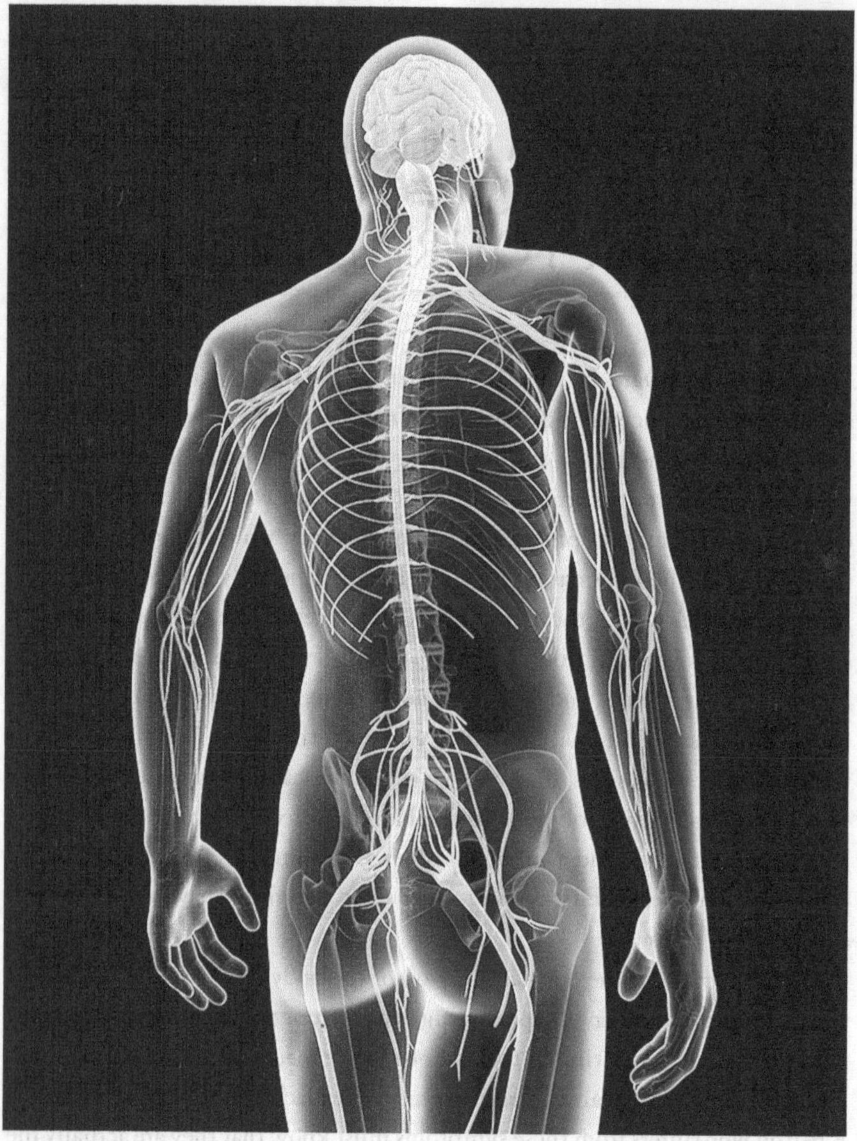

progresses to more intense and severe symptoms.

For others who look beyond the pain, frustration is also felt when they try to discover the cause of the symptom, and fail to find it. They wake up with back pain but do not realize that they are using an inappropriate mattress; they complain of neck pain and dizziness but don't realize that when they lie in bed and watch television, they are putting their necks in hyperflexion, a position that overloads their cervical region. They fail to relate their lumber pain or sciatica or the fact that they limp on their right to the fact that their pants are longer on one side than the other, showing a difference in leg length and hence causing overload. They may even consult a medical specialist in the hope of

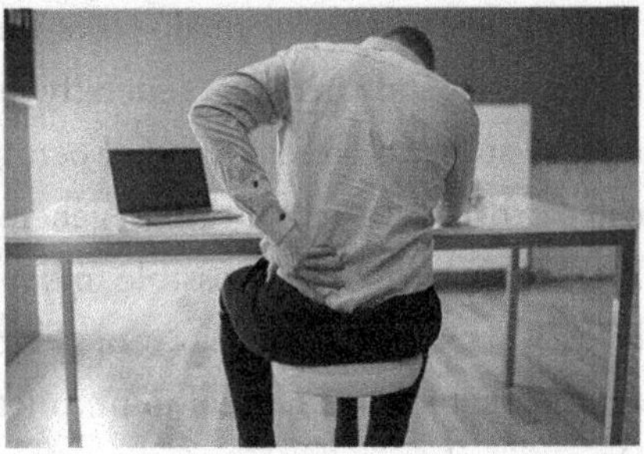

rectifying the problem but fail since the paradigm of that specialist is focused on symptom relief and not the restoration of normal physiological function. In other words, correcting the problem.

> *"What good is remorse if it does not change anything that has happened? The best remorse is to simply change."*
> JOSÉ SARAMAGO

If, as children, we had received and read an instruction guide detailing how to correctly use our spine and our bodies, we would have learned from the beginning of our lives what should and should not be done to help them function correctly. Knowing that the function of our spine directly affects the function of our body, we would be better equipped to make important decisions about our health, and obviously, avoid unnecessary suffering.

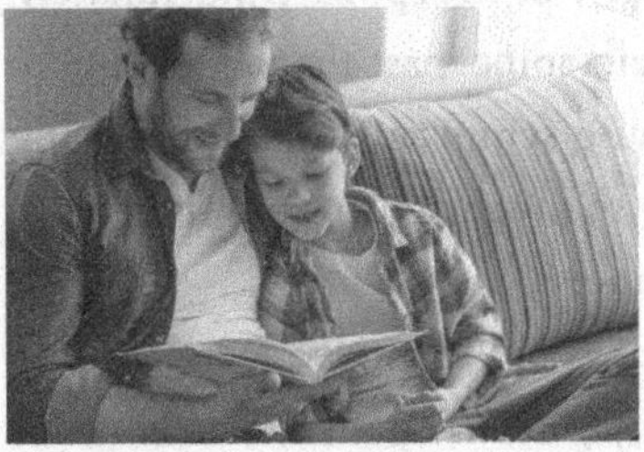

It would not be necessary to first notice a deterioration in our health and feel the unpleasant effects of pain and sickness for us to realize that something was not right. We would know beforehand because we would have learned good habits from early childhood.

Correct posture would always be maintained, as we would obviously know the serious consequences of poor posture on our spine and subsequently our body. We would exercise regularly and perform our domestic duties in a way that would favour correct spinal function. We would drive our car and use our kitchen more efficiently, with less wear and tear on our spine. Above all, we would know that the most important rule would be to take any pain or symptom seriously, to never ignore it, and always look for the underlying cause first. This knowledge would be used to avoid compromising our body's innate function and we would enjoy greater longevity and quality of life, thus slowing the ageing process.

There is no better time than now to start caring for yourself.

Most people take a lifetime to learn about how their body works and how to adequately care for it, however, there are some things that we really need to know from the start, so that we may be able to avoid so many of the afflictions that we end up suffering from. The fact is that we are not born with an instruction manual – like the ones we receive when we buy any new appliance – and therefore generally only learn how to treat our spine when it already starts to present signs of permanent damage, such as reduced mobility, osteoarthritis, vertebral disc degeneration, or joint dysfunction. The problem is that it is virtually impossible to live in this modern world, with the majority of us working sedentary jobs or performing repetitive movements and other actions that inhibit normal joint function and posture, without compromising the optimal functioning of our spine. We can't expect to move less than the amount that our body innately needs without having serious effects on our health. That is the reason why I wrote this book. Our spine is like any other machine that needs to be understood, respected, and taken care of continuously from the beginning of our lives if we are to enjoy its full potential and see it fulfil its optimal longevity.

In contrast to our teeth which are visible, the spine cannot be seen, which is why we often forget this vital structure. Dentists have educated the general population extremely well about the importance of brushing our teeth at least three times a day, but the role and importance of the teeth (sorry dentists!) do not come close when compared to the importance of the spine. Unfortunately, most people only understand this when their spine has already begun to degenerate, a process that may or may not cause symptoms (the latter being the most frequent scenario). Why do we allow so much time to pass before we start to even think about taking care of our spine?

This book is an instruction manual to your spine, a guide on how to use it, understand it, and take care of it, helping you maintain it in the same state, or as close as possible, to what it was the day you were born, functioning as it should. Any vintage car can be driven a whole lifetime as long as it is well maintained from the moment of purchase. Why should your spine be any different?

This book will help you avoid spinal problems before they arise and teach you how to resolve them when they occur. You'll learn that your back pain is actually a positive, normal reflex, that it deserves attention, and should be seen as an opportunity to search for the underlying cause of the problem. You'll discover the danger of focusing exclusively on your pain and relieving it without first discovering why your body intelligently caused it.

I have been a chiropractic sports practitioner for twenty-six years (a quarter of a century) – and have consulted thousands of people in various countries, with different professions and from varying social classes. I have also been a part of the World Surfing League's Medical team for twenty years, working with their elite athletes. Spinal problems do not discriminate against race, gender, or social status. Most problems are caused by a simple lack of information and understanding of how to use and care for the spine. Throughout my career, I have been continuously frustrated to see that most of the degenerative problems that we suffer from, such as arthritis and disc degeneration, result from apparently innocuous activities or bad habits repeated daily, month after month, year after year. These problems could generally have been avoided if people had access to information about the future health dangers resulting from these activities. It truly is frustrating to encounter so many people during my career that had absolutely no idea that they were damaging their spines while they were doing it. Equally frustrating for me was seeing patients (most commonly elderly patients) with advanced degeneration that occurred without them knowing, as there was no pain or symptoms and they simply did not comprehend the concept of caring for something that wasn't already symptomatic. Our body does not always communicate to us through pain or obvious symptoms that some particular aspect of our health is not right (think about how many people have cancer for years without knowing and then get told that they have only months to live).

Many health professionals traditionally miss the golden opportunity to restore the health of their patients by focusing on their symptoms and not searching for and identifying the underlying cause. In the following chapters, you will learn that many of these causes are surprisingly simple to rectify by actions such as learning what good posture truly means and how it greatly contributes to spinal health, replacing a soft mattress with a firmer one, organizing your workspace more ergonomically, or walking. The list of simple modifications is extensive and the positive ramifications on the health of the spine and a person's general health even more extensive.

We must understand that while we could get by without an arm or leg or some of our organs, we cannot live without our spine. The spine is absolutely vital for the normal functioning of your body and the fact that it is not visible does not mean that it can be forgotten. Learn as much as possible about it now. You need to nurture it now, as tomorrow it may be too late. Your activities and daily routine will not change, but after reading *The Secret to a Healthy Spine* (your spine's instruction manual), the way you perform your activities will! As is the case with any other machine, wouldn't it be better to read the instruction manual before you attempt to use it? This book will help you decide for yourself.

"The body, if properly treated, will last a lifetime."

NOEL CLARASÓ

HOW TO GET THE MOST BENEFIT FROM THIS BOOK

The Secret to a Healthy Spine is a comprehensive book containing vital information on the care and maintenance of your spine. It's an instruction manual guiding you in how to use your spine correctly and, as such, has two principal goals: giving you the secrets to a pain-free life and teaching you how to ensure the longevity of your spine.

You will learn that the real definition of health is probably not what you always thought it was. You will be challenged to learn that back pain and other unpleasant symptoms are actually positive, deliberate reflexes of bodily communication. Unlike other material previously written on this subject, this book will teach you that it is extremely dangerous to simply focus on the pain, concentrating on its relief. To understand this, you must recognize how your body works. You'll find a questionnaire for PHYSICAL, CHEMICAL AND EMOTIONAL CAUSES of back pain that will help you to pinpoint the root cause of your pain and symptoms. It will then be easier to read through the book and will allow you to further research potential causes. Even if you are tempted to uncover the cause of your problems quickly, please resist doing so, as you will get a limited understanding of your very unique situation and all of the other possible factors influencing you. Pain and other symptoms are generally caused by multiple factors, especially when the problems are chronic (long-standing).

You will learn about the three main causes of back pain: PHYSICAL, CHEMICAL AND EMOTIONAL.

Information about PHYSICAL CAUSES applies to everybody since everybody 'uses and abuses' their spine every day. The spine is a machine that can be bio-mechanically compromised through so many of the activities and postures that it endures day after day, year after year. The principal causes of these PHYSICAL problems will be discussed and you will learn how to correctly execute these activities, many of which are probable causes of your present or future symptoms.

The focus will then be shifted to CHEMICAL CAUSES of pain and you will learn how what we eat and ingest can influence our physical and emotional health. Inflammatory foods, drinks and other substances as well as cigarette smoking, alcohol and sugar add to the inflammation caused by the pre-existing physical problems in your life. Why aggravate this inflammation and accelerate damage by unknowingly ingesting substances that will worsen your back pain and other symptoms? This chapter will help you recognize and avoid these silent aggressors.

Lastly, in the chapter EMOTIONAL CAUSES of back pain, you will discover how the power of our mind and the quality of our thoughts and emotions influences our health and the pain we feel. We are all subject to the effects of stress, poor sleep patterns and alterations in the level of happiness. As such, it is very important to recognize when symptoms appear and understand how our emotional state influences our levels of inflammation and consequently, our health.

Imagine revealing to someone who had never brushed their teeth the concept of preventative dental hygiene. Initially, it would be difficult to accept since this habit had never been practiced. However, shortly after commencing with this new habit, it would not only make perfect sense but the results would be observed quickly, validating the decision to change. The concepts that will be presented in this book will leave you with the same degree of satisfaction in regards to your spine. They will empower you with the knowledge to care for your spine yourself instead of relying on someone to relieve your pain when spinal dysfunction finally manifests itself. Some of them may seem ineffective or unnecessary, however, please read with an open mind as they offer the opportunity of a pain-free future if you are accustomed to pain. If you are one of the lucky ones who hasn't suffered back pain until now, these concepts will help you have a healthy, fulfilled lifestyle and the guarantee of a future without being restricted by pain or disability.

The Secret to a Healthy Spine is all about human health optimization on all levels, and in this book, this starts with the spine. You will learn about basic spinal anatomy, and how this relates to the optimal function of the whole body. Covering topics such as flexibility, the definition of health, posture, the role of the nervous system in instructing the body on how to perform basic tasks that you've performed your whole life without actually being told how. This book is a user's guide to the spine and it contains the information necessary to not only keep your spinal health in its actual state but improve its function on all levels. With an optimally functioning spine comes true health (homeostasis), which means 100% cell function.

Understanding the effect of CHEMICAL factors such as your diet, hydration, inflammation, smoking, drinking alcohol, and medication combined with understanding the effect of EMOTIONAL factors, such as stress and psychological pain from the past is imperative. It is only when these factors are considered alongside the more obvious, traditionally recognized PHYSICAL causes of back pain, such as posture, impacts, falls and accidents, and more, that we can start to actually recognize the CAUSE of your back pain or limitation, and consequently resolve it. This allows your body to naturally diminish pain and other symptoms itself.

Have you ever considered that your DIET and SLEEP may be negatively impacting your body and contributing to your spinal dysfunction and/or resultant symptoms? While a dentist at some point has probably instructed you on how to brush your teeth in a way that will guarantee dental health and longevity, more than likely nobody has ever shown you how to correctly EXERCISE, stretch, and strengthen your spine to maintain its optimal function. *The Secret to a Healthy Spine* will guide you through these vital tools.

So, get ready for the journey. Whether you are feeling pain or simply want to get your spine to its best possible state of function, in the following chapters *The Secret to a Healthy Spine* will take you on a journey of transformation, one that will help you deal with any challenges better than ever.

Look forward to finally learning the pillars of spinal health, guaranteeing you a life without limitations, a higher quality of health, and the ability to fulfil all of your goals.

HEALTH = 100% FUNCTION

Health is only possible when your body is functioning 100% correctly! In other words, when every cell of your body is working at its full potential.

We start to lose our health when our body starts to function less than 100% correctly. It's as simple as that. As most pathologies affecting our quality of life are degenerative, there are various grades and stages in the degenerative process caused by lack of health. Pain and other symptoms that warn us of these conditions are often only activated when there is much less than 100% of normal function, for example, as we see often in cases such as cancer, arthritis, and other degenerative illnesses, where people only find out they have a disease when obvious symptoms appear. Undoubtedly, their state of health has been less than optimal for much longer than when their symptoms first appear.

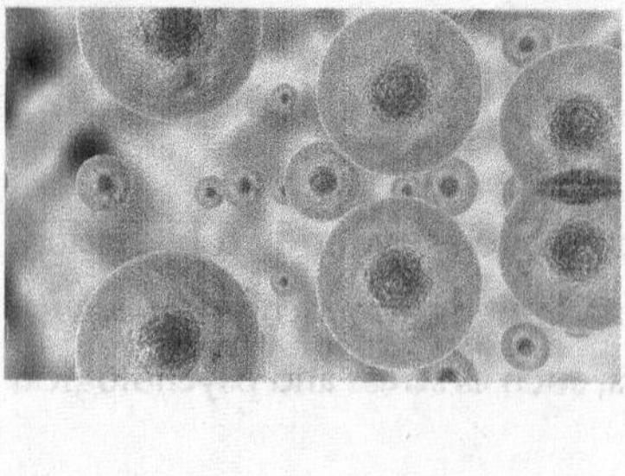

If you eat something rotten and your body intelligently recognizes that and rejects it via the gag (vomit) reflex, you are healthy! You may not feel very well at that moment, but this reaction is totally healthy and necessary. One can say the same thing for fever, coughs, or hiccups, all signs that your innate intelligence is functioning as it should. Our traditional concept of 'health' is related to the suppression of symptoms and resolving emergencies in times of crisis or illness.

Dorland's Dictionary, one of the world's most well-known medical dictionaries and a reference for many doctors and specialists, defines health as "mental, physical and social well-being and not simply the absence of disease and infirmity."

True health is when your body is functioning at 100% of its mental, physical, and emotional potential. If something in your body, a cell, tissue or organ, is not functioning 100% optimally, you are not 'healthy'. You would have degrees of dysfunction and so therefore degrees of sickness, even if you may not be made conscious of it via obvious symptoms such as pain.

Too many people judge their health by how they feel or how they look in the mirror. Sadly, this incorrect definition can result in not only a reduction in the quality of their life while they are alive but also in a death that may be sooner or more painful than what their body was genetically programmed to experience. Therefore, learning the true definition of health is key. It will not only prolong your life but also allow you to enjoy the highest quality of life possible.

WHY DOESN'T THE SYSTEM WORK?

> *"If someone is searching for health, ask them first if they are willing to avoid the causes of disease in the future; if not, refrain from helping them."*
>
> SOCRATES

It is a sad fact that we as humans only worry when there is already a problem. We may have eaten sugary food for years and only worry when the doctor tells us that our insulin levels are dangerously high and that we are pre-diabetic. We may suffer from stomach problems such as gastric reflux or ulcers as a result of an inadequate diet, but only really worry about it when the discomfort is so strong that it prevents digestion. Many cases of cancer could have been avoided had early symptoms been recognized and taken seriously. Sadly, over 85% of all degenerative illnesses happen as a result of poor lifestyle choices. When we stop to think about it, it is not only our health that we are careless with. Who in their life hasn't driven a car past the date that the mechanic recommends for its next service? Or when the oil or tire air pressure only end up being checked when the temperature is already too hot or the tire is so bald that it's no longer providing traction? And what about our personal relationships? How often do we ignore a problem with a spouse, co-worker, or friend simply because we prefer to avoid the unpleasant possibility of conflict, letting the problem grow to a possibly unbearable or destructive stage? Ignoring these sorts of problems will always result in much more serious consequences somewhere down the line.

As humans, we are simply not accustomed to thinking about prevention nor do we care for what we have while we have it. Without pain or unpleasant reminders, we simply follow the pain-free path, often oblivious to the direction that it is taking us in.

The level of pollution in our world is another example. We have polluted the environment so much and for so long that we're almost to the point of no return, possibly leaving us unable to reverse the situation. There are countless examples of human neglect, where we become conscious of the situation only when it is too late. How many more can you think of?

How many of us are eating greasy, sugary, salty foods and only worry when we become obese or hypertensive (high blood pressure) or, even worse, after a heart attack? We may smoke for decades and understandably believe that, because nothing serious has ever happened, or because "my friend's grandmother smoked her whole life and died at the age of 98" that everything is fine. That is until we are informed by our doctor that we have lung cancer. Many of us live stressful lives, depriving ourselves of sleep, suffering from insomnia and other problems resulting from low immunity such as constant colds and cases of flu, or recurrent allergies but only stop to examine the situation when there is a serious problem. When we reach this stage of neglect, is it really necessary to do the standard medical tests to 'officially' confirm that we're not healthy? Why do so many people abuse their health for so long and use the results of diagnostic tests to supposedly define whether they are healthy or not, as the tests only warn them if they have finally arrived at a measurable level of dysfunction? These diagnostic tests are not a measure of our health, but rather a confirmation of whether we are in a state of disease or not. We must understand that DIS-EASE starts with cellular dysfunction and that this commences way before it gets to measurable levels via pathological exams. DIS-EASE starts when we lose EASE.

There are no diagnostic methods to measure the exact percentage of health or EASE we have, so we should not have a false sense of confidence when seeing that our DIS-EASE test results 'were not so bad' and continue repeating the same mistakes with our health. This is unfortunately how it plays out for most people.

It is no different when addressing spinal problems since a large percentage of the population misuse their spine without consciously knowing they are doing so and assume that they are fine simply because they feel fine and are symptom-free.

CASE STUDY

David was an apparently healthy, symptom-free 42-year-old who accompanied his wife to a consultation. After hearing that her problems had been developing for decades, despite the pain being very recent, he decided to get examined and take some X-rays. He said that he'd never felt any back pain and, therefore, assumed that there were no problems. During his physical examination, I noticed that his spine was very rigid, with thoracic kyphosis (increased curve of his upper back). He then said that he'd always had difficulty maintaining an upright posture. When we looked at his X-rays, we discovered osteophytes (bone spurs) throughout his whole dorsal spine! David was shocked when he saw the X-ray results and how advanced his arthritis was. His first reaction was, "But I never felt anything".

I have witnessed similar situations happen literally hundreds of times in my twenty-six-year career. The patient is generally astonished when they discover that they have a degenerative problem that has been occurring for decades without any obvious signs such as pain to advise them and allow them to change the factors and environment that are causing the degeneration.

TIP

There is a common misconception about X-rays and how unnecessary radiation may be harmful to our health. It is important to understand that the radiation emitted from microwave ovens, mobile phones and even the amount we receive on a plane during an overseas trip, are all damaging. It simply depends on the dose. Similarly, a one-off set of X-rays, despite having a very low dose of radiation, offer an opportunity to observe the bio-mechanical effects of years or decades of spinal dysfunction, such as Osteoarthritis (bone/joint degeneration), Degenerative Disc Disease (wear and tear on our discs), or structural anomalies such as scoliosis, etc. Almost always the degeneration discovered in the X-rays shows that the problem has been present for way longer than the patients' symptoms. It is my opinion, after more than 26 years of clinical experience and seeing tens of thousands of people and their X-rays, that X-rays are an imperative tool to both doctor and patient. Problems discovered in an X-ray can motivate somebody to take continual care of themselves as well as help their practitioners provide the most appropriate stretching and postural advice.

MYTH – Spinal problems always cause pain

Although many of my patients come to the clinic with back pain or some other symptom related to the spine, most of them have problems that began long before the onset of their pain.

Changes in the bio-mechanical function of the spine unfortunately take months or years to manifest themselves as pain and other symptoms. Most patients over 35 years of age have some kind of structural 'surprise' when we study their X-rays, as the accumulation of decades of spinal dysfunction results in wear and tear on bones, joints, cartilages and intervertebral discs. This is not totally unexpected, since we are subjected to many PHYSICAL factors such as bumps and traumas, falls, bad postural habits, and other harmful influences that alter the alignment of the spine. If we don't correct the resultant spinal dysfunction of these impacts soon after occurring, our situation will be much like that of a misaligned wheel when it goes over a bump or a hole in the road – the resultant uneven load on the tire wears it out faster.

With this type of degeneration, X-rays literally show the black and white reality of what is occurring.

It is possible to identify areas of the spine or a certain vertebra that have been subjected to excessive forces and therefore manifested bone degeneration in the form of osteoarthritis. I recommend that everyone over 20 years of age get examined by a spinal specialist who understands how to analyse X-rays to determine how their habits and physical traumas have affected the structure of their spine.

After seeing their X-rays many people say, "But I've only been in pain for a week!" or "But the cause of my pain was the fall and that only happened a month ago" and forget the 'other' fall or falls from thirty years ago that inevitably contributed to the bone degeneration they observe on their X-rays. They may also forget that they carried their backpack on the same shoulder for their entire school lives, slept face down their whole lives, played contact sports and many other activities that negatively affect spinal function. This process is similar to the accumulative lung damage that smoking causes, repeated and insidious, as chronic smokers suffer relatively little during the process and most don't stop to relate the cough to any serious bodily warning sign of the damage they are causing.

Except for acute pain caused by trauma, back pain in most cases appears long after the normal bio-mechanics of the spine were disrupted.

> *"We feel the pain, but not its absence."*
> ARTHUR SCHOPENHAUER

CASE STUDY

Brendan came to my clinic with severe lumbar pain on his right side. He was convinced that the pain had started when he bent down to pick his baby up off the floor. He said that he had never felt a pain like that before and could not remember any previous trauma. Upon examination, I asked him to stand on two scales, with a foot on each one, and discovered that he was 5 kilograms heavier on the right side of his body. During the observation, I realized that his right shoe was also notably more worn out than the left. On his X-rays, I observed that his right leg was 7 mm shorter than the left. There was significantly more load going through his right side. No wonder his spine finally made it clear that it needed attention!

These structural problems had obviously been present for many years, perhaps since he stopped growing or possibly even since he was born. This accumulation of load over the years resulted in a bio-mechanical compromise that overloaded some areas of his spine more than others. When he bent down, it was simply the straw that broke the camel's back. The body reacted with muscle contraction and inflammation of the lumbar spine and the sciatic nerve, causing extreme pain. This was a perfectly normal reflex caused by the brain to protect him from damaging his spine any further until the brain had the time to access whether his problem posed a threat to the normal function of the nervous system. He was pain-free after receiving a month of chiropractic adjustments, deep tissue massage, and using a heel lift to balance the load between each side of his body.

Our health system is unfortunately partly responsible for cases like Brendan's. We are encouraged to visit a doctor usually only when we are already symptomatic. We are accustomed to losing our health and then having somebody else pay for it. Health funds don't generally pay for health maintenance and as such, we aren't accustomed to paying for it out of our own pockets. It's the same as any other insurance. Car insurance is relevant for paying for damages after an accident or when the car is stolen but does not cover the cost of anything that ensures the longevity of your car, like servicing your car and the regular change of oil and air filters etc.

MYTH – If I am sick, I will feel sick.

Most disease processes develop without any symptoms. Let's consider the case of heart disease. For 80% of people that suffer from cardiac disease, their first symptom is cardiac arrest. Of these people, 12% will die (Statistic from the Centre of Disease Control and Prevention (CDC)).That's really sad. Most of these people are examined regularly for the standard markers of heart disease, such as blood pressure and cholesterol, but they still ended up suffering from cardiac arrest. So, what's the problem? Where are we going wrong? Have you ever heard of someone who everyone considers as being 'super fit' and 'the healthiest person I know', dying of a sudden heart attack whilst practicing the sport that they loved? Did that person simply develop a problem just before they died? Probably not. They more than likely suffered from heart problems asymptomatically and therefore understandably thought that they were 'healthy'.

Health insurance companies and government health programs, such as Medicare in Australia or the National Health Service in the United Kingdom, cover costs when we are already sick or where there is a suspicion of a disease process occurring. Whether it be a hospital bill for surgery, blood tests for insulin or cholesterol, a visit to an allopathic doctor, or diagnostic imaging to enable a diagnosis of the disease process that the person is already suffering from. Allopathic medicine literally means something that treats the symptoms of disease and not the underlying cause.

TIP

Focus on the key elements of health (diet, exercise, sleep, and emotional state), before you are obliged to treat the consequent lack of health – disease.

Thankfully we have allopathic medicine when we suffer serious accidents, have cancer or cardiac arrest, and during other emergencies, however, we must not confuse the role of the medical doctor with someone who has studied health and specializes in restoring it. My observation is that the general public confuses the definition of health with disease, or in other words, ease with disease, and also confuses the role of the allopathic doctor. As sick people can receive allopathic medicine and 'feel' well after it, they may be excused from confusing how they 'feel' with how they actually 'are'. You'll read more about this in the chapter about the true definition of health. Our doctors don't confuse this sickness or dis-ease paradigm with a health or 'ease' paradigm. It is the rest of society that does this. Their medical course specializes in subjects related to disease and how to diagnose it. They have a negligible amount of information on subjects related to health such as nutrition, exercise, psychology, and emotional health, the action of vitamins, minerals, and fatty acids, etc. I often compare an MD to a fireman who saves our house when it is burning but plays absolutely no role in the reconstruction of the house after the fire has been put out. Please don't take this as criticism of the medical establishment, it isn't. It's an observation of reality. Most MDs are responsible, dedicated professionals doing what they were trained to do, that is, diagnose and treat disease. They are definitely not trained to restore health when it has been lost or maintain it while we still have it, as their paradigm doesn't include this scope of practice. Health Insurance companies follow this allopathic paradigm and we must realize that by the time we consult a doctor or make a claim with the insurance company that we have already lost our most valuable asset – our health or EASE. As such, too many people are accustomed to ignoring their health until DIS-EASE develops and then have someone else PAY for the treatment of disease, instead of INVESTING in their health to maintain it and obviously avoid the unnecessary suffering that disease causes. Investing in their health would include such things as a healthy diet high in nutritive value, avoiding toxins of any type such as processed food, cigarettes, alcohol, etc., and adopting healthy practices such as regular exercise, good sleep habits, avoiding toxic thoughts, etc.

CASE STUDY

Carol had suffered from back pain for twelve years before visiting my clinic. She had been to several specialists and had been taking anti-inflammatory drugs on and off for five years without any results. After thirty sessions of physical therapy recommended by an orthopaedic surgeon, she went to another orthopaedic doctor who had told her to do an MRI to investigate the possibility of a herniated disc or some other kind of degeneration. There was no arthritis or disc degeneration detected. She returned for 20 more physical therapy sessions and was treated with anti-inflammatory and anti-depressant drugs. Understandably worried by the fact that she was still symptomatic, her Orthopaedic surgeon even recommended a simple surgery, where superficial nerves would be severed to impede the painful stimulus. Since Carol did not want surgery, she consulted three other specialists, and each proposed a different treatment: ranging from therapy with a psychologist (because the problem was thought to be psychological), to trying chiropractic to simply living with the pain and accepting that there was no solution. During her first visit to my clinic, I examined her and asked when the pain was more intense. Carol said that she always felt more pain in the morning than during the day. After asking her about her mattress, I found out it was very soft and over twenty years old! When I explained the importance of a good quality firm mattress for spinal health she was surprised. She had never stopped to consider that possibility and initially rejected the idea since she had consulted so many specialists and tried so many different treatments over the years. She questioned, "But how could something so simple have such an impact?" I asked Carol to buy a firmer mattress, and until she did, to sleep on the floor with blankets as padding. She felt a difference the very first night! Her pain began to subside and after a week on the new supportive mattress, she was pain-free!

MYTH – Just because the cause of your pain has not been identified by a health professional doesn't mean that there isn't a cause that is responsible for the unpleasant symptoms you are feeling.

The factors that cause disease and pathology can be present for many years before causing pain and other symptoms. These factors are often inconspicuous and apparently 'insignificant' to most of us and usually right under our noses. We cannot rely on the absence or presence of these symptoms to gauge our health. The fact that this happens is understandable since we have never been instructed on how to correctly use our spine or our body.

TIP – It must be understood that, like any machine with its moving parts, our spine needs care and continual maintenance. As I mentioned previously, this is a concept that we all understand very well when it comes to our teeth.

Dentistry has done an excellent job in teaching us the importance of brushing our teeth, flossing regularly, and having preventative check-ups. Today, it is rare to see people with bad teeth. Most people, regardless of their economic status, know how to take care of their teeth. This is as basic as taking a bath to keep the body clean and is virtually automatic. Couldn't spinal care also become as easy and widely practiced? Imagine the impact on the way we age, the amount of medication we take for back pain, the resultant absence of chronic side effects related to medication, and the incredible feeling of flexibility and mobility that this habit would bring to our lives. When was the last time you met a healthy elderly person with terrible posture or a sedentary lifestyle? That's right, they don't exist. Poor posture and good health simply don't go hand in hand. Lack of physical activity and poor posture are not congruent with maintaining health and we need a healthy spine to allow both.

Unlike the pharmaceutical industry who invests billions of dollars in drug research and allopathy, there has been no financial investment made in creating the content of this book. *The Secret to a Healthy Spine* is the result of over twenty-six years of clinical experience with over one hundred thousand patients from all economic classes, educational backgrounds, and ages. By simply listening to them, examining them, and joining the dots I was able to find the real cause of their symptoms and accumulate solid information on the actual cause of their spinal dysfunction and resultant back pain.

I made a habit of asking my patients over these years: "Why?" "Why does the pain only appear on the right side of the body?" "Why do the headaches always start at the end of the day?" "Why do you have lower back pain in the morning, just after getting up?" "Why have you been pain free your whole life until last week?"

Unlike allopathic treatments for pain and disease (which don't include finding the root cause of the problem), I learned that focusing on my patients' past experiences was a great tool in answering the question 'why?' This is how I helped them resolve their pain and symptoms, while also saving them from any other more dangerous conditions that could have resulted if the problem was left uncorrected.

By using just a little common sense and being relentless in finding the real reason 'why?', you will observe that everyday activities such as getting in and out of bed a certain way, the choice of high heels that you use, the food you eat and the quality of your emotions can have harmful effects on your health and consequently, your spinal health. I didn't learn this at university or read it in a medical journal. I simply listened to my patients. It's simply common sense. Listen to the complaint, identify the cause and remove it. When we combine these findings with a basic knowledge of anatomy and bio-mechanics, health, and physiology, we can see that the contents of this book make perfect sense without needing to spend billions of dollars on scientific research.

Similarly, it is not necessary to teach your body how it works. Since pain is 'painful' and unpleasant, your body's intelligent warning system innately warns you of potential danger. As such, it is not the intention of your body to have you treat and relieve the pain when it manifests, it simply wants you to remove the cause that you yourself created.

When we speak of spinal-related problems, pain doesn't always manifest itself when it should with many activities and influences in our lives harming our spine, without us being aware of it.

In conditioning yourself to ask 'why?' you'll do your own 'research' regarding what is and what isn't favourable for your spine. You'll begin to listen to the symptoms of your body, relating them to your lifestyle, and consequently preserving your spine and your health with the added benefit of living pain-free!

If you suffer from back pain, you are not alone, as it is one of the most common and least understood conditions of modern times. Back pain is so common that many people think it is a part of normal life. Fortunately, this doesn't have to be your reality. If you are willing to find out what is causing it, you will not only relieve your back pain by yourself without the use of drugs or surgery, but you will also lay the foundation for exceptional health and longevity.

THE BASICS – UNDERSTANDING HOW YOUR BODY FUNCTIONS

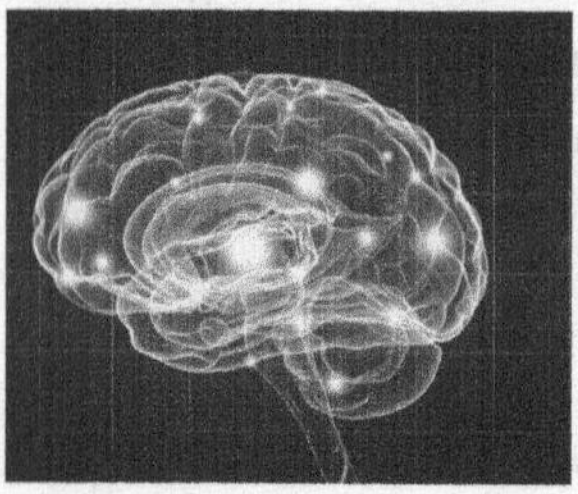

THE BRAIN IS THE MASTER CONTROL CENTRE FOR THE BODY

The brain controls the function of each cell, tissue, organ, and system in our body. One of the keys to good health is a healthy nervous system. Blood circulation, blood pressure, and heart rate are all controlled by the brain via the nervous system. Your hormones, digestion, elimination of wastes and toxins, skin, movement, when you feel hungry or tired, etc. are all controlled by your brain's communication through nerve impulses via the nervous system. Absolutely everything is coordinated by your brain. What then is the driving force behind the brain? What life force activates the brain and all of the cells in the body to be able to work and give us the life we have? The answer is innate intelligence.

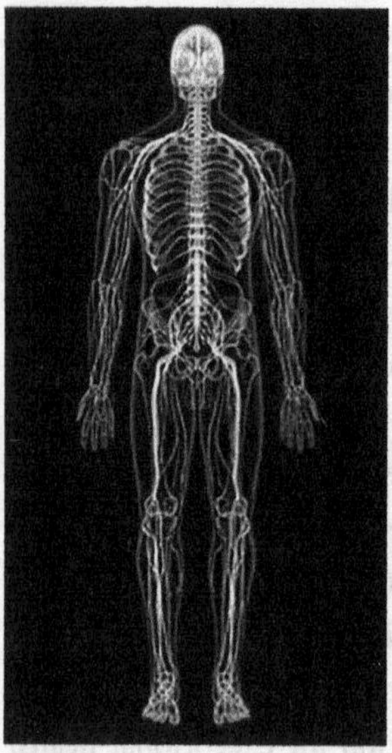

THE NERVOUS SYSTEM

The Brain and Nervous System make up the Central Nervous System.

This incredibly important bodily system is a network of nerves and cells that transmit messages from the brain to every cell, tissue and organ in the body and relay equally important information from these organs back to the brain, so that it may control how the body functions.

INNATE INTELLIGENCE – The power that made the body, heals the body

"True knowledge comes from within."

SOCRATES

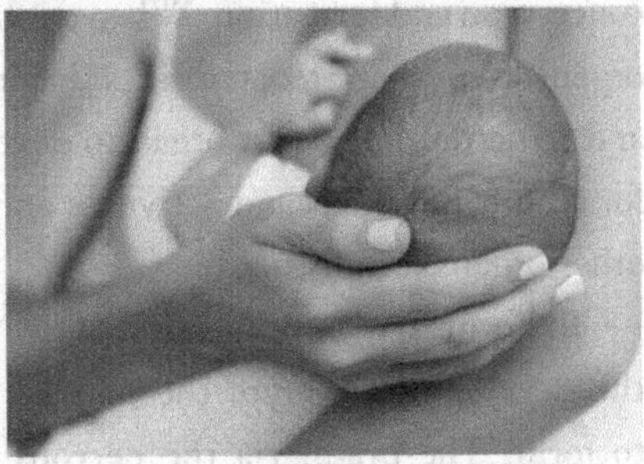

A baby is born already knowing how to feed.

So, what drives our brain to be able to coordinate our bodily functions and our health?

There is nothing in the world, no machine, computer, or example of technology that is as complex as our body. Humans have conquered space, can communicate across the world in a second, and even view live images via the Internet, but still do not fully understand how our brain functions.

The brain possesses intelligence that governs the way it functions and how it coexists with the other cells in the body. There is an extreme organization behind any living being, whether it be a single-celled organism like an amoeba, or one of the largest organisms on the planet, the giant sequoia tree that grows up to 90 meters and lives up to 2000 years. These organisms obviously do not have a brain or a control centre that coordinates the basic functional necessities required to stay alive. However, they still have an intelligence, active from the day they became living organisms. A living being needs a highly organized system coordinating all of its cells, or even parts of its cells, to maintain life. In the case of the human body, this innate, inbuilt intelligence is what keeps our brain active and enables it to perform its job as the master control centre for the human body.

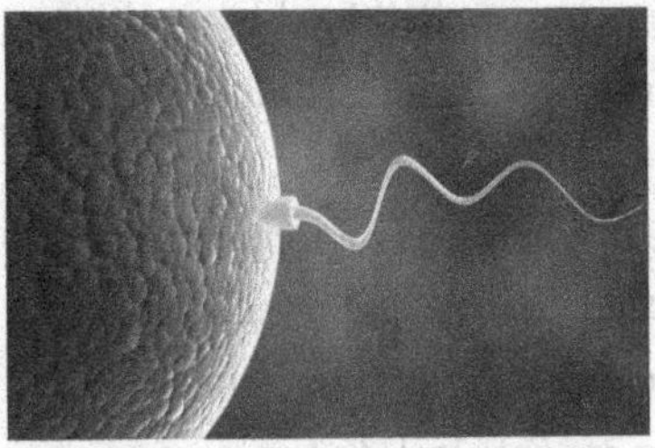

When male cells (sperm) and the female cell (egg) come together at conception, there is an intelligence that directs the order of cell development, making it split into two, four, then eight cells, and so on. This intelligence is the engine that allows our body to function until the end of our life. It is even working right now, as you read this page, with your eyes passing images to your brain, where each word is automatically deciphered. It is also responsible for hunger when your body needs to be nourished, or tiredness when it needs rest, and of course, responsible for pain and symptoms when your body is not working at 100%.

All these processes are unconscious, which means that even if you wanted to control these functions, it would be impossible. Your innate intelligence is more powerful than you or your conscious mind. It only stops working when you die.

How is this innate intelligence stored? Let us return to the embryo's conception and formation. When a cell begins to divide and develop, there is an organization that predetermines the order and position of all our organs, limbs, and structures. The first organ to develop is the brain because it is responsible for all our functions and activities and as such needs to exist before any of the other organs it will coordinate.

To form a communication network between the brain and the rest of the developing embryo, the nervous system is the second important organ to form. The brain, via the nervous system, is responsible for transmitting developmental information to every cell of the embryo's rapidly growing body. Our body does not need to be instructed or taught how to function, we are simply born with the innate intelligence that instinctively guides and controls all of our physiological functions.

While the word innate is not one that is commonly used in day-to-day life it has a very important connotation. It literally means 'inborn, unlearned, instinctive'. When conferring with the *Webster* dictionary we read that it is "existing in, determined by factors present in an individual from birth".

Our innate intelligence is responsible for:

- directing growth;
- regulating body functions such as blood pressure, bodily secretions, menstruation, hunger, tiredness;
- coordinating the function of all of our organs;
- protecting us by controlling the immune system, causing fever when there are organisms that threaten our health, rejecting spoiled food by evoking the vomit reflex, healing injuries such as fractures, sprains, and lacerations;
- our metabolic processes;
- causing pain when necessary and relieving it when it is no longer needed;
- causing inflammation of the spine and related tissues, and organs when necessary and decreasing inflammation when there is no more threat;
- causing reflex muscle contraction when bio-mechanical dysfunction of the spine may threaten the normal function or put us at risk of long-term harm; and
- hundreds of other processes that we are unaware of while they are occurring.

Pain, inflammation, muscle tension, and other symptoms such as thirst, hunger, numbness, tingling, weakness, cramps, vertigo, arrhythmia, tinnitus, and chills, among others, are warnings from our innate intelligence that there are problems inside our body that need attention.

HOW YOUR SPINE WORKS

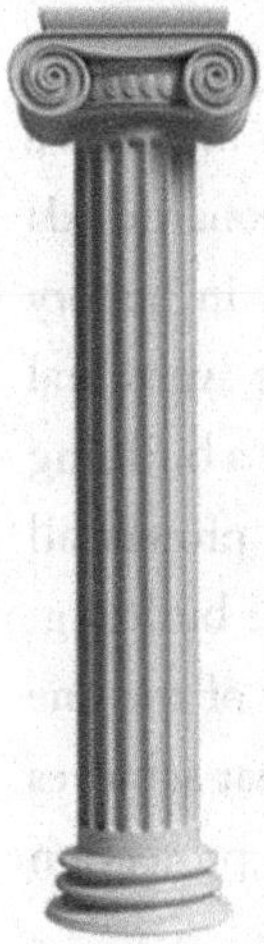

The Vertebral Column

COLUMN is a word of Greek origin, and it means to "support and protect".

To understand how our health can be negatively influenced by our spine, it is first necessary to recognize the relationship between the nervous system and the bony structures that protect it.

An organ as important and delicate as the brain needs protection, the same way that an eggshell must protect the delicate yolk, giving the chicken the best chance of life. The SKULL acts as our eggshell, comprised of a layer of bone 4–6 mm thick. It is an effective armour against potential trauma that may damage our brain.

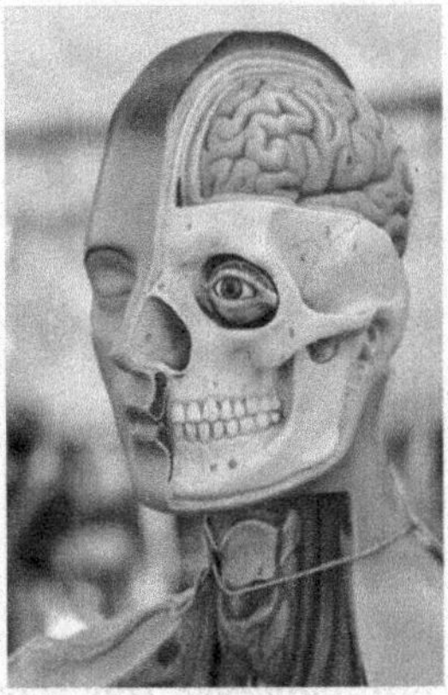

The spinal cord runs almost the entire length of our vertebral column, housing the billions of nerve fibres that carry the information that our innate intelligence sends from the brain to the body, and back from the body to the brain.

The spinal cord must also be protected, and this protection is provided by the VERTEBRAL COLUMN. In the same way that the skull surrounds and protects the brain, the vertebral column (also known as the SPINE) envelopes and protects the SPINAL CORD. However, there is another very important function of the vertebral column that invariably ends up compromising its ability to fully protect the spinal cord as effectively as the skull protects the brain. This relates to its fundamental role of also being mobile and allowing the body to move.

Look at the intimate relationship between the vertebral

column and the spinal cord. Can you imagine having the electrical component of a car encased inside the wheels? Obviously all of the bumps and potholes that the wheels encounter would threaten the ability of the electrical system to do it's job, that being transmit electrical impulses that allow you to control the car. Unfortunately our electrical system is encased inside something that suffers an equal amount of physical forces that threaten it's function on a daily basis.

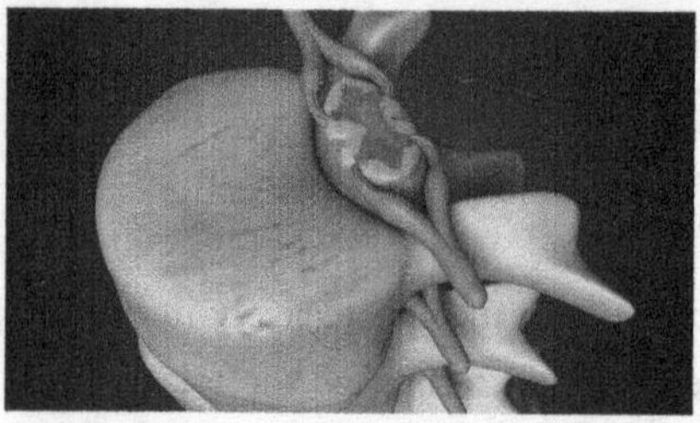

The vertebral column is a fascinating structure. Leonardo da Vinci was the first person in history to accurately depict the vertebral column. He referred to it as a "masterpiece of engineering". Imagine a building that bears its weight against the weight of gravity and manages to protect all of the rooms and inner installations from the elements outside the building, while at the same time allowing each floor to move independently of the one above and below it. Our spine is the only structure that I know of that achieves this union of support and protection with movement.

Vertebral column: Posterior view

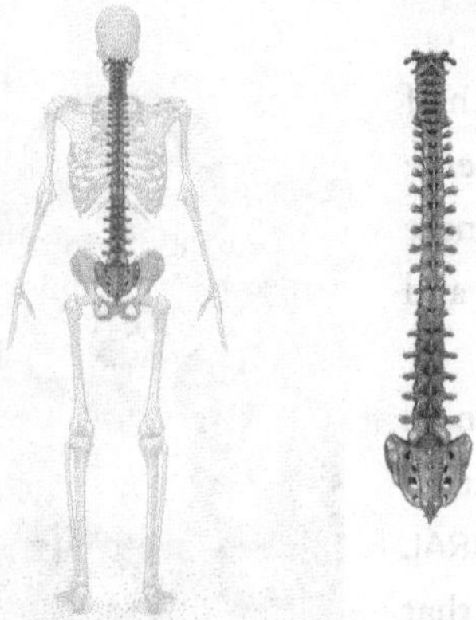

If the bones around the spinal cord were fused similar to the bony plates of the skull, we would not be able to move, bend, or have the free range of mobility that we take for granted. The VERTEBRAE are separate bones, each articulating with the vertebra above and below via an encapsulated articular surface. They do this while also protecting the delicate spinal cord. However, this is only made possible when they are all perfectly aligned, which is no surprise as the spine is, of course, a column.

The vertebral column is divided into four regions, the cervical spine (neck) with seven vertebrae, the thoracic or dorsal spine, with twelve vertebrae, the lumbar spine with five, and the sacrum comprising five fused vertebrae joined to the movable, but not freely articulating, coccyx.

VERTEBRA

The vertebra of each region of the spine have different shapes according to where in the spine they are and the bio-mechanical requirements of that particular area. However, they do have some basic structural similarities in common:

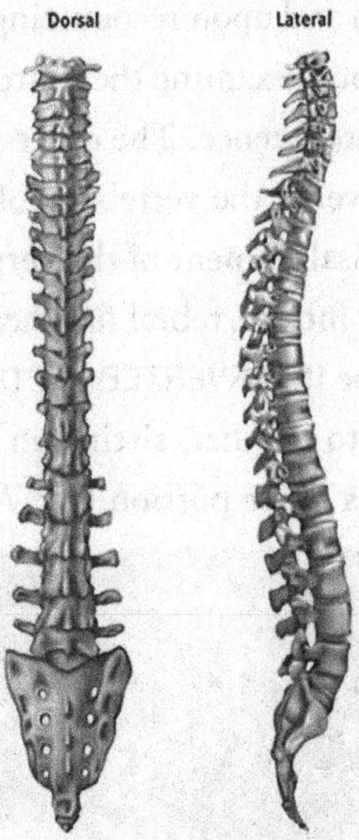

1 A rounded anterior portion called the VERTEBRAL BODY.
2 An oval hollow portion called the spinal canal which encases the SPINAL CORD.
3 A posterior portion formed by three processes, two lateral processes, called the TRANSVERSE PROCESSES, and one posterior process called the SPINOUS PROCESS, all of which vary in size and shape depending on the region of the spine. These processes serve as structures for the insertion of important back muscles that move the spine when they contract or relax.
4 The INTERVERTEBRAL FORAMEN (or NEURAL FORAMEN), is an opening between two vertebrae through which the NERVE ROOT passes. The vertebra above has an indentation that compliments the indentation of the vertebra below, allowing the nerve to pass between them while still freely articulating with each other.

The aperture of the intervertebral foramen can open or close, depending on the position of the vertebrae. A reduction in aperture would obviously be a potential problem if it were to affect the communication of nerve impulses from the brain to the body or even back from the body to the brain. This could be compared to standing on a water hose. The root of the problem is obviously where the break in the water flow occurs however the effect is felt far from the cause. If that flow is used to water a garden, the garden

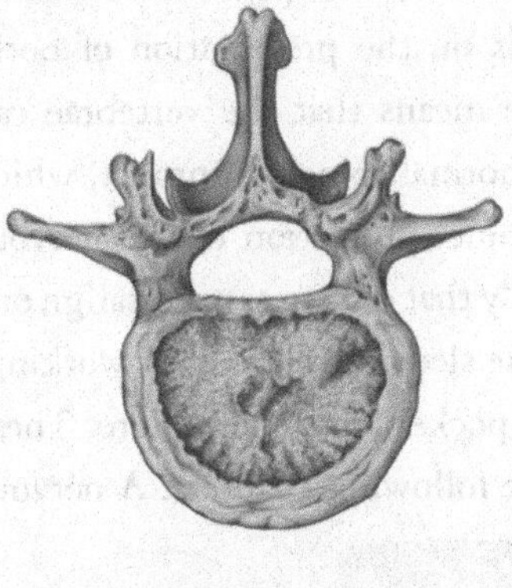

would obviously die if it doesn't receive water. If we were looking for the cause and wanting to solve the problem, we wouldn't be focusing on the garden and just treating that. We would look for possible causes of ill

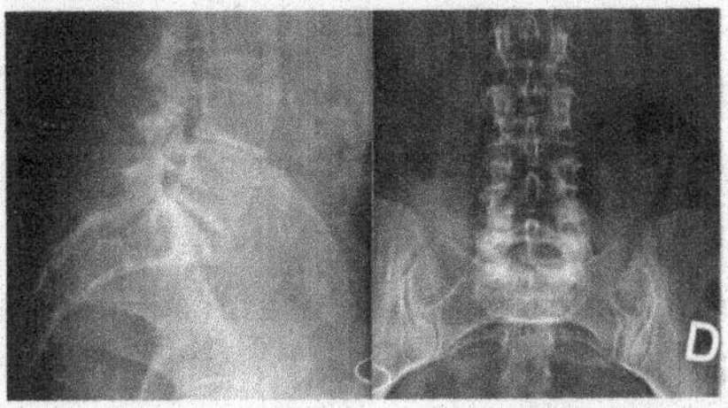

health and upon recognizing that water isn't arriving to the flowers and plants, we would examine the source, finding what is impeding the flow and removing the interference. The exact same situation can and does happen in our body at the level of the vertebral column and specifically the intervertebral foramen.

Misalignment of the vertebral column can cause a reduction in the aperture of the intervertebral foramen.

The INTERVERTEBRAL DISC is a pad of cartilage that connects one vertebral body to another, sitting in between each vertebra. It consists of two parts: a fibrous outer portion (the ANNULUS FIBROSUS) and a more gelatinous inner portion (NUCLEUS PULPOSUS). The nucleus pulposus, which consists of around 80% water, absorbs loads that are transferred outwards to the fibrous ring, the annulus fibrosis.

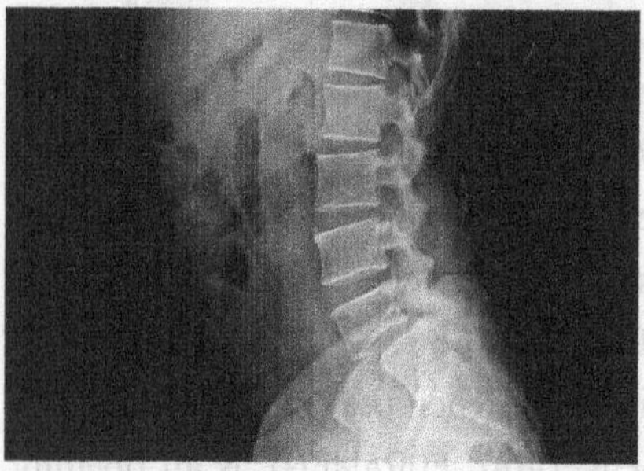

When the vertebral column is correctly aligned, the intervertebral disc manages to protect the nerve root, preserves joint integrity, and contributes to the mobility, protection, and support of the spine. These functions can be performed together because of the ingenious design of the spine and its ARTICULATIONS. When we review the structure and function of the spine, it becomes obvious that it is a complex machine, containing articulating components that can be misaligned and as such, needs continual maintenance, as does any other machine.

Our spine has two important purposes, mobility and protection, and by virtue of its design, normal function depends on the preservation of both. The fact that the spine is a mobile structure means that the vertebrae can also move out of their correct position, out of normal spinal alignment, which compromises the secondary purpose of the spine, protection of the nervous system. We perform dozens of activities every day that can stress or misalign one or more of these bones, from poor posture while sleeping, sitting, or working, high heels, keeping your wallet in your back pocket, and many more. These and many more causes will be discussed in the following chapters. A nervous system without adequate protection represents an enormous threat to our body's health because it is the main form of communication between the brain and body. When the bio-mechanical function of the spine has been compromised to the point of

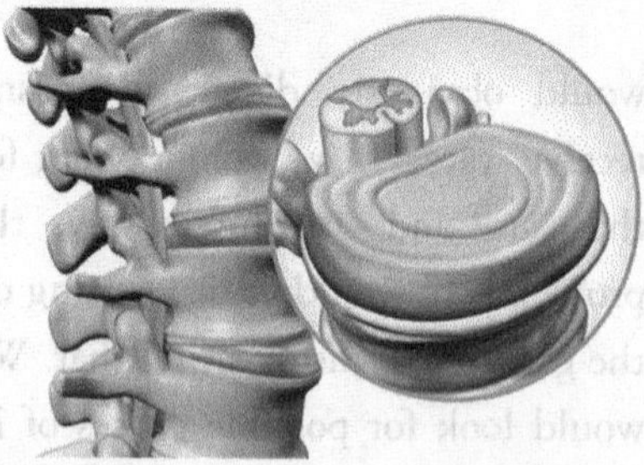

affecting the transmission of nervous impulses, it forms a dysfunction called a SUBLUXATION.

THE PELVIS

In the same way that a building needs a firm and stable foundation, our spine also depends upon its reliable base, the pelvis. The pelvis absorbs the effects of gravity and distributes the force between the two sides of the body whilst articulating with both the spine and the legs simultaneously.

To perform this challenge, each leg must be of the same length and each foot must have the same bio-mechanical function. Small differences in leg length or bio-mechanical problems in the ankle or arch of the foot can cause profound effects on the normal function of the spine. The pelvis itself can also have bio-mechanical dysfunction at the level of the SACROILIAC JOINT, an area that is poorly understood in regards to treatment. The junction of the sacrum and the ilium (lateral pelvic bones) is an atypical articulation, bone on bone, with a small degree of movement. It can easily become compromised through activities such as falls, lifting loads that are unevenly distributed between each side of the body and more. This is the reason why the pelvis, legs, and feet should never be forgotten when searching for the cause of any back pain. I have consulted many patients over the years for headaches or problems with the Temporomandibular Joint (TMJ or jaw) that were actually caused by problems in areas far away from the head, such as the foot or pelvis.

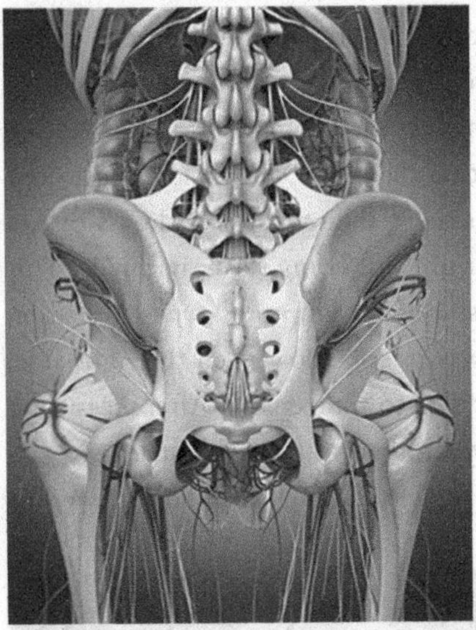

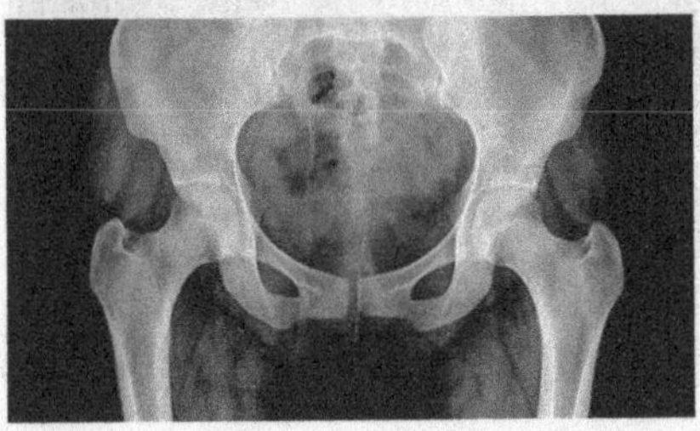

The spine, pelvis, and legs form a kinetic chain and therefore problems in any part of this chain can produce effects in any other region.

MYTH – It hurts here, so this area must be where the problem is

It is quite common that a patient asks their practitioner why they are not doing their manual work over the symptomatic painful area. The example of the car wheel is useful when answering this question. If the wheel of the car is misaligned enough for it to shake the whole car, including the steering wheel, where should we focus? On the vibration of the steering wheel under our hands as we drive or the wheels in contact with the road that are actually making the steering wheel vibrate? Nobody would simply focus on the vibration of the steering wheel without actually correcting the cause of this vibration. Why is it then, when our body is concerned, that we accustom ourselves to just looking at the site of the symptom and not the other possibilities of what could have originally caused it?

CASE STUDY

Andrew, thirty-four years old, is a marathon runner and has been suffering from back and sciatica pain on his right side for fifteen years. Physical therapy helped him to continue running with some degree of relief. When this treatment and painkillers were no longer relieving his pain and his right knee started to hurt as well, he visited my office. He had also been to an orthopaedic surgeon who had suggested knee surgery, since years of treatment had not resulted in relief, and therefore "there was nothing else left to try". When Andrew asked for my help, he simply wanted a second opinion.

When new patients are being examined, I ask them to step on two scales, with one foot on each to measure the weight difference between each side of their body. There should be no difference as the weight falling on one leg should ideally be the same as the weight on the other. The patient's feet need to be perfectly aligned with the lateral side of the scale. In Andrew's case, a difference of 8 kg was observed with the right side being the heavier side. This finding pleased me as it correlated to the side of his symptoms. On examination of his standing pelvic X-ray, his pelvis was inferior (lower) on the right side, and the lumbar spine was leaning to that side to compensate. After measuring the height of each leg at the level of the femoral head, the right leg showed a 6 mm difference and was shorter than the left. This clearly showed why his right side was being overloaded!

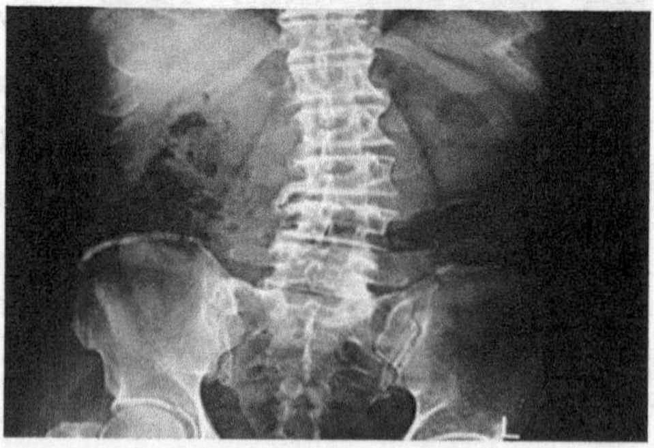

I suggested he use an orthotic in his right shoe and receive 3 chiropractic adjustments for three weeks to see how his body would react. I also asked him to receive deep tissue massage in the areas of his spine, gluteal muscles, and hip that had been overloaded during this time. After the 3 weeks, he reported a complete cessation of the pain he had been feeling. I asked him to stand on the scales again while wearing his shoes and orthotic and was happy to see that there was no difference in weight between right and left sides. I suggested a couple more weeks of chiropractic sessions and deep tissue massage, and some form of regular stretching. He chose yoga. After 2 months of preparation, he was back running at the same intensity as before our consultation.

Andrew's example is a typical one. Many people suffer from pain on one particular side of their body, sometimes for decades, and find it very difficult to discover the root cause of the problem. Many are told by their doctors that the problem is psychosomatic (in their 'head'), or that it is caused by stress.

However, if this is the case we must ask. "If the pain is on the left side of the neck and was supposedly caused by stress, why didn't the stress, (which affects the whole body), not cause pain on both sides? Does stress favour a particular side?"

When it comes to problems with our health, we all have our distinct 'health puzzle' to be solved. It is up to each one of us, with the assistance of our chosen specialists, to decipher the cause of this puzzle and take the appropriate steps to change the situation. Focusing on the root cause instead of treating and suppressing it's resultant symptoms is obviously the most favourable strategy for our overall health and longevity.

SPINAL ALIGNMENT AND THE SPINE'S NORMAL CURVES POSTURE

Optimal posture = Optimal health

Our posture is a window to our spine, and as the spine directly influences our health, we can also conclude that our posture greatly influences our health. When most people think of posture, they have flashbacks to their childhood with their mum or dad nagging them about standing up straight and not slouching with their shoulders forward. Despite our parents probably being

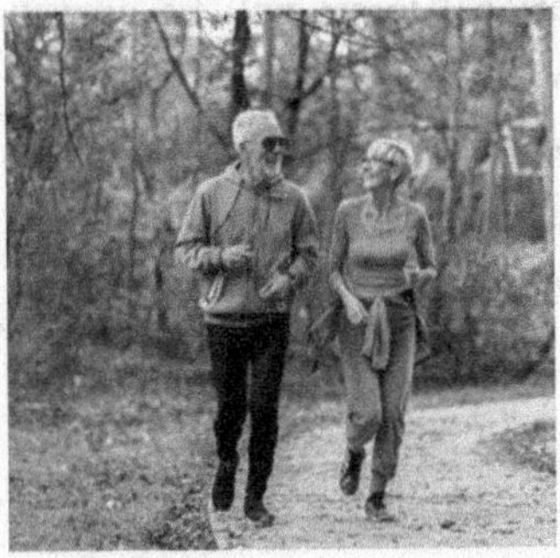

more focused on the aesthetics of bad posture (and not knowing just how much our health is affected), if we as children followed their advice, we'd all be better off for it. While a tall, straight-standing person is perceived as being a more confident, self-assured person, their posture actually indicates an optimal situation for their nervous system, and therefore it's ability to carry unimpeded messages to the rest of the body.

Correct posture enables the body to stand, walk, sit, or lie down in positions where a minimal load is placed on the muscles and ligaments that support the spine and joints.

A correct posture:

- prevents muscle fatigue because muscles are used more efficiently, allowing the body to use less energy;
- helps reduce abnormal wear and tear of the joints;
- leaves bones and joints in correct alignment, and thus allows antagonistic and protagonist muscles to function properly;
- helps avoid back pain;
- contributes to a confident looking aesthetic appearance.

To maintain a correct posture, we must be conscious of the spine's position in two different angles: frontal and lateral.

FRONTAL

When viewing the body's posture from the front we should note that the head is straight, with ears maintained at the same level. If the head is tilted to one side, articulations of the neck are being overloaded, and as a result, muscle tension and pain can result. The nerves of this region go to the head, neck, and surrounding organs like the thyroid, throat, mouth, ears, and eyes, therefore structural problems in this area can result in headaches, vertigo, torticollis, and even problems with the thyroid, ears, and eyes.

The shoulders should also be level, at the same exact height. A height difference could mean an increased load on the neck, upper dorsal region, or shoulders. Many nerves leave this region going to the shoulders, arms, and fingers. Structural problems in this area can result in pain and numbness of the upper limbs and fingers or even carpal tunnel syndrome.

Similarly, the hips should also be level. This can easily be checked by observing the lower fold of the buttock. Both sides should be the same height. If one side is lower, it is expected that gravitational forces will be uneven between each side. This can result in excessive load falling on the ankle, knee, and hip of the same side of increased load, accelerating arthritic degeneration and dysfunction. Uneven loads through the pelvis can also cause scoliosis, increased loads on certain lumbar discs, and even problems in other regions such as the temporomandibular joint (TMJ).

LATERAL

If we look from the side, correct lateral posture should show 3 predominant curves, one in each region of the spine (cervical, thoracic, lumbosacral). The articulations of each vertebra have precise angles that change according to where they occur in the spine. These angles should be maintained to allow normal mobility. Preservation of the curves in each area of the spine will guarantee this. These curves allow each vertebra to move in perfect harmony with the vertebrae above and below and as such permit the load in each region to be distributed to each vertebra and each joint equally.

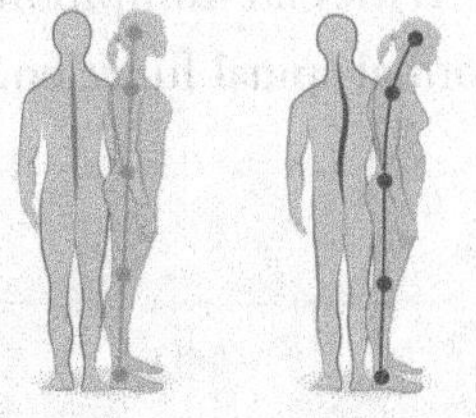

THE NORMAL CURVES OF THE SPINE

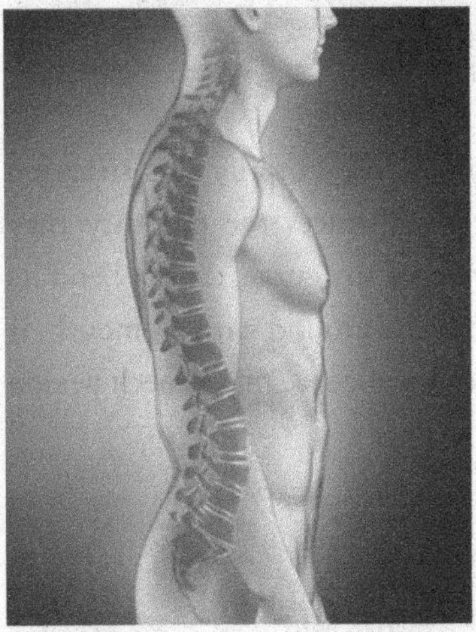

Very different from the problematic curvatures of scoliosis, these spinal curves are absolutely vital for optimum spinal function. These curves can be seen when viewed laterally and normal spinal function cannot be achieved if they are not maintained. Our ever-increasing sedentary lifestyle combined with the postural demands that technological advances are placing on our spine is making this increasingly more difficult. If we go back as little as one hundred years ago, we would find that we were more active, both at work and in day-to-day life. Desk jobs were far less common than manual labour and without the widespread ownership of motor vehicles that we see today, people were obliged to be more active. In the last 50 years, many factors have contributed to the fact that there are far more people now required to sit to perform their work tasks. We are spending much more time sitting, whether it be in our cars or on public transport, whilst eating, watching television, or playing video games, etc. We are also looking down at smartphones, working on

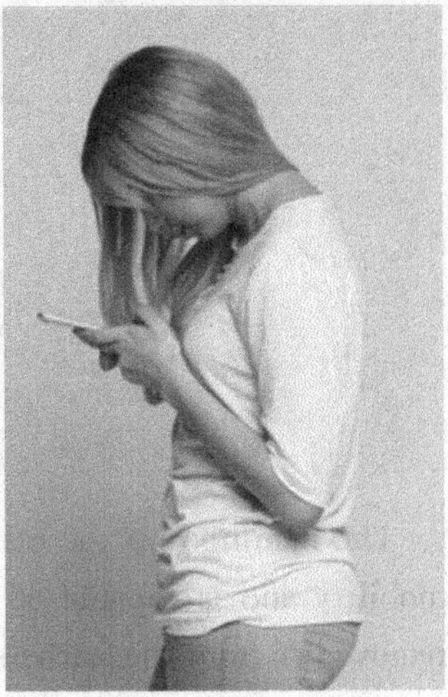

laptops, or watching television lying down in bed or on a sofa. All of these activities are compromising the angle of these curves and therefore modifying normal spinal function.

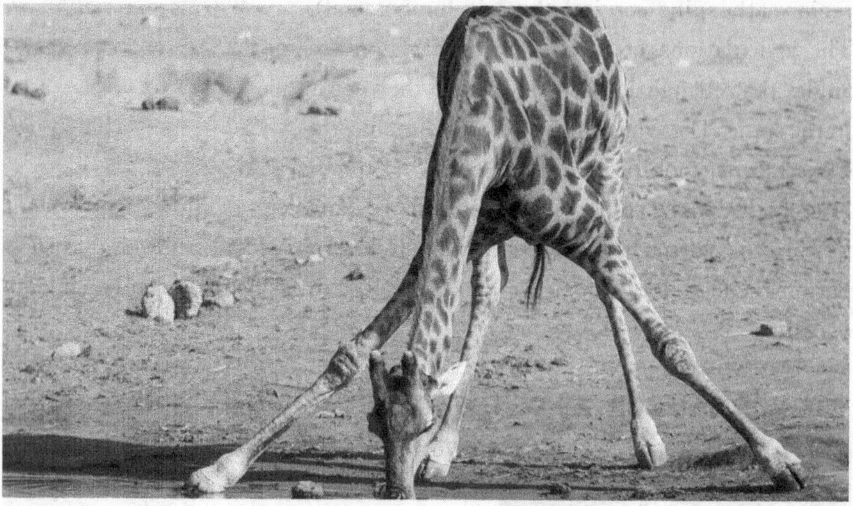

We can use the necks of two familiar animals to exemplify this situation and how the formation of their neck directly influences the mobility they possess. The giraffe, with its straight neck devoid of any curve, cannot bend its neck. When the giraffe picks something up from the ground with its mouth, it needs to open its legs and bend over. Lack of a cervical curve makes neck flexion (bending forward) impossible.

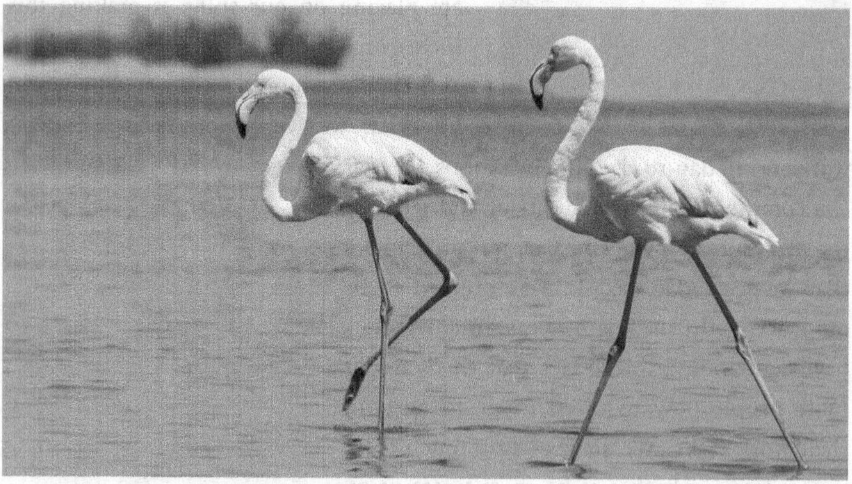

The flamingo on the other hand, with two curves in its neck, has great mobility and is capable of turning its head 360 degrees, and can actually remove lice from the feathers behind its neck!

So where does the importance of correct posture come into play? A correct posture in any position, whether it be sitting, standing, or lying, will maintain the curved form of the spine, helping to avoid factors like gravity that influence its rectification (straightening). The loss of these curves drastically accelerates bony, arthritic degeneration, and excessive load on the discs which also promotes their precocious degeneration. When the vertebral column has it's curves preserved, the distinct orientation of its articular facets is also preserved. These facets need to move as a vertebral unit with the vertebral facets above and below. When their angles change due to the alteration of spinal curves, the facets cease to function in the way that they were bio-mechanically intended to, increasing the load on them and speeding up wear and tear. Correct posture maintains the alignment and preservation of normal spinal curves, and therefore the correct bio-mechanical angles of the facet joints. The majority of my patients with bio-mechanical problems suffer those problems due to alteration in posture and these postural errors will be discussed in the chapter PHYSICAL CAUSES of back pain.

When we suffer pain as a result of actions that compromise our normal curves, we often do so without relating the pain to the action that caused it. Many who wake with neck pain do so because the pillow that they use, or the position that they sleep in, flattens the curve in the neck while they are sleeping. This overloads the articulations, inflaming them and promotes contraction of certain muscles. In these cases, when a suitable pillow is used or the correct sleeping position is assumed, the pain disappears. I can attest to this fact due to the hundreds of patients I have witnessed that showed improvement just by following this advice.

Other people will suffer pain and other more worrying symptoms like paresthesia (pins and needles) in the hands or headaches for years due to the loss of neck curve simply because they have the seat of their car reclined too far back or are sitting too far away from their computer screen. In these positions, their head is too far forward from their shoulders, which also results in a straightening of the cervical curve. Frequently when they correct their posture, the pain and symptoms disappear. When you lose the normal curves of the spine, you compromise its normal function, overloading it, accelerating degeneration and promoting pain and other symptoms. For this reason, recognizing correct posture and learning how to keep it is fundamental for a healthy spine and good health.

Almost all of the structural problems referred to in this book are caused by loss of posture and alignment resulting from normal daily or job-related activities. These problems are easily avoided if we respect the structure and the function of the spine and understand how these two elements are interrelated.

In the diagram below it is clear that poor posture that promotes a forward head position leads to flattening of the neck (cervical) curve. As the joints become overloaded they lose their ability to maintain normal function. The pain and symptoms are the brain's way of calling out for your help to change position, return it to normal and minimise the risk of danger to the spinal cord.

Office workers, dentists, architects, and drivers, among others, are professionals who must remain seated to perform their activities. This creates a huge bio-mechanical challenge for their spine since these activities create a stooped posture, with shoulders slumped and head forward (anterior). Many of us know what correct posture is and even feel better when we can keep it, but we are either overcome by laziness or simply obliged to maintain an unhealthy posture due to the demands of our profession. When this happens, gravity wins; our posture gets worse, parts of our spine start to manifest dysfunction and many other symptoms, and pain begins to be felt. Hopefully now, with a deeper understanding of the importance of the spinal curves, you will be more vigilant in maintaining correct posture and consequently investing in the longevity of your spine.

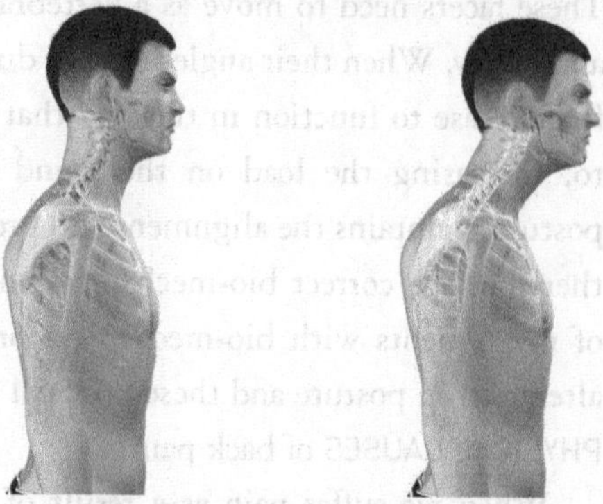

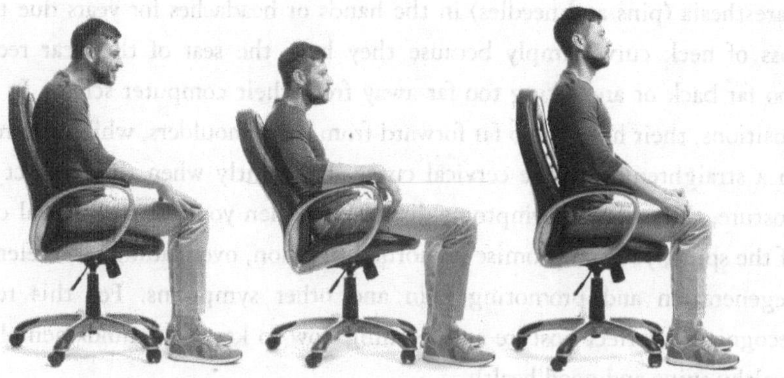

"Overcoming laziness is the first thing that a man should look at if he wants to own his future."

THOMAS ATKINSON

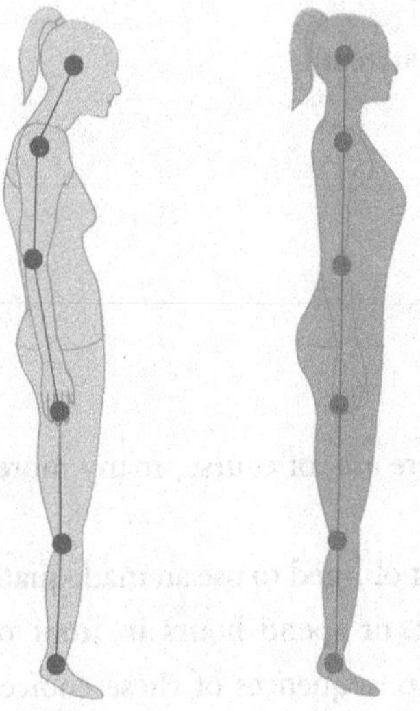

When observing a person in a standing position from the side, a correct posture would show a line we call the CENTRE OF GRAVITY LINE, falling down perfectly through the ear (external auditory meatus), shoulder, hip, knee, and the lateral malleolus of the ankle. When the human body is maintained in this position, the forces exerted upon the body due to gravity are minimal. Should the body shift from the alignment of these key points, the excessive load will fall on areas that are too far in front or behind the line (think of modern-day scenarios like people looking down at their phones with their heads down and necks bent forward). As mentioned, with time, the excessive load will compromise normal joint bio-mechanics, subluxation, muscle tension, pain, and arthritic wear and tear.

POSTURAL CORRECTOR

TIP – The correct use of a postural corrector can warn a person when their posture is compromised.

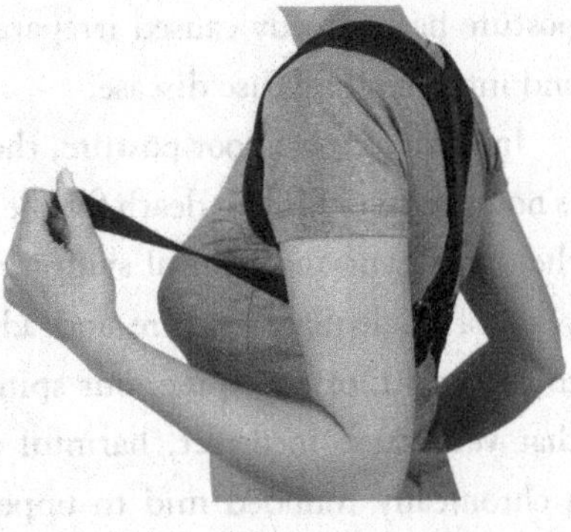

Living on planet Earth means never being free of the gravitational forces. The effects of gravity are always acting on your body in a compressive form. We as humans are bipedal, which means we walk on two legs instead of four. When we are standing, the forces of gravity are transferred through the spine and then to each side of our body through the pelvis, hips, and legs. When there are bio-mechanical problems on one side of the body, these forces can concentrate on the muscles and joints on one side more than the other.

Some of the most common activities that promote bad posture are:

- accidents, injuries, and falls;
- obesity;
- emotional problems;
- problems with our sight;
- inadequate support during sleep (pillow or mattress);
- foot problems or improper shoes;
- watching television or reading in bed;
- poor positioning while sitting or standing;
- occupational stress;
- poor posture while driving;
- large breasts.

These are some of the most common causes. There are, of course, many more, and most are covered in this book.

You have control over your posture. You are not obliged to use an inadequate mattress, sleep on your stomach, be overweight, or spend hours in front of the computer. All these choices are yours. The consequences of these choices generate profound effects on your health and begin the same day that you strayed from your normal position, whether you feel it or not. They can be present every day with changes so subtle that they are almost imperceptible. They accumulate progressively throughout your life until they stimulate your brain to cause symptoms like a stiff neck, tight muscles in the lower back, tightness between the shoulder blades, headaches, etc. Unfortunately for many, by the time obvious symptoms start, these slowly developing changes in posture have already caused irreparable degenerative changes such as arthritis and intervertebral disc disease.

In most cases of poor posture, the body simply adapts because poor posture is not a matter of life or death for the brain and therefore doesn't always provoke the unpleasant and painful symptoms that it should. Through the successive years of inadequate posture and adaptation to positions that are deleterious to the health of our spine, our spinal column ends up assuming the form of that very same incorrect, harmful posture. This is most commonly seen as a chronically rounded mid to upper back, resulting in straightening of the cervical curve, loss of flexibility, and the inability to fully straighten (extend) one's spine. Look at childhood photos of anybody who has assumed this posture later on in life and you will see that they had perfectly normal, healthy postures as kids most of the time. Whether it be years of knitting or sewing on the couch, years of working with the head bent forward or years looking down at a computer (now a smart phone of tablet), these postural changes are 100% avoidable. Please don't wait until it is too late to think about the importance of a correct posture on your health and well-being.

As our posture is a window to our spine with the ability to directly influence the nervous system, poor posture can most definitely result in reduced health and the serious consequences that this poses.

CORRECT POSTURE = GOOD HEALTH

THE IMPORTANCE OF SPINAL ALIGNMENT

Let's imagine that the building in which you live is lopsided. Would you feel safe whilst inside it? Or if one of the tires of your car was deflated. Would you feel safe driving the car? Obviously not, as we associate alignment with stability, correct function, and safety. And alignment starts with a solid base. Now observe how many people have their bases unbalanced. On a sunny day at the beach, you will observe people's bodies. It is common to see that many have one buttock lower than the other when they are standing. How many are supporting themselves more on one leg than the other? You may even notice yourself predominantly favouring one side of your body by leaning on one particular leg when in a queue or in a line for a prolonged period of time. You will also observe that many people have one shoulder lower than the other or even lean their head to one side with an ear lower than the other. When you really start to pay attention, you will see that most people show these signs of misalignment. The fact that it is common to see doesn't mean that is it normal. Quite the contrary.

Our legs (hips, knees, ankles, and bones of the feet) must share the weight of our body equally between the two sides to allow the forces of gravity to fall evenly on each side of our body. If any one of these joints or bones falls out of position in relation to the bones around it, the normal bio-mechanics of that joint will be disrupted and loads will be distributed unevenly. Thanks to our spine, we can maintain ourselves upright. The fact that we are also mobile, with 24 movable vertebrae in our vertebral column permitting its mobility, means that these vertebrae can misalign. Mobile structures must function with even loads being exerted upon them, otherwise, they will wear and tear at a faster rate than normal. Vertebrae can easily misalign due to physical forces such as falls and traumas or even less obvious ones like incorrect sleeping posture or prolonged sitting. Additionally, chemical and emotional factors can also affect spinal alignment by causing inflammation and affecting the way that certain muscles interact with the spine. When muscles and ligaments lose their bio-mechanical integrity, uneven forces exerted by the muscles can cause subluxations. The resultant imbalance between the two sides (left and right) can contribute to an altered bio-mechanical state. The spine can also misalign if any of the other bones of the lower limbs become bio-mechanically compromised. Can you imagine the consequences of having uneven forces continually acting upon our vertebral articulations and the joints of our knees and hips? Yes, those joints would wear our faster, however before this occurs, the gradual loss of function would affect or body and our health in many ways.

When our spine is straight, all joints are aligned perfectly one above the other. Only with this alignment can correct function occur. When the spine loses its normal alignment, the resultant subluxations can lead to a decrease in the aperture of the intervertebral foramen affecting communication between the brain and the other 3 trillion cells of the body.

CASE STUDY

Lachlan was an eight-year-old patient who came in complaining of mid-back pain that had been present for one year. His mother explained that the pain began after he fell from a tree. She said that she witnessed the fall, and although there was some bleeding from a scratch on his back, she was greatly relieved when Lachlan stood up without pain. She understandably thought that "nothing serious happened" as Lachlan wasn't crying or complaining. She treated the abrasion and forgot about it.

After a couple of days, Lachlan began to have hiccups and indigestion after eating foods that he previously ate without causing any problems. A month later he started complaining of back pain. His mother took him to a doctor who recommended an analgesic and said he should come back again if the pain persisted.

He took the medication for 2 weeks and the pain slowly subsided, however, his digestive problems continued. After another 2 weeks, he woke up again with pain and returned to the doctor, who recommended a stronger analgesic and antacids for the stomach. He took the painkiller for two months and the antacid for six months. After this period, during a football game, his spine started to hurt again and at this time his mother brought him to my office.

During the physical examination, I noticed a misalignment (that appeared like a small lump) in the area of the spine where he felt pain. There was a small scar on the top. I asked for X-rays of the spine and found a subluxation between the fifth and sixth thoracic vertebrae, with slight scoliosis.

Lachlan was then adjusted, and by the third adjustment, he felt no more pain. Soon after, the hiccups and indigestion also improved and he stopped taking the medication.

Lachlan's case is very common. When he fell, he suffered a subluxation of the spine where the nerves exit to the stomach and liver, causing a disturbance to normal nervous communication between the brain and these organs and therefore contributing to the digestive problems that he experienced after the fall.

The vertebral column can only function correctly when it is perfectly aligned, and a fall like Lachlan's can cause subluxations. Lachlan's symptoms were his body's innate alarm system warning him that there was a reduction in nervous communication resulting from the subluxation. In this case, hiccups, indigestion, and persistent pain were the vital alerts that the brain was used to warn him that the messages to the stomach were being interrupted by the spinal misalignment.

When functional problems occur in childhood, they may affect the alignment in a more severe form as the muscles of the child's body don't have the 'muscle memory' that an adult's body has due to the years of use that seem to protect the adult spine more efficiently. The deviation in alignment also results in the shortening of muscles, tendons, and ligaments at the subluxation site. In general, this occurs on one side of the spinal column, while on the other side, the muscles can be lengthened. As the child's spine is in its growth phase (the most active phase), the muscle shortening can cause the spine to become even more misaligned, sometimes causing scoliosis. This condition is very difficult to reverse once they become an adult as dysfunction and chronic muscle shortening has been sustained for many years. Subluxations caused at this phase of life can have profound consequences on the child's life and should be corrected as soon as possible after the incident that caused them. Simple acts such as carrying a backpack always on the same side or sleeping on your stomach should be observed and avoided in the growth phase for this reason.

WHAT IS SCOLIOSIS

> *"There are many varieties of curvatures of the spine, even in persons who are in good health; for it takes place from natural conformation and from habit, and the spine is liable to be bent from old age, and from pains."*
>
> HIPPOCRATES

In Greek, the word skolios means 'crooked'. Scoliosis is a word that describes the lateral curvature of the spine when viewed from behind. Some of the factors that cause it are still not known, though many causes are identified but rarely

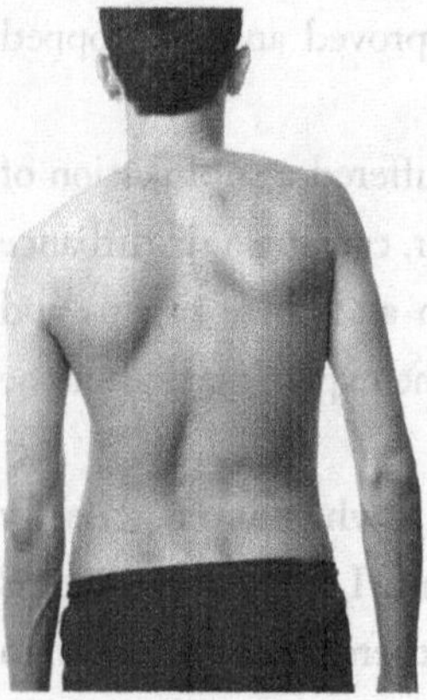

considered in the majority of scoliotic patients. A spine can be compared to a growing tree, which should be upright and straight when young if it is to grow straight. When the tree is in it's growth phase and becomes crooked for some reason it will grow crooked and become a deviated adult tree if not corrected beforehand.

Even though this condition understandably frightens many people, our body actually has a logical reason for causing the compensatory scoliotic curves. Our eyes should always be parallel with the floor to perform our daily activities and must receive and process all of the visual information correctly. When the vertebral column is misaligned sufficiently to threaten the position of the skull and therefore the angle of the eyes with the ground, it creates compensatory curvatures to maintain the eyes parallel with the ground. The spine creates these curvatures to compensate for deviations in the spine from its normal alignment. It is important to remember that most deviations of the spine do not cause scoliosis, especially when they are caused in adulthood, and are compensated for by segments above and below, before they manage to affect whole regions of the spine.

There are two types of scoliosis: STRUCTURAL and FUNCTIONAL (non-structural). A simple test, easily performed at home can tell you if scoliosis is functional or structural.

Start with the person being analysed standing with their feet together. Ask them to look down and run their hands down the front of their legs, looking down as they go. They should bend as if they were bending over to touch their toes. Instruct them to just bend as far as they can without straining themselves to do so, whether they touch their toes or not will not affect the results of the test. Stand behind the person being examined and observe the symmetry and shape of their back through this whole process. In a normal, non-scoliotic case, both sides should look the same the whole time. When someone has scoliosis, one side will be more pronounced, often higher than the other when they have fully bent over. This indicates that there is structural scoliosis, which is generally the most aggressive of the two types of scoliosis and most common in young women during adolescence, with the incidence of 9:1, girls to boys. Its cause is still unknown and that is why it is referred to as IDIOPATHIC SCOLIOSIS. Adolescents in the age group of ten to sixteen years who have this type of scoliosis must be monitored with x-rays every three months, as structural scoliosis can worsen suddenly and aggressively at this stage of life. When adolescent growth ceases, further worsening of the scoliosis is unlikely. Other causes of structural scoliosis include trauma, degeneration, infection, radiation (resulting in deformation of the vertebrae), neuromuscular diseases, and congenital.

The majority of cases of scoliosis are of the functional variety and are less aggressive. They are generally related to identifiable causes such as falls, excessive weight on one side of the body (think of a backpack being carried on one side only), sleeping face down, a difference in leg length, or pain due to other spinal problems such as a herniated disc. This type of scoliosis actually corrects itself while doing the standing test described above for functional scoliosis. In other words, a spine that visibly shows asymmetry whilst standing then 'appears' to straighten when the person bends down.

Spinal curvatures are measured in degrees, and the higher the degree of curvature, the higher the risk for the scoliosis. The greater the degree of scoliosis, the greater the impact on somebody's health, due to the compromise of nervous communication. This occurs due to the fact that nerve roots exit between vertebra and become nerves that supply every cell, tissue and organ of the body.

It is important to remember that due to the bio-mechanical configuration of the vertebral column, it will only function correctly when it is perfectly aligned. Any degree of scoliosis will alter normal spinal function and higher degrees of curvature will increase the rate at which it degenerates, also compromising the transmission of nerve impulses from the brain to the body. There are three principal options in respect to the management of scoliosis: observation, use of a corrective brace, and surgery.

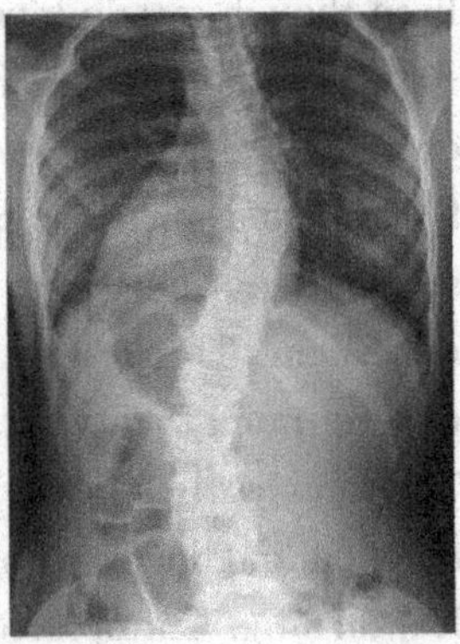

If the curvature is less than 20°, it is considered mild and medical interventions like surgery are not recommended. These cases should be monitored regularly, especially during the major growth phase (10 to 15 years of age) to check if it is getting worse. If there is a worsening of 5 degrees (or more) in a period of 3 months, the use of a vest may be considered. This is a frustrating situation for parents who feel like they are looking at the problem and waiting for it to worsen, without being able to be more proactive.

The vest is also often recommended in cases where the curvature is between 20 and 40 degrees to prevent the scoliosis from becoming more pronounced, though its use doesn't guarantee this. In general, it is used for 23 hours a day until skeletal maturity. Receiving regular chiropractic adjustments, physical therapy, and exercises are also recommended at any phase of curvature. This is because they promote movement, both specific articular movement and global movement of the spine, therefore minimising the load that certain areas of the spine receive. Chiropractic adjustments help improve nervous communication by reducing the effect the scoliosis has on the nerve roots at the level of the intervertebral foramen. These same areas also degenerate at an accelerated rate since the degree of misalignment increases the load on the articular facets. During this period, X-rays should be taken every three months to monitor possible progression.

Parents should be sure that the scoliosis is getting worse before deciding to use the vest, because its use at this stage of life can cause profound effects on the child, both physically and psychologically. Besides the limitation in the mobility of the spine caused by the brace, there are psychological effects similar to those that children with corrective orthodontic braces on their teeth encounter. They are uncomfortable to wear, limit movement, and make practicing sports and other activities with other children quite difficult.

If the corrective brace is unsuccessful and the scoliotic curvature continues to worsen, surgery may be recommended. Two of the most common procedures include using metallic rods to physically straighten the spine (Harrington Rods) or a system of wires and screws (Dwyer procedure) on each side of the spine to stabilize it. In cases where surgery is necessary, operated patients should remember that their spine is a dynamic structure and needs movement. Even though certain segments of the spine have been physically fused by the surgical technique, all of the others still possess their normal function. Many operated patients don't realize the importance of movement for normal spinal function and make the mistake of not doing regular physical activity. Fused segments can no longer participate in the normally shared action of spinal movement. This leaves adjacent segments to receive more load, as they are moving more than what they should to compensate for the fused segments. The muscles, ligaments, and tendons that act on these joints also have their function modified, with some tissues contracting (shortening) and others lengthening. Chiropractic care focuses on distributing the load as evenly as possible between all of the articular facets, promoting movement at a segmental level. Exercises such as swimming, yoga, stretching, or simply walking will help maintain normal functional loads between the muscles and other soft tissues. Anybody that has been operated on for scoliosis must continue physical activity throughout their whole life to minimise or avoid unnecessary premature arthritic or disc degeneration of their spine. Regardless of the severity of the scoliosis, spinal mobility must be maintained continuously to enable the transmission of nerve impulses between the brain and body, thus minimising the risk of health complications.

Many young patients with lower degrees of curvature have noticed significant improvements in curvature measurements simply by doing some sort of exercise and receiving regular chiropractic care. In the case of severe scoliosis, such measures can help prevent a worsening of the scoliosis but are not alternatives if surgical intervention is required.

Cases of severe scoliosis can have serious consequences on a person's health and as such should be taken seriously. More advanced cases can cause cardiac, pulmonary, digestive, and reproductive problems, which usually worsen in later years, sometimes well into adulthood.

Changes in certain daily habits can have an enormously positive impact on the way that a person's scoliosis affects their life. I have observed countless patients in my career with the same degree of curvature have extremely different levels of comfort. A person with scoliosis that has a sedentary lifestyle would be expected to be compromising the function of their spine much more than others and therefore suffer more symptoms for this reason. Similarly, those who have unhealthy spinal habits such as sleeping face down, wearing high heels, and carrying heavy loads definitely complain more of back pain than those who don't have these types of habits. Scoliotic spines do not respond well when they are left in the same position for prolonged periods of time, especially when these positions are detrimental to the normal function of the spine (think sitting or lying incorrectly). People with scoliosis who choose this kind of lifestyle will usually end up suffering serious pain and other symptoms, while others with the same degree of curvature but with proper posture and an active life, will suffer significantly less or even not at all.

MYTH – Having scoliosis means tolerating a life of pain

If you have a painful scoliotic spine and take medication to 'treat the problem', please focus on the real problem. Learn about your scoliosis (it may not be as severe as you imagine), do exercises, take advantage of any opportunity you have to move the spine, and have regular chiropractic adjustments. Maybe you, like thousands of others, can avoid the unnecessary consumption of pharmaceutical drugs to relieve the effects of a detrimental lifestyle rather than the effects of a scoliotic spine. If you have scoliosis and have to choose between living a healthy, active lifestyle and taking medication to calm its effects, I strongly recommend trying the former option first.

TEXTER'S NECK – FORWARD HEAD CARRIAGE

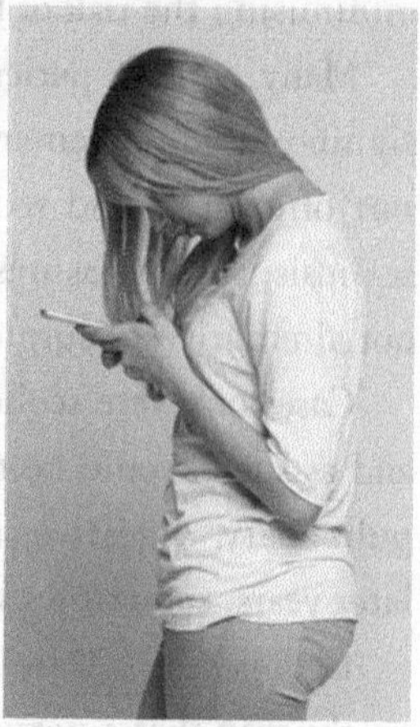

The human head is roughly the same weight as a bowling ball (5 kg/11 lbs). For the neck to correctly function, it is necessary for the curve and all of the precise angles of the articulations to be maintained. This is only made possible when the head is in the correct position, with the ears exactly in line with the shoulders when viewing it laterally (refer to the previous section on posture).

With the constant effects of gravity, we are continually challenged to keep our head in position. Whether it be while we are driving, working on the computer, reading, or walking – gravity influences us to succumb to its effects and allow the head to move anteriorly, in front of the shoulders. This is of course if we let it. If we are not conscious of the necessity to avoid this tendency and therefore do not pay attention to the orientation of our head, gravity will win this constant war.

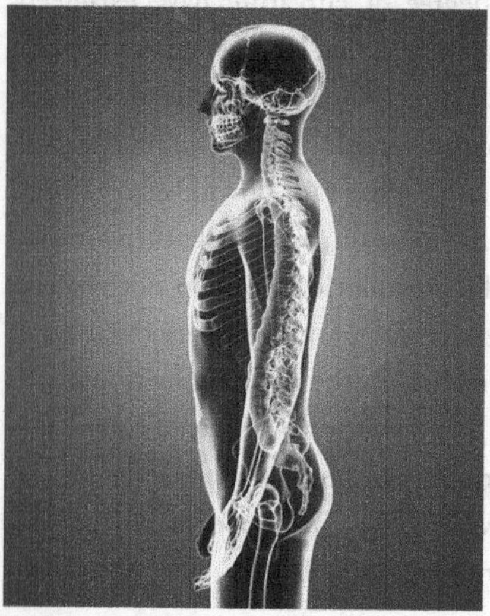

The forward head is a perfect example of one of our habits that usually worsens with time. Have you noticed that lumpy protuberance at the base of the neck of many elderly people? It's called a Dowagers hump. They weren't born with it. It progressively worsened with time because that person wasn't successful in resisting the constant effects of gravity. Young people often come into my clinic complaining about the appearance of a small lump in the same area. They are pleasantly surprised when they see that it improves as soon as they restore their normal posture. Unfortunately, it is not this easy for people who have left it too long, where chronic muscle shortening and arthritic bone degeneration make complete improvement of this lump almost impossible. Certain professionals like hairdressers, accountants, and dentists

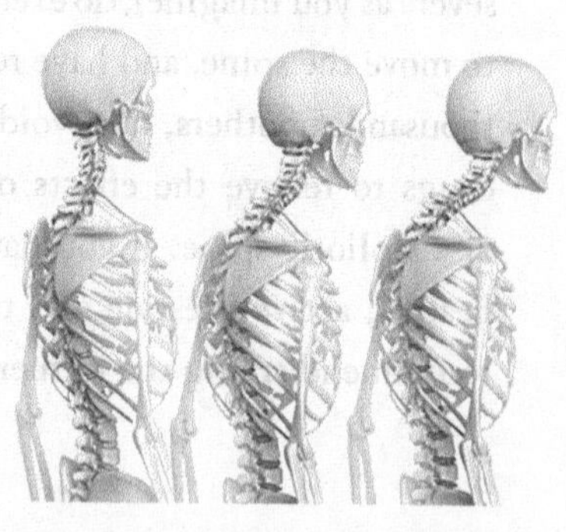

are especially prone to this since they have to look down to be able to work. Accordingly, they should do preventative exercises to compensate for the time that they are looking down with their head forward of the centre of gravity line previously described in the section on 'Spinal Alignment'. Most of these professionals report periods of their life where they have suffered pain or other tell-tale symptoms like headache, vertigo, tinnitus, insomnia, muscle tension in the neck and shoulders, tingling in the arms and hands, and TMJ pain. Most people who listen to their body at this point and look for the cause instead of focusing on simply relieving its effects (the symptoms) will be able to avoid serious, long-term consequences. Those who don't, however, may be suffering from the effects of their profession long after they retire.

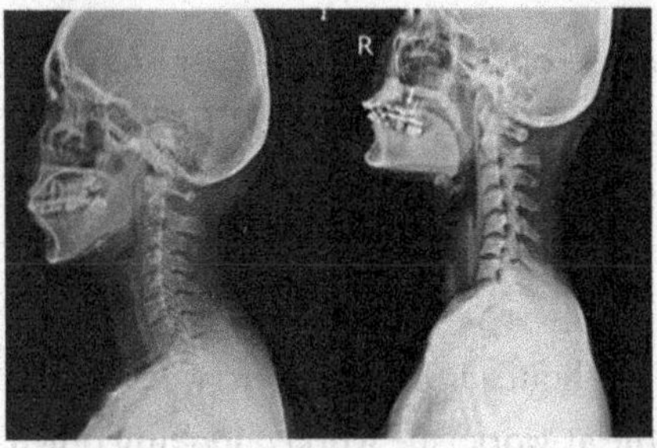

Always seek the cause and ask yourself 'why?'

- Why is there a lumpy protuberance at the base of my neck?
- Why am I suffering headaches or neck pain when I use the computer?
- Why am I dizzy?
- Why is it becoming more difficult to turn my head to the left or the right?

These are just some of the questions that you need to ask yourself to be able to recognize the true cause of your problem.

With the head in its correct position, there are no additional external forces transferred to the spine, muscles, or ligaments. They are not working any harder than necessary to hold the head where it is. However, when the head moves forward, additional compressive forces are transferred to the cervical spine, muscles, and other soft tissues because the forward shift of the head obliges the muscles of the neck to resist it and support the spine by contracting. It is estimated that for every 1 cm that the head moves forward, the muscles and joints of the neck receive an additional 5 kg (11 lbs) (the weight of the head) of tension. It is for this reason that bony and or disc degeneration is way more common in the vertebrae and discs of the lower neck (C5/6, C6/7), due to it being the area that receives the majority of the load when the head is forward.

Sitting with an incorrect posture can be as equally harmful for the neck as it can also be for the thoracic and lumbar spine. One of the most common actions that causes loss of lumbar curve is simply sitting with your buttocks in the middle of the chair and not at the back of it and supported against the posterior, vertical support that a good chair should have. Those who are accustomed to keeping a good posture whilst sitting will usually notice that this incorrect sitting

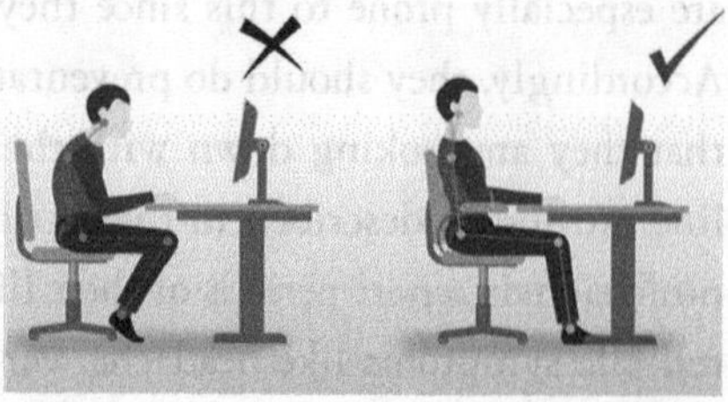

posture will cause low back pain and a sense of stiffness when they stand up after prolonged periods of sitting. So remember, if your head is forward and your shoulders are slumped, your low and mid backs are suffering also.

CASE STUDY

Cindy, a 54-year-old seamstress, worked 12 hours a day for over twenty years sewing t-shirts. For the majority of her time at work, she worked looking down to feed the material through the sewing machine. When she presented to the clinic, she complained of severe headaches that had been worsening in the last three years. She had suffered neck pain for the last 15 years but "got used to it". She took painkillers and anti-inflammatory medication prescribed by her doctor so that she could work with a degree of comfort but the pain would always reappear if she stopped taking the medication. She had noticed that in recent years, her posture had worsened considerably and she felt considerable difficulty in maintaining a straight, upright posture. By the time she had come to me, she was unable to turn her head past 45 degrees on each side.

When I examined her, I noticed that the base of her neck was quite pronounced (she had a bumpy protuberance) and the muscles of her neck and shoulders were very tense. She also complained of vertigo (dizziness) that would come on strongest after changing from a lying to a sitting position, reporting that she would need around a minute for the vertigo to stop before she could walk without falling. At this stage, it was almost impossible to work, which gave her even more anguish because she worked for herself and was not financially secure enough to be able to take time off work. When I looked at her X-rays, I noticed that there was a complete loss of cervical curve. The curve was actually inverted in the opposite direction to what it should have been (refer to the photo on the previous page of the X-ray showing normal and inverted cervical (neck) curves). Her work posture was obviously the aggravating factor so I asked her to interrupt her activities for two weeks and evaluate the results. I showed her specific stretching exercises and suggested chiropractic adjustments. After a week, the symptoms started to improve. A month after these changes, she was symptom-free for the first time in 15 years!

When she returned to work, I suggested that she lift the sewing machine as close to eye level as possible to minimise the degree of flexion in her neck and therefore minimising the rectification of the cervical curve. Cindy also began to interrupt her work activity every hour with stretches for the muscles of the neck and upper back. She continued doing her home exercises and compensate for the fact that her work posture was still not ideal with fortnightly chiropractic adjustments and myofascial massages. She has been symptom-free for three years now simply because she managed to break the 'vicious cycle' of the forward head carriage that her work had promoted, and found new strategies and work postures that weren't compromising the spinal function of her neck.

WHY BEING FLEXIBLE IS IMPORTANT

> *"An elderly person who is flexible is limitless while a young person who is rigid is limited."*

The healthiest elderly people I know are those with the most flexibility. Those people are usually also the most active. Is this just a coincidence or is there a relationship between flexibility and the state of our health? I must say that some of the unhealthiest elderly patients I treat are also the stiffest (least flexible). FLEXIBILITY is defined as having a full range of mobility of your joints and integrity of your muscles so that they can function at their optimal potential and without restriction. We lose our flexibility for many reasons, however, one factor stands out above all of the others – when we adopt incorrect postures (this includes sitting!) for prolonged periods of time. Think of someone you know who has worked at a desk job all of their lives (maybe a lawyer or an accountant), who hasn't compensated for their sedentary job by doing regular exercise. Or someone who has slept face down their whole life and consequently has lost full rotation to one side due to chronic muscle shortening. This problem can further be worsened by other factors such as inadequate muscular nutrition or dehydration.

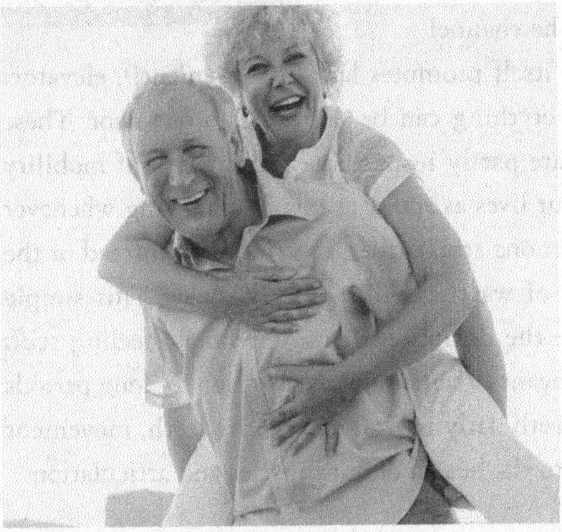

Here are some of the other most common causes of loss of flexibility:

- dehydration (affects muscle function)
- use of high heels (chronically shortens the calf muscle)
- poor muscle nutrition
- favouring strengthening exercises and not compensating by adequately stretching
- doing exercises that don't demand the full range of motion of the joint
- body type
- previous traumas that permanently compromise joint function and therefore muscle function Arthritis and chronic inflammatory joint conditions

Flexibility is vital for us to be able to function the way that we were intended to. With time, flexibility becomes harder to maintain and therefore we need to work harder at maintaining it. Changes in our metabolism and the integrity of muscle and connective tissue fibres change with time, meaning that we must focus more and more on our flexibility as we age. Flexibility allows the maintenance of a correct posture so if we are inflexible, we will use more energy to maintain basic postures like sitting and standing. With time, this can result in muscle fatigue, bio-mechanical dysfunction, and consequently muscle and articular pain for many people.

Flexible people are able to maintain physical activity throughout their lives, which has a direct influence on the state of their health. Another important benefit is that they experience less pain and few or no symptoms resulting from spinal problems, precisely because they have maintained correct posture.

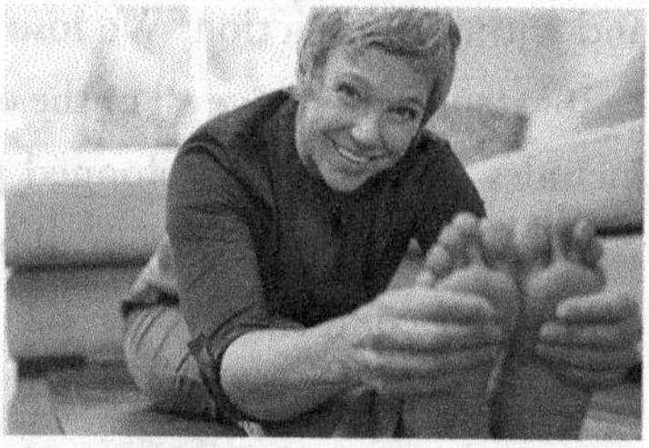

Modern life is promoting laziness and reducing the necessity for us to move. We use remote controls to change the channel on the TV (even the television itself promotes lack of movement!), elevators instead of stairs, and almost everything can be delivered to our door. These factors as well as many others are partly responsible for our lack of mobility and flexibility. We must keep our lives as active as possible, moving whenever possible. Get off the bus or train one stop earlier, use the stairs instead of the elevator, go for a walk instead of watching TV. Simply move! This simple change will drastically improve the flexibility of those who are feeling stiff. Our skeleton and spine are not meant to remain in one position for long periods of time. Just as brushing your teeth daily is vital for healthy teeth, movement and regular stretching are vital to the health of our muscles and articulations.

Most people avoid stretching because they incorrectly think that it takes too long. Just 5 minutes a day will already be enough to improve all levels of flexibility. In just one month, you will notice a huge difference. Of course, the more time you dedicate to stretching, the better the results. You must be patient and consistent in doing stretching exercises. There should be no pain as this is a sign that you may be injuring the muscle fibres, which can end up causing even more stiffness. Be careful if you are not in the habit of stretching. If you have any doubt on how to do it, find someone who can guide you in a safe manner, such as a yoga or Pilates instructor. Get your kids into stretching with you as this will help them form healthy habits from a young age, avoiding many of the problems that we adults suffer, like back pain and degeneration. Remember to consider the other factors mentioned above, like general movement, nutrition, and hydration when focusing on improving your flexibility. If muscles are poorly nourished or hydrated, they lose their ability to relax and contract and therefore considerably influence our level of flexibility.

THE VERTEBRAL SUBLUXATION

A VERTEBRAL SUBLUXATION occurs when the spine cannot adapt to a certain stress that it has been exposed to, whether it be physical, chemical, or emotional. Subluxations act as short circuits that deprive tissues and organs of the body's innate intelligence. When this happens, a vertebra misaligns with the vertebra above or below, affecting the transmission of nerve impulses between the brain and the body. It is not fractured, dislocated, or luxated, it is simply misaligned and consequently affecting vital nervous communication. The term subluxation is not a medical entity and therefore is not recognized by allopathic medicine. On a spinal X-ray report, a subluxation will not be cited even though they are very easy to recognize. This may be because there are no tools in modern medicine to correct or realign it. This is easy to understand when we consider that an MD or Orthopaedic Surgeon is a specialist in identifying and treating disease. Treatments such as medication and surgery are the most common tools of medicine. Sadly, over 95% of all complaints of spinal complaints seen by a medical doctor will be of a bio-mechanical origin, where chemicals (medication) and surgery are irrelevant until the problem degenerates to a symptomatic or pathological stage, many years or decades after the bio-mechanical problem first appears.

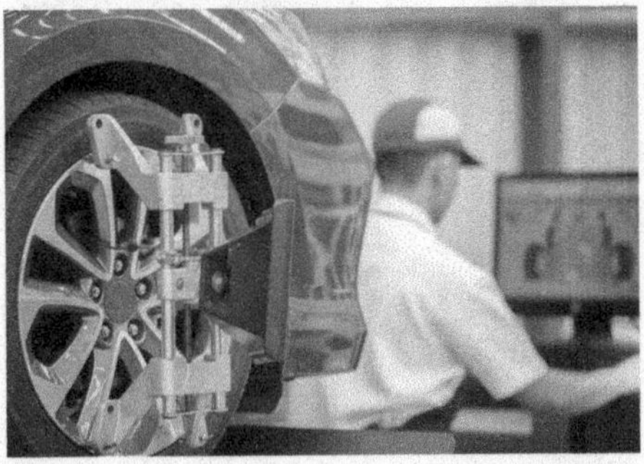

A common metaphor that I use with my patients compares the mechanic and what he/she does with a car's wheel out of alignment to the treatment approach of both the chiropractor and the MD. If a car's wheel is left misaligned after going over a bump, it will start to wear the tyre out faster, due to the increased load that that wheel will carry. This could be compared with the intervertebral disc when a subluxation occurs. The load on the disc is increased significantly due to the misalignment, and with time causes dehydration of the disc and subsequent degeneration, both in the surrounding bones and the discs. What makes more sense? Waiting and then operating the disc and fusing the articulation (one of the principal tools of medicine) or simply correcting the subluxation before it degenerates? The other main tool used in allopathic medicine is the use of pharmaceutical drugs, which are obviously composed of chemicals. Is there a chemical in the world that you know of that is capable of a physical action, such as restoring function to a bio-mechanically compromised vertebral segment? Of course there isn't and this is why pharmaceutical drugs fail miserably with the correction of bio-mechanical (physical) problems of the spine. Their purpose is to relieve pain or relax contracted muscles but they do not focus on correcting the root cause of the problem. They are incapable of physically restoring function to the vertebral segment. Professions such as chiropractic, osteopathy, and physiotherapy however utilize manual manoeuvres to restore vertebral function and improve nerve communication.

Refer to a normal spinal segment in the following photo with the vertebrae aligned and a clear, unblocked passage for the nerve root to transmit messages.

Now refer to the diagram on the following page of a misaligned thoracic spine. Remember that these misalignments occur in day-to-day life, from childhood onwards, due to falls, incorrect posture, sporting impacts, and even bad diet, stress, and other chemical and emotional factors.

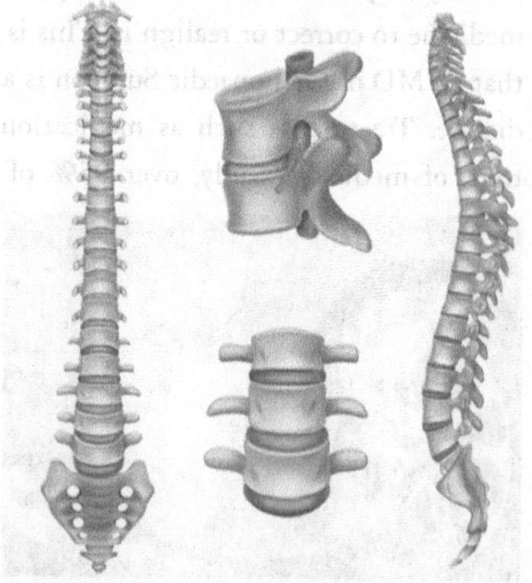

An intervertebral disc hernia is an example of a subluxation, where a compromise in bio-mechanical function has been present for a prolonged period of time resulting in wear and tear of the disc and subsequent interference to nervous system communication between the brain and the rest of the body.

When an asymptomatic

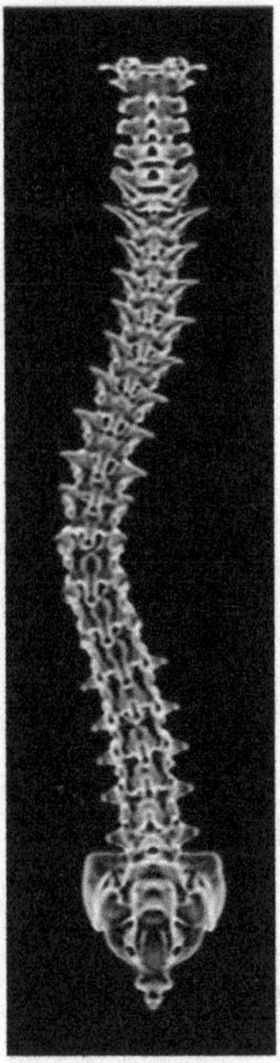

subluxation is present for an excessive amount of time, it can result in permanent wear and tear of the elements that absorb impact in our spine, compromising their function. Tissues such as discs and articular surfaces are the most susceptible and the majority of people who have degeneration in these areas are genuinely surprised when they find out. This is of course is due to the fact that subluxations contribute to bone and disc degeneration in an asymptomatic, silent manner.

STRUCTURAL CONSEQUENCES OF A SUBLUXATION

When a vertebral subluxation has been left uncorrected for a sufficient amount of time for the change in biomechanical function to alter the actual structure and form of the vertebra, the following changes may occur:

- Weakening of the fibres in the annulus fibrosus
- Dehydration of the disc
- Bony wear and tear of the vertebra resulting in osteoarthritis – growth of osteophytes (bone spurs) in areas of greater load
- Degeneration of the disc (protrusion or hernia)
- A reduction in the size of the intervertebral foramen called FORAMINAL STENOSIS
- A reduction in the size of the actual vertebral canal, called CANAL STENOSIS. When such changes occur, they can result in permanent, physical interference of the transmission of nerve impulses with the consequence varying depending on which level of the spine is affected
- Muscle and ligament shortening
- Fibrosis of soft tissues in surrounding regions, such as the capsular ligaments surrounding the articular facet.

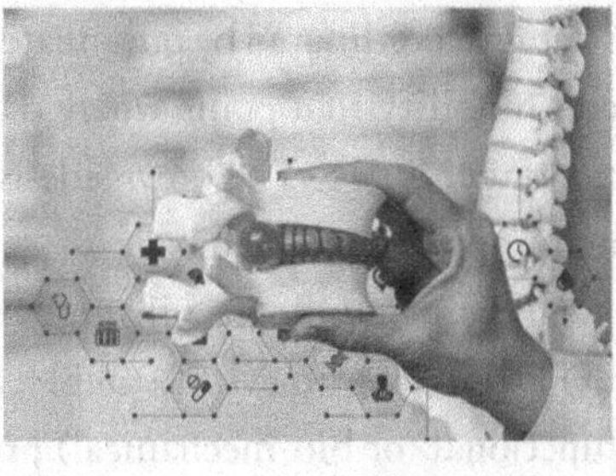

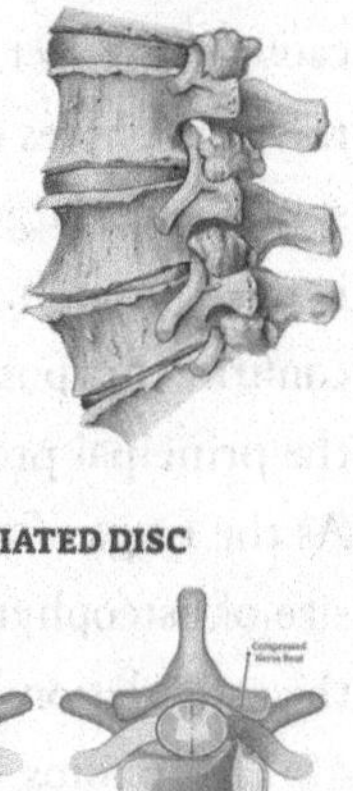

HERNIATED DISC

OSTEOARTHRITIS, BONE SPURS AND MORE

BONY DEGENERATION – OSTEOARTHRITIS

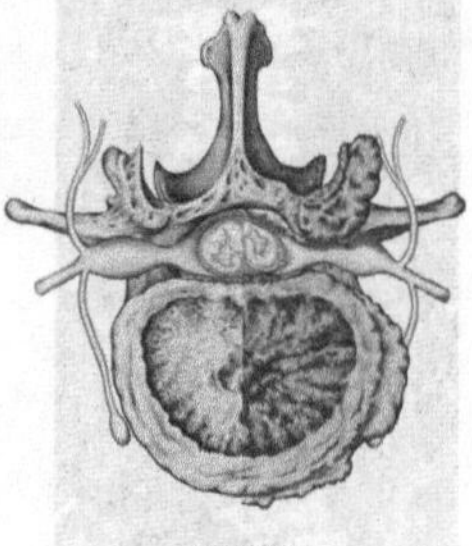

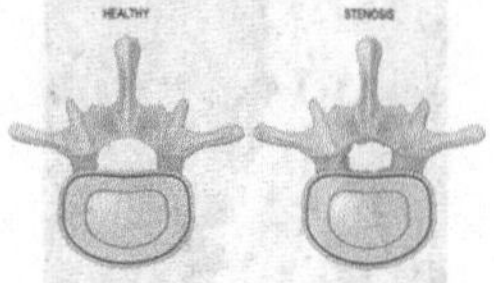

This degenerative process occurs when bony areas of the vertebra or joint are overloaded for extended periods of time, usually by being placed in a state of altered spinal bio-mechanics. The body reacts by depositing calcium (calcification) in the affected, overloaded region, either in the intervertebral joint or in the external margins of the vertebrae. Bone spurs called OSTEOPHYTES may grow, either minimally or substantially, to the point where they are fusing the whole joint or two adjacent vertebrae. Also known as OSTEOARTHRITIS, this process is extremely common as it is almost impossible to live our lives and maintain our spines perfectly aligned, avoiding the traumas, poor postural habits, and other forces that may contribute to compromising its function.

Calcification can also occur in ligaments and, less frequently, in the tendons where the excessive load may also subject these tissues to histological (cellular) changes in their composition. This process, surprisingly, is an intentional strategy coordinated by our innate intelligence in an attempt to limit movement and mobility to a point where damage to the nervous system is minimised or no longer a risk. The downside is that it takes decades to actually fuse a joint and impede its movement.

As pain, numbness, pins and needles, and other symptoms are the consequent EFFECTS of a primary PROBLEM, osteoarthritis is similarly the effect of a spinal functional (or bio-mechanical) problem. It is understandable how people who suffer from pain and also have an osteoarthritic process occurring, confuse this cause-and-effect relationship and actually believe that their pain is caused by the osteophytes (bone spurs). While advanced arthritis can result in these bony spurs being large enough that direct contact with the nerve roots can occur, it is not common. A Magnetic Resonance Image (MRI) can easily and quickly confirm this possibility. More commonly the osteophytes are being caused by the principal problem, just as the pain is a consequence of this same problem. As the rings of a tree can be used to identify the age of the tree, so too can the size of osteophytes be used to approximately identify the amount of time that the articulation has had its function compromised.

The photos of X-rays on the following page clearly show bone spurs (osteophytes) occurring on the anterior (front) margin of the cervical (left

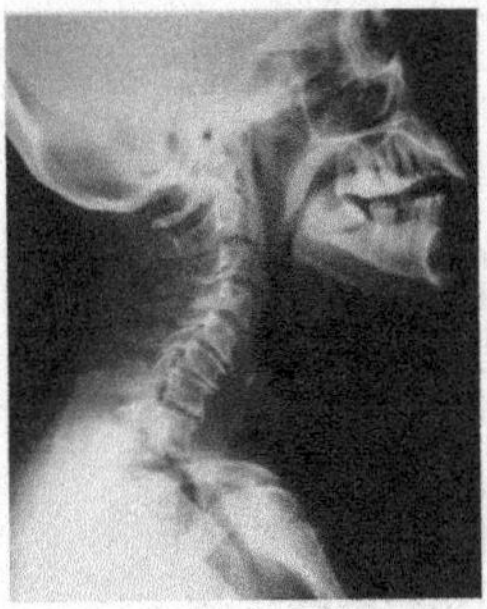
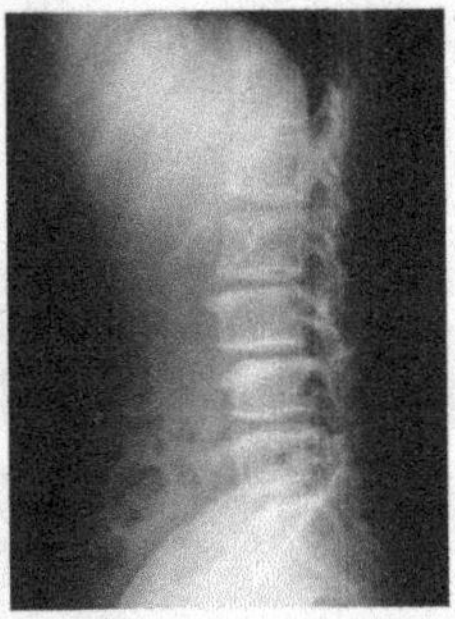

photo) and lumbar (right photo) vertebrae.

Many patients come to the clinic with pain of recent onset (sometimes after only a few days), however, their X-rays show that bony degeneration in the form of osteoarthritis dates back to two, three, or four decades. In many cases the painful symptoms also associated with spinal dysfunction simply manifest themselves too late when the irreversible damage has already occurred.

INTERVERTEBRAL DISC DEGENERATION/DISEASE

Alteration in the structure of the intervertebral disc poses serious risks to the integrity of the intervertebral foramen and thus, the nerve it encases. Vertebral subluxation is the most common cause of disc degeneration. Contrary to popular belief, intervertebral disc degeneration in the form of disc prolapse or disc hernia is not necessarily age-related and can be avoided by following correct spinal hygiene procedures.

As previously mentioned, the intervertebral disc is composed of approximately 80% water.

With the excessive load on the disc caused by the subluxation, the fibrocartilage of the annulus fibrosus can rupture.

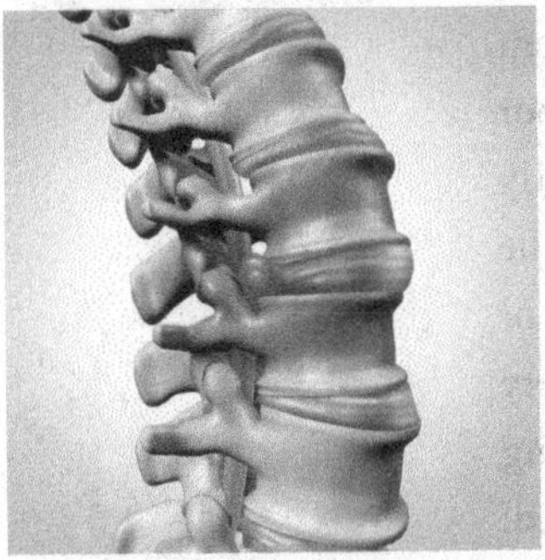

With time, untreated bio-mechanical dysfunction and uneven loads, the inner central nucleus pulposus bulges, causing a DISC PROLAPSE, also known as a DISC PROTRUSION.

If the causative factor/s involved is/are removed, the collagen rings may heal. If the spinal bio-mechanical dysfunction is not corrected and excessive load and dysfunction are allowed to continue, the central nucleus may herniate even further, passing the outermost layers of the annulus fibrosus, forming a DISC HERNIA, EXTRUSION or even a SEQUESTRATION (where a piece of the disc breaks off).

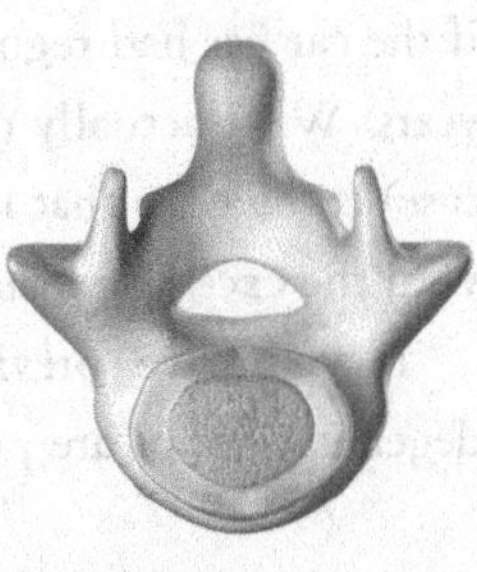

Unfortunately, most people do not change the conditions in their lives that originally caused the disc prolapse, even after suffering one or more

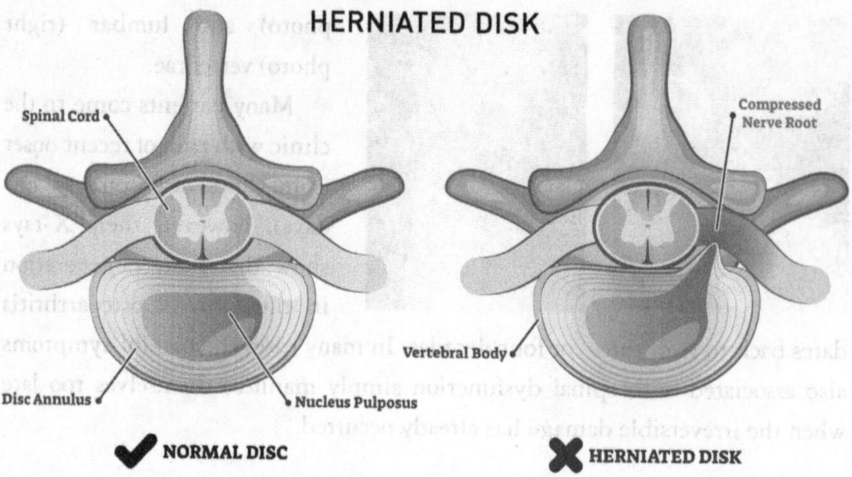

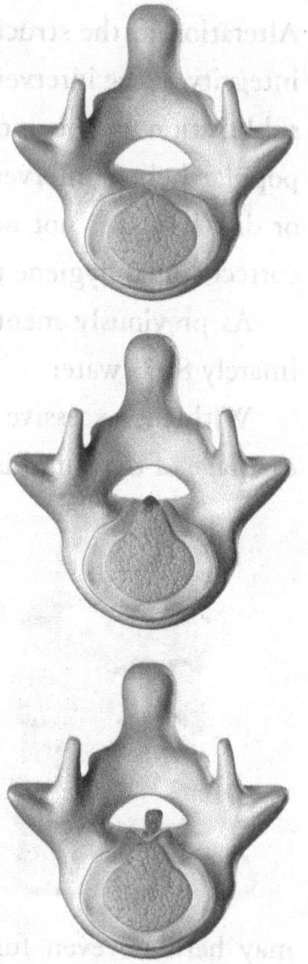

painful crises. As a result, most disc prolapses will continue along the degenerative path and end up as disc hernias. Once again, this is due to a lack of understanding of the problem and how to prevent it worsening as opposed to an inevitable pathogenesis of the degenerative process. Disc degeneration is generally related to the amount of time the person has had the subluxation, in other words, the actual time that the disc has been under excessive loads. This is contrary to the most common belief that a certain fall, twist, or heavy weight that was lifted is what "blew the disc out". I hear this excuse from my patients all the time and I use another metaphor to explain to them in layman's terms what really happens. Once again this could be compared to the example of the car wheel and tire. A large hole or bump could blow out a tire, however, this is very rare. The most common reason for a tire wearing out is prolonged use while the wheel is misaligned. The tire may actually be quite old but still be intact if the car has had regular wheel alignment over the years. What actually degenerates the rubber on the tire (disc cartilage in our case) is the time that it was left to driving out of alignment and consequently with the excessive load that misalignments cause.

If you have previously been diagnosed as having some sort of disc degeneration, or are presently suffering from back pain and know you have a

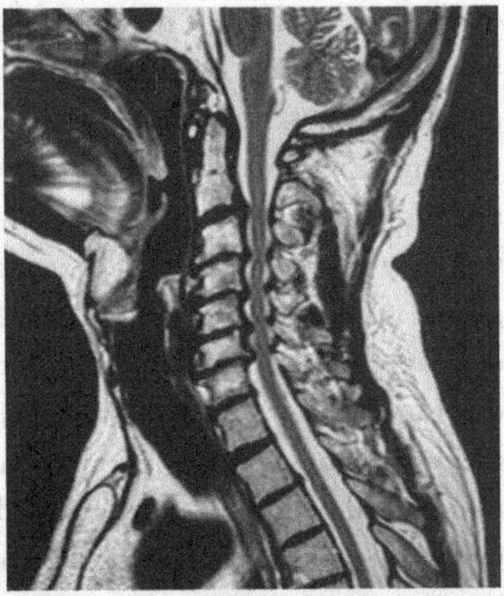

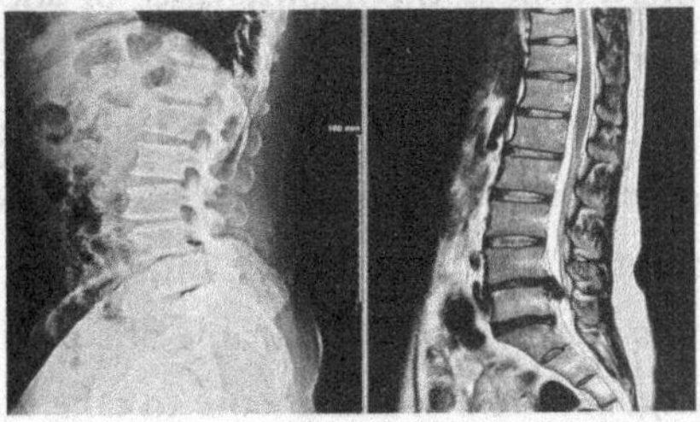

disc hernia, please don't despair. You are not necessarily condemned to a life of suffering.

MYTH – I am condemned to suffer because I have a disc hernia

As in the case of bony degeneration (osteoarthritis), most people with disc degeneration have no symptoms because the nervous system is not yet compromised, i.e., their disc degeneration isn't affecting nervous communication between the brain and their body (yet). A study conducted by the *New England Journal of Medicine*, one of the most respected medical journals in the world, presented 98 asymptomatic people (without pain or other symptoms) who underwent a study using Magnetic Resonance Imaging (MRI): 64% of them showed some sort of disc degeneration and 28% disc hernia! Most would understandably think that the degenerative process would cause some sort of painful symptoms however, no individual in this group felt any back pain at all!

Many people who suffer from back pain and also have a herniated disc think that the hernia or protrusion is the cause of their pain. However, it is more logical to recognize that the degeneration and pain are both the result of joint dysfunction caused by subluxation. In cases where disc degeneration is well advanced, compromising the neurological function, the disc degeneration can then become an independent source of their pain.

Frequently people endure pain and numbness in their arms and legs for years but only start to take it seriously when an MRI 'officially' confirms that they have a herniated disc, even though the intensity of their pain had not worsened. In cases like these, the disc hernia was obviously present for some time, but the subluxation that caused it even longer.

Intervertebral disc degeneration can occur in any disc of the spine, but the most common areas are the lower cervical region (C5–C6 and C6–C7) and the lower lumbar region (L4/5, L5/S1). This is because these areas have a propensity to being subluxated due to their location in the spine (L5/S1 is at the bottom of the spine at an angle of 35–45 degrees, and so receives a larger load). The lower cervical spine receives the load of the head, especially when it migrates anteriorly due to bad posture (see Forward Head Carriage).

In my 25+ year career, I have diagnosed literally thousands of patients with disc hernia who didn't even know they had it. Remember that disc degeneration will only cause a problem if it is compromising neurological function. The greater majority of intervertebral disc hernia cases occur in areas of the disc that don't approximate important areas of the nervous system (nerve root and spinal cord) and therefore don't affect nervous communication between the brain and the body. This is why they lay apparently dormant. This should not be a reason to relax and be passive in regards to how you care for your spine. The spine, just like every other organ of the body, needs to be cared for regularly and this includes the maintenance of adequate posture, regular exercise, and the correction of subluxations when they occur. Specific segmental movement of the vertebrae removes excess load from the disc, spreading the load evenly over the entire disc and not just in one focal area (where the prolapse or hernia forms). The chiropractic adjustment provides such movement and it is for this reason that it is capable of slowing down or even preventing further disc degeneration. If you choose to take medication for the pain, that is, of course, your choice. However, please do not take painkillers or anti-inflammatories believing that they will resolve your disc problem, simply because these drugs may have relieved your symptoms. In the example of the car wheel, a mechanic would be required to physically re-align the misaligned wheel. Only a physical intervention capable of restoring function to the vertebral segment and removing the excessive load from the disc will truly help the body cure the real cause of your problem. Chemicals simply mask its effects.

CASE STUDY

Doris, a 72-year-old woman, came into the office with severe bilateral sciatic pain, which had begun seven weeks before. When I asked why she thought she was suffering, she replied that she thought that the pain had started at that time, but could not identify any potential causes. She said that she had not worked in the garden, had not fallen or suffered any trauma, and that she had practised regular physical activity in her life with daily 40 minutes walks over the last fifteen years.

Her mattress was firm and comfortable. During the consultation, she remembered a fall from the first floor of her house fifty years ago, but according to her "it could not be due to that fall because she had spent all these years without pain". When asked about the fall, she remembered that she had been unable to move for four days after falling and had felt considerable pain and discomfort for at least 6 months. When the pain disappeared, she understandably concluded as many people do, that her problem had been cured in the same way that the body cures itself of the flu with time.

After X-rays were taken, we were surprised to see that the disc L5–S1 had been worn down completely with advanced osteophytes (bone spurs) growing into the vertebral foramen. With surprisingly little treatment, her pain had been greatly reduced, however, the degeneration that had already occurred meant that she would have to take great care and be more focused on regular maintenance to avoid more intense pain.

Doris's case is not isolated. For the past 20 years, I have consulted patients with advanced bone or disc degeneration but little pain or other short-term symptoms, at least once a week. If we use our 'machine' and wait for the warning light to appear to worry about the bio-mechanical state of the spine, then it may be too late and we risk having permanent irreversible structural and functional compromise.

Many people suffer from falls throughout their lifetime or work in positions that alter the normal function of the spine. Many people who feel pain choose to take painkillers to mask the pain and other symptoms, and others choose to ignore the pain and let the body adapt to the bio-mechanical alterations (see 'Adaptation'). Others lead stressful lives that result in the body simply not activating it's warning signs, such as pain, numbness, tingling, stiffness etc., allowing them to live years with structural abnormalities and continually degenerating joints, without being conscious of this fact.

"The only way to predict the future is to have power to shape the future."

ERICH HOFFLER

THE PURPOSE OF PAIN

"All of science started from pain. Pain is always looking for the cause, while the well-being is inclined to be quiet and not look back."
STEFAN ZWEIG

Our brain decides whether or not we feel pain. **If you are feeling pain or any other unpleasant symptom it is because your brain has ordered that command.** As every single action that the brain participates in is intelligent and has a physiological intention behind it, it is therefore easy to understand that your pain is actually a positive entity, even though it makes us suffer. Pain is unpleasant, uncomfortable, and inconvenient however it needs to be. Can you imagine what would happen if pain was as enjoyable as the feeling you have after laughing, having an orgasm, or that post-exercise buzz? These pleasant feelings are 'reward' type feelings based upon the fact that your body wants/needs you to exercise or reproduce and therefore rewards you with satisfying sensations that will motivate you to continue. If pain was pleasant, we would never be inclined to investigate its cause and may even deliberately repeat the damaging action that caused such pleasure! Pain must be unpleasant, and sometimes even disabling, modifying our behaviour to make us stop doing activities that cause and exacerbate the problem. It's as simple as that.

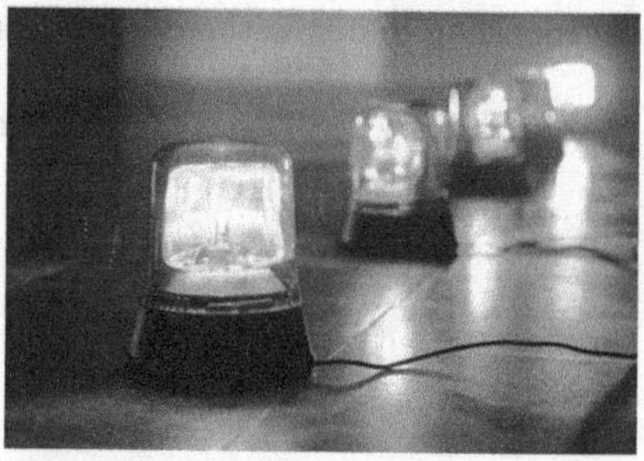

Pain is a completely necessary sensation, as is the light in the car that flashes to warn us when there is almost no oil or fuel in the tank. Without it, the dysfunction occurring in our body that needs attention would obviously progress to a much worse state, possibly compromising its physiological function to a point where it may never recover. If you are suffering from pain, please be grateful for the fact that you are being warned and respect your body by not ignoring the signs. Many others are not this lucky.

TIP – If we focus on the root cause of the problem, we have the opportunity to correct it and allow our body to continue to function the way it was intended to.

If we suppress the symptoms with analgesic drugs or worse still, ignore them, we must accept the fact that this decision will distract us from the cause and the completely normal signal that our body has communicated to us. It is like ignoring a fire alarm in a house by turning off the electricity. Obviously, the fire will continue to burn and the damage will be costly and possibly irreversible. Unlike a house, which can be rebuilt, when the damage in the body passes a certain point, normal function may never return.

CASE STUDY

Steven was suffering intense lower back pain accompanied by left leg pain due to a herniated lumbar intervertebral disc. He had worked as a manual labourer for 15 years. He had been suffering lower back pain for 10 years and would relieve the pain by taking anti-inflammatories and pain killers during times of intense pain. An MRI scan that he had taken 10 years ago showed that, despite the pain that he was feeling, there was no intervertebral disc degeneration. A more recent scan (taken two years ago) showed a moderately sized intervertebral disc hernia protruding towards the intervertebral foramen (the space between each vertebra that encases the nerve root exiting the spine) on the left side. Unfortunately, while Steven was masking the pain by taking medication, the load on his lumbar spinal joints continued and caused degeneration in the intervertebral disc.

TIP – Don't ignore the obvious signs that your body uses to advise you that something is not quite right. They represent a golden opportunity to avoid unnecessary suffering and more serious consequences in the future.

MYTH – The intensity of your pain or symptom is proportional to the severity of your problem.

The disc is a gelatinous cushion that sits between two vertebrae and keeps the nerve that exits between them encased in a protective opening. As any disruption in communication between the brain and the leg may be a serious threat to our health, people who have a degenerated disc affecting the nerve root may end up feeling intense pain in the course of the sciatic nerve (radiating from the spine into the leg). I have personally suffered from this condition and can attest to it being the most excruciating pain I have ever endured. Even though I was in constant agony I knew that the pain was there to prevent me from overloading my spine and possibly damaging my spinal cord, which would obviously worsen the situation that I was in. I was totally aware that if I had have taken painkillers and continued my normal activities that I risked permanently damaging the nerve root and possibly end up with a loss of bladder or bowel control, or sexual organ function, as the same nerve supplies these organs as well.

There are many other examples of signals that the brain uses to advise us that there are threatening problems, such as headaches, shoulder pain, chest pain, numbness, etc. Each one is a distinct sign that something is not right and needs immediate attention. The problem is that we are not educated to interpret every pain, sign, and symptom of our body and, unfortunately, the pain may be ignored or, worse still, erased with painkillers, fooling our bodies and allowing the problem to degenerate and affect our health even more.

In situations where pain would not be 'advantageous', it is often not activated by the brain. For example, it is common that soldiers at war do not feel pain until they leave the battlefield. I have treated many people over the years shortly after they had lost a loved one who they had been caring for. Even though they obviously had the condition that was causing their pain for many years beforehand, their bodies had suppressed the sensation due to the stress that they were under caring for their family. Many of these patients reported the onset of the symptoms after the person who they had been caring for passed away. The brain analyses all the information it receives from our sensors and receptors to determine if the pain you feel will be 'advantageous' or not in that particular moment.

So, if you're suffering, your brain somehow concluded that creating the pain is necessary – that biological tissue is being threatened and that your brain needs you to change this situation before damage, possibly permanent, occurs. Therefore, if you're feeling pain or any other symptom, it is your responsibility to find out why your brain made that decision and remove the threat.

Contrary to what many people think, the intensity of pain that we feel is not necessarily related to the severity of the injury or damage suffered by the tissue. This can be quite confusing. For example, a relatively harmless tissue injury, such as a paper cut can be extremely painful. At the same time, many other serious conditions such as vertebral disc hernias, advanced arthritis, and even cancer remain asymptomatic in many cases.

When pain is severe and debilitating, we can easily forget that this symptom is an order from our brain and we naturally worry since we believe that the intensity indicates that the injury is more serious than what it actually may be. Can you remember any similar situations that you have experienced, where you thought that your problem was much worse based on the fact that the pain was intense or even excruciating? If you have, it's normal, as most have us have been programmed to be afraid of pain from a very young age. When a child falls and cries, the concerned and sometimes horrified expression on the parent's face associates this common impact with something to be feared. Obviously when they know that the child is OK their expression changes but the horrifying image has often been etched into the child's subconsciousness and pain will understandably never naturally be associated as a positive entity.

The intensity and quality of pain that an individual suffers also depends on several other factors such as gender, culture, age, knowledge about the cause of pain, and how much the person depends on the affected area.

Similarly, the amount of time that someone has been in pain also has no relation to the severity of the problem. People commonly mistake the fact that "it's only been hurting for a week or so" with the idea that it is a new problem and therefore can't be too serious. I see this every day when I question new patients about their symptoms. However, almost always, after persisting and repeatedly asking when it was they first felt pain, they will conclude that it was years or decades before. A common response would be "Oh, yes, I did feel lower back pain many years ago. It was that bad that I was taken to the hospital, carried in by my son, but that was years ago and it never came back". The flu goes when the body's immune system deals with it and 'comes back' when the same immune system is weakened, however back pain that 'goes' almost always has a underlying problem beneath it, and if left uncorrected, will come back stronger and more frequently with time.

It is common, after examining many of these cases and studying their X-rays, that we identify some type of degeneration, such as osteoarthritis or a herniated vertebral disc, which takes years to develop. The extent of the disc and/or bony degeneration frequently shows that the process has been active for decades. It is easy to understand how some people have difficulty believing that the process has been occurring for years if they have not felt significant pain, either in intensity or duration. In the following section, I will discuss motives as to why we may not feel a degenerative process evolving. We must remember that we are all created with a unique body and the way we perceive our world and feel certain sensations such as pain is subjective. This not only applies to spinal-related problems but also other health-related conditions. We can ingest harmful substances every day for many years, damaging the tissues of our body continually as we do, but have no pain or symptoms until cancer or other degenerative illnesses appear. We can smoke for decades, damaging our lungs and other cells of our body with little or no warning of the damage and only find out when the first symptoms are followed by a diagnosis of heart disease or cancer.

We must remember that our body has an amazing ability to adapt and that it is the brain that decides when and how it will emit signals. Sometimes this decision apparently does not make sense, but when we analyse other factors, it is easy to understand why. The body may adapt because many stressful factors 'distract' our brains from the problem. Stress, sleep quality, pharmaceutical drugs, diet, dehydration, the amount of sugar we consume, and many more factors can influence our brain to adapt to a certain problem and fail to transmit pain signals. The pain perception of an alcoholic or a diabetic with poor circulation may be drastically reduced due to their illnesses, which is why many do not feel the damage caused by falls or blows to the feet and, as a result, frequently show extremely advanced arthritic degeneration without even knowing.

It can take years to feel the pain and consequences of a past fall, trauma, or incorrect posture.

There are numerous cases to illustrate that the duration and intensity of pain have no relationship to the severity of the problem. Similarly, the length of time needed for somebody to potentially feel pain relief for a serious problem after commencing treatment may surprise many people when it 'disappears' in a short amount of time. Someone who has cancer will not give up treatment or their regular follow-up appointments simply because the symptoms have decreased or are absent. Most would know that they'd still need to follow certain lifestyle changes after going into remission even if they now feel good. When we refer to pain, we must always remember that your brain's decision to provoke it does not always seem to make sense and that every reflex that your brain provokes has an intelligent reason behind it.

We can either go years without feeling pain or just experience tolerable and occasional aches and pains and understandably think that everything is OK. Then unexpectedly we could suffer a crisis that affects our body in a very sudden and strong way, scaring us, as everything was 'apparently' fine until a short time ago. Most of us neglect our spine and posture for years or decades (obviously unintentionally) without compensating for the harmful activities of daily living (falls, trauma, and even the effects of gravity) and hope that our spine will remain in perfect condition, as it was the day we were born. The fact that we do not feel pain or do not have any other warnings does not mean that our activities are not damaging the spine.

Generally, we do not wait until we have cavities or dental problems to start taking care of our teeth. Otherwise, at some point, we would have to deal with serious tooth decay or periodontal disease, and at that moment, the brain would warn us that something needs to be done.

There are many examples of situations where a lack of care has continued throughout a person's life, obviously compromising their health, yet the symptoms are slow to appear. The continuous consumption of sugar may occur for many years or decades before it causes obesity, diabetes, hormonal disturbances, or heart disease. Alcohol consumption takes time to have obvious, measurable effects on the liver, with liver function tests or cirrhosis not appearing for some time. Such illnesses take a while to become apparent and receive attention as the symptoms are also slow to appear. This does not mean that a particular organ has not been in a state of dysfunction simply because there have been no obvious signals to advise us.

A smoker does not show signs of cancer with the first puff of a cigarette, but the lung dysfunction has already begun on a cellular level and it commonly takes fifty years or more for signs to appear that lead a person to investigate what is happening. The pain process is no different from these examples or many others where the body, unfortunately, does not tell us that something is not working as we would imagine it should.

Stop for a moment and consider whether you really want to wait to have back pain, leg numbness, headaches, or other symptoms before you start taking care of your spine and body? Will you need to get to this stage of dysfunction before you start to focus on caring for the spine and body that you were born with? Of course not, because by this stage the damage may already be irreversible, with the possibility of permanent degeneration affecting the bio-mechanical function of the joints.

When referring to duration, PAIN can be divided into two groups: ACUTE and CHRONIC.

ACUTE PAIN

This type of pain results from RECENT tissue damage and is usually short-lived. Acute pain almost always has an identifiable cause (like a fall, impact, or action already known to be painful, such as cutting your finger with a knife or bumping your knee on a table). The purpose of acute pain is to discourage repetition of the activity or factor that generated it to avoid more serious damage, while the brain is analysing the severity of the problem. It frequently stops the person in their tracks and does so to enable the person to avoid further tissue damage. If the cause of the acute pain is not removed and therefore further aggravation of the biological tissue continues, it may one day reappear or progress to the form of chronic pain. When the pain disappears, it is due to the body's normal self-healing processes that occur when there is no aggravating factor to slow this healing down.

CHRONIC PAIN

Pain that persists for six months or longer is referred to as chronic pain. Most people with chronic conditions have symptoms for months, years, or decades and therefore causative factors present for much longer still. When related to spinal dysfunction, chronic pain can result from a specific spinal lesion. More than 95% of these lesions are of a physical (bio-mechanical), chemical, or emotional nature where normal vertebral joint function has been altered by one or more factors. Chronic pathological conditions like cancer, autoimmune diseases, etc. may also be a source of chronic pain, however, it is important to highlight that these causes account for a minority of chronic pain cases, with some authors citing less than 3% of cases.

For those who suffer from chronic pain, it can appear to occur without any 'apparent' reason, which can be confusing. This is because the factors responsible for this chronic pain may have been present for quite some time, are more likely to be multi-factorial and cause pain long after the tissue was originally injured. It is for this reason that the cause of the pain in these cases is usually much more difficult to identify and often even more difficult for the patient to accept upon identification.

Chronic pain may be constant or intermittent. It limits the normal activity of everyday life and often leads to other consequences, such as sleep disturbances, reduced work performance, side effects due to medication used to control the pain, financial problems, and even relationship problems.

As traditional allopathic medicine 'seems' to be successful in those cases where intervention results in pain relief, it can shift the focus of the patient and the doctor to symptoms and not the actual cause of the symptoms, the pathology. Of course, in these cases, 'success' is measured by how the patient feels and not actually how their DIS-EASED tissues are functioning.

A responsible doctor will understandably not want to see their patient suffering. Any person who is suffering from pain or other symptoms will also understandably want relief. Unfortunately, this desire distracts us from the real, original purpose of the painful signal.

PHYSICAL (BIO-MECHANICAL) factors that result in chronic pain are the product of activities and situations that compromise normal spinal bio-mechanical function, such as falls, poor posture while sleeping, sitting, or working, and bad lifestyle habits acquired early in life that were never corrected. I compare the effects of these factors to a car wheel when it goes over a hole in the road, resulting in the misalignment of a wheel.

CHEMICAL factors increase the levels of inflammation in the cells, tissues and organs of the body. If articulations of the spine or other joints of the body already have a degree of bio-mechanical compromise, chemical factors tend to exacerbate the underlying inflammation, triggering the body to cause symptoms. These factors include the ingestion of certain inflammatory foods like sugar, soft drinks, alcohol, or drugs, environmental pollution, etc. I compare these chemical causes to filling a car's petrol tank with dirty petrol instead of clean petrol. Your car will run OK for a while before the dirty petrol ends up affecting its function and eventually causing the motor to seize. As well as causing problems for your spine, these factors also obviously contribute to devastating degenerative problems all throughout the body.

EMOTIONAL factors such as stress, sleep disturbances, negative thoughts, and psychological problems also have a surprisingly negative effect on spinal function and are frequently overlooked by both the patient and the health practitioner treating them. When emotional influences disturb hormonal balance, particularly the hormone Cortisol, levels of underlying inflammation can elevate significantly also.

You'll find a summary of the most common causes of pain detailed in this book. It is essential to understand that they can be avoided or managed in a way that minimises their impact upon the function of your spine and that only *you* can control these factors.

MYTH – I feel good, therefore I am healthy.

Health is an interesting paradox; for most people it is probably what they desire most and certainly the most important, although rarely understood by those who desire it. When people are asked if they want to be 'healthy', they will certainly reply 'yes'. However, if you ask that person to define what health means or what it means to be 'healthy', you will more than likely find that they never actually stopped to think about it. One of the most common answers would be "health means to feel good".

This is, indeed, the concept of health for most people: to feel good. However, many people feel good now and are still very sick. Some people have woken up in the morning feeling great and died of a heart attack during the day. These people obviously had heart disease before they died but were oblivious since they were feeling fine. Health, therefore, is something more than what most of us think it is, as a mere absence of symptoms does not mean you're a healthy person.

Your pain can save your life.

"It's good to learn to be wise in the school of pain."

ESQUILO

How many times have we considered a spine-related problem when we have indigestion? If a woman is not menstruating or if someone is constipated, would dysfunction of the vertebral column be considered as one of the possible causes? The organs that influence these conditions and every other cell of the whole body receive the energy needed to function via nerve impulses sent from the brain. For the organ, tissue, or cell to receive 100% of the message emitted by the brain, it must flow down through the spinal cord and transmit out through nerves to the organs. If one of these nerves were severed, a blockage in that transmission would occur, and the organ, tissues, or cells attached to this nerve would understandably be left without nerve impulses. Cell death would probably result unless the organ was receiving nerves from some other level as well. Similarly, if nerve impulses were interfered with at any location within the pathway, while the impulses may still flow to the cells and organs, they could be reduced. If less than 100% of any communication is consequently occurring due to this blockage in communication to that particular cell, tissue, or organ, it would not be expected to function at 100% of its potential. What percentage of nerve impulses from your brain to your heart would you like to be receiving? 100%? Or 70%? I'm sure that you'd say that you wouldn't want any less than 100% of this intelligent and vital communication to arrive at your heart. These impulses can, unfortunately, be interfered with. The vertebral column is the most common source of blockage and also the most overlooked by allopathic medicine.

What would happen if the stomach, bladder, sexual organs, liver, heart, and lungs, could not function at their 100%? You may reply that gastric reflux or indigestion, incontinence, impotency or menstrual problems, cirrhosis, arrhythmia or cardiac disease, and difficulty breathing may be the result. But do these symptoms occur just to make us feel bad? Why would the brain stimulate these unpleasant signals if there wasn't an intelligent reason behind it? Would it make sense to simply try and relieve these symptoms, making us feel good while at the same time distracting us from the actual cause behind them?

There are of course numerous reasons for pathology in these organs but one of the most obvious is the spine by virtue of its intimate relationship with the nervous system.

Hippocrates in 300 BCE stated, "look well to the spine for the cause of disease".

Your spine should be one of the first areas of your body that you consider when looking for the cause of your symptoms or disease. This is even easier to understand when we acknowledge that our lives are more sedentary than ever and that pathologies such as bony arthritis or disc degeneration are more and more common.

Numerous cases of disease have improved after the structural problems of the spine were corrected, as any organ can suffer when it receives fewer nerve impulses from the brain. Let's consider the intense pain felt in the sciatic nerve as it leaves the spine and goes down the leg and to the foot. A blockage in communication anywhere along its course will result in fewer nerve impulses arriving at their target cells and tissues, principally the foot and muscles of the leg. Those who have suffered the intense, burning and aching pain of sciatica (I am one of those people) will be able to relate to the assumption that the problem was in the leg, especially if there was no lower back pain accompanying it. These people would also be able to attest that the relief of their symptoms was only achieved after intervening at the level of the spine or gluteal muscle of the buttock, in other words, much higher up the leg. This pain is usually caused by a bio-mechanical dysfunction of the lower segments of the lumbar spine that consequently interfere with the normal nerve communication between the brain and the leg or foot. We experience this pain because muscle and skin tissues in our leg have nerve RECEPTORS to stimulate these symptoms and sensations. That said, most of our organs do not have nerve receptors to be able to advise us when they are not receiving the normal, healthy quantity of nervous impulses. So how do we end up knowing in these cases? It's quite a scary thought to consider that our heart, stomach, or any other vital organ may be in a state of dysfunction without us knowing about it. But this is actually the case since these organs do not possess receptors for the transfer of painful impulses as do the cells of the back, legs, arms, head, and thorax. If we are lucky, we may receive some other form of neurological communication in the form of unpleasant symptoms. Yes, being lucky to suffer pain really does sound strange but a person who has the chance to discover and cure the cause of their sickness before it silently and unexpectedly makes them sick, or worse still kills them, is undoubtedly lucky.

Nobody enjoys feeling unpleasant symptoms generated by spinal dysfunction such as muscle ache, back pain, headaches, or even indigestion. Taking analgesics or other drugs to deal with this discomfort is a personal and understandable choice. But after taking medication to relieve these normal warning signs emitted by the body, doesn't it make sense to search for the root cause of the problem?

Investigating why your body has given you a warning sign means listening to it and finding the cause of the suffering.

Our health is arguably the most valuable asset we possess. Stop to consider what your most important priorities are. Priorities such as family, your partner, your work, or even the sport that you love. Now imagine how those things would be if you did not have sufficient health to fulfil them. Or if back pain impeded you from fulfilling them. There are thousands of bodily functions occurring every day without us being conscious of them. Less than optimal health negatively affects these functions which may or may not cause obvious symptoms. When symptoms do occur, they can severely impact everything important in our life.

Up until only a short time ago, the number one cause of death was old age. Now it doesn't even get a place on the list of the ten most common causes of death. The majority of the list is now occupied by degenerative (avoidable) illnesses, such as heart disease, cancer, diabetes, obesity, etc. According to the World Health Organization, these are the top ten causes of death.

1. Ischemic Heart Disease
2. Stroke
3. Chronic Obstructive Pulmonary Disease
4. Lower Respiratory Infections
5. Alzheimer Disease and other dementias
6. Trachea, Bronchus, and Lung Cancer
7. Diabetes Mellitus
8. Road Injury
9. Diarrhoeal Diseases
10. Tuberculosis

Degenerative means that they are progressive, worsening with time until the physiological function of the biological tissue ends up incongruent with the healthy function necessary to sustain life. Degenerative also means that we have total control whether they happen to us or not. In a very short amount of time in human history, something significant and drastic has occurred to show that the common causes of death reflect our decreasing quality of health. Where accidents, food shortage, predation, and infectious diseases once would have predominated the list, non-communicable diseases such as cancer, obesity, diabetes, and hypertension, all a product of poor lifestyle choices, now feature as the main causes of death.

Could it be the fact that we in the Western world now worry about the symptoms of the disease and relieving them to make us feel better, rather than focusing on the causes of the actual disease? Could the fact that medication is frequently used for the sole purpose of relieving symptoms, be an important contributing factor in this shift? What about self-medication where the patient doesn't even bother consulting a general medical practitioner and takes it upon themselves to decide how much of a certain type of over-the-counter pain killer, anti-inflammatory, or muscle relaxant their condition requires?

The wonders of modern medicine in the treatment of the effects of serious diseases are unquestionable, especially those that some decades ago would have led to intolerable suffering and sometimes death. I do not want to be misunderstood when I talk about the rationale behind the use of certain drugs such as pain killers or anti-inflammatories. My point is that the cause of the problem needs to be identified and solved even when those patients who receive pain relief from these drugs feel that they have been cured. Only the human body is capable of curing itself. The drugs suppress the symptoms while the body is left to do its work. Once again, I am referring mainly to chronic disease processes and not acute conditions like bacterial infections where antibiotics are useful to help the body's immune system combat the infection. While the antibiotics may kill the bacteria, it is the body that has the capacity to boost its own immune system and keep future bacterial infections at bay. If a body is receiving all of the prerequisites of health, to begin with, it may not even need antibiotics. Now let's reconsider the symptoms already mentioned: the agony of constipation or menstrual pain, the unpleasant sensation of indigestion or gastritis, disabling sciatic pain, or headaches. What do these symptoms have in common? They are all unpleasant. Even though the tissues causing them are different, the rationale behind the signalling system is the same. By being unpleasant, they are intended to direct our attention to the actual cause of the problem and fix it as opposed to ignoring it by trying to feel better through symptomatic relief.

ADAPTATION

Our body has an incredible capacity to adapt to a variety of conditions and situations that we may subject it to. Let's stop to think of a few. If our body was unable to adapt to the temperature on a hot summer's day, the brain would overheat, or similarly, freeze on a cold winter's night. Without being able to adapt to all of the pathogens that we are exposed to daily, each breath would result in massive infections. We often place our body in situations that may be deleterious to our health, and our cells generally adapt to that new environment. Many cancerous substances stimulate the receptors on our cells to switch from using oxygen to sugar as an attempt to give our body time to adapt to that toxic environment. If this didn't happen and our cells were deprived of oxygen, they would die quickly. By converting their receptors to take glucose as fuel, they cause a healthy change in our environment. Many forms of stress threaten our physical, chemical, and emotional homeostasis (more on the meaning of this word shortly). These include bacteria, viruses, fungi, cancer cells (which reproduce irregularly and are constantly appearing in our body), pollution and chemicals, lacerations and trauma, excessive work, noise, kids, the pressure of school, the strain of personal relationships, and hundreds of other factors – and we constantly adapt to them without being conscious of it.

Despite the low levels of oxygen at extreme heights, our body adapts to the changed conditions.

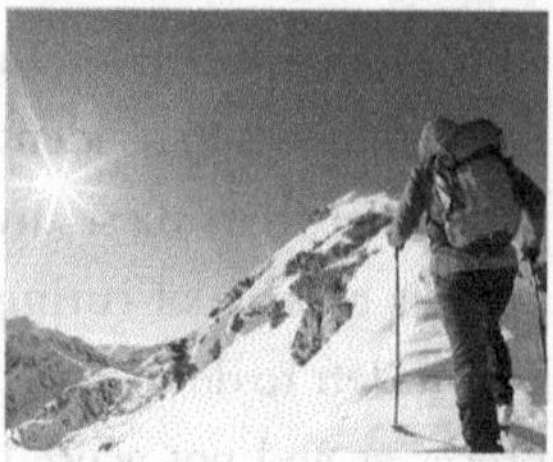

While adaptation is vital for our body to maintain homeostasis (correct function), there is a downside, as the body often accustoms itself to certain situations that threaten the correct function of our body and our vertebral column.

Knowing that stimulating pain and other symptoms is our body's way of alerting us of a potential threat to our wellbeing, it would obviously be detrimental to our health if our body did not provoke these reflexes. However, when the body adapts to a harmful stimulus, it stops causing or decreases the intensity of the pain and symptoms, even though the threat of danger and damage to cells continues.

Think about the times you put your body in an abnormal position, whether it be when you stretch out to change a lightbulb or take clothes off the line. Similarly, if you fall asleep on the arm of your couch or in a plane or car with your head leaning against the window. Likewise, when you use a computer or laptop that's positioned differently from the one you are used to using. These actions usually result in some sort of unpleasant sensation, whether it be a warning sign in the form of fatigue, pain or stiffness, a headache, or contracted muscles. These sensations are obviously warning us, because they are unpleasant, that that particular posture or position doesn't favour the health of a certain cell or biological tissue. Your body doesn't want you to continue, it actually needs you to stop, so that it may avoid the risk of more serious damage. What an efficient way to guide our behaviour!

So, what hope does our body have if we ignore the signs that try to induce a change in our behaviour, for example from an inadequate posture to the correct one? Or the incessant smoker's cough, trying to discourage us from inhaling the smoke of another cigarette. Our body adapts to harmful situations for many reasons, and one of the principal reasons is when it perceives that behavioural changes are not occurring and consequently the risk of damage is not lowering. Therefore, painful, unpleasant, and tiring symptoms are no longer serving their purpose. For many people, the symptoms cease despite the problem remaining and 'appearing' to lie 'dormant', sometimes for many years or decades. When the cells and tissues leave a homeostatic point for long enough and tissue damage and pathology have occurred, it is common that the person will feel a reoccurrence of the symptoms that they originally experienced, often in a stronger, even incapacitating form. For many at this point, permanent tissue damage has often occurred. Most people will understandably reason that this is a new problem, as no apparent symptoms have been felt for long. Take the example of the smoker again. The tissue damage has been continuous since the day they started smoking, with that violent cough being a reaction to the harmful substance being introduced into the lungs. As the majority of smokers spend their whole lives with little or no continuous cough, they have no obvious continual signal from the body advising of the degree of danger that the act of smoking is putting their body in. A huge percentage of these people will only discover that they have lung problems when the pathological process has already advanced to the point of irreversible lung tissue damage, such as cancer or emphysema. Similar situations occur when the body is subject to a diet lacking in nutrients or excessive toxins. Our body is capable of ingesting inappropriate food for years and years and 'appears' to function well, based on how a person is feeling. As we lose our health gradually in these situations, we forget how it felt to be healthy and understandably think that we are well because we feel well. In the same way that gasoline is the correct fuel for a car, nutrient-rich food is the most appropriate fuel for our body. No one would doubt the harmful effects of using contaminated petrol in their car. Even though it still may 'function' it would not function anywhere near its potential and slowly but surely contribute to the degeneration of the engine. We eat what pleases our palate or what satisfies our hunger, without considering what the cells of our body actually need to function optimally. This invariably results in a decline of the level of our health, happening imperceptibly most of the time.

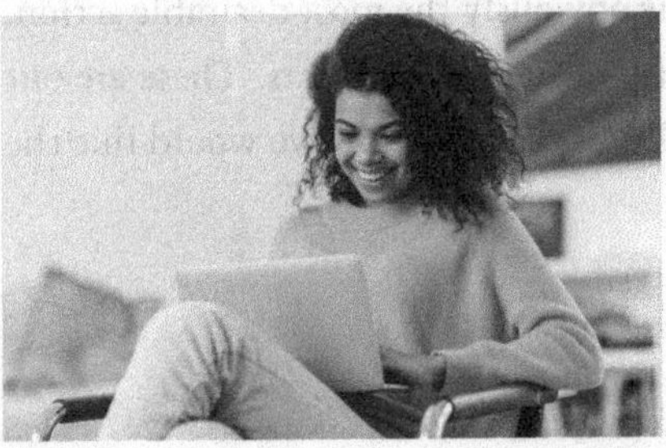

Our spine has its function continually compromised by many factors, including incorrect posture, bumps and falls during childhood or whilst playing sport, accidents and repetitive movements at work and even our sleeping posture. Similar to any other machine, our spine can continue operating in an 'apparently' normal, healthy way however be totally compromised in it's function. Since it adapts to harmful stimuli and is extremely durable, the spine can also degenerate gradually over time without causing pain in most cases. People will commonly observe that they suffered a bout of pain years or decades ago, with the occasional ache or pain before discovering that they have major irreversible arthritic changes. I like to compare these changes to the ones that occur to the tire of the car when a wheel is misaligned. After going over a hole or a bump, the wheel may easily be misaligned. To avoid degeneration of the tire, we would ideally feel a vibration or even a warning light advising us that we should take the car to a wheel alignment centre. As the tires are made to be durable, we drive for months or even years before even thinking about our wheel alignment. At this point, it is often too late for our tires and they generally have to be replaced with new ones.

Adaptation has its obvious advantages but it also sets the scene for advanced pathology and irreversible changes when it prevails for long enough. Different from the example of the tire used above, most organs and tissues of the body cannot be replaced, and notable changes to human health and the quality of our lives result when we 'wait for symptoms to appear'.

It is extremely important to understand the concept of adaptation as many examples will appear in the following chapters. Whether it be in reference to degenerative disc disease, degenerative joint disease or any one of several other degenerative illnesses you must understand that they are exactly that, degenerative. Doctors estimate that up to 90% of the diseases that kill us are degenerative, avoidable, and a consequence of our lifestyle choices. As such, they are pathological processes that occur gradually, imperceptibly and if you are lucky, you will feel warning signs such as pain, a stiff neck or lower back, or swollen joints sometime before degeneration has occurred. Our body's power of adaptation is what permits these conditions to occur slowly and without our knowledge. We have choices. We can ignore the pain and wait until it passes. We can ignore the pain and take painkillers before it passes or we can maintain healthy practices during our lives and correct problems as they occur. Acting before irreparable damage occurs is obviously the most desirable action, especially if we would like to enjoy quality of life in later years. These are our personal choices and we decide in over 90% of the cases how we would like the story of our health to play out.

"Optimal health is a process of continuous adaptation to microbes, irritation, daily pressures and problems that challenge the human being."

RENÉ DUBOS

MYTH – I don't feel any more pain, so my problem has been resolved.

I feel that this way of thinking is one of the principal reasons why we continue with bad habits that are repeated over years and decades, causing degenerative, irreversible conditions. If we wait for pain to appear before we consider whether we have any problems or not, we are actually playing Russian roulette. It's quite simply a game of luck.

HOW WE USE OUR POWERS OF ADAPTATION TO AVOID FEELING PAIN

Besides our brain's innate adaptive mechanisms to suppress pain, there are other factors that we consciously control that also hinder our body's ability to advise us when there are problems or threats to our health. Nonetheless, there are many effects that, while seeming to work 'magic' on our body, actually interfere with the natural processes, intentions, and desires of our innate intelligence. When adopting these measures, we should bear in mind that our body may not necessarily be capable of expressing itself in the way that it should and successfully alert us of any problems and possible threats to our health. Some of these factors include:

- using medication such as painkillers;
- consuming alcohol and illicit drugs;
- eating artificially processed foods, with preservatives, artificial colouring agents, and stabilizers;
- sleep deprivation;
- worrying too much or occupying our thoughts with negative, destructive emotions;
- suffering from emotional conditions such as depression;
- breathing contaminated air;
- drinking contaminated water;
- dehydration.

THE 3 CAUSES OF BACK PAIN – PHYSICAL, CHEMICAL AND EMOTIONAL

In the following chapters, you will learn about the three principal causes of back pain and the symptoms associated with spinal dysfunction. There are three main categories, however, in most cases, resultant symptoms are a combination of various factors.

PHYSICAL

Physical causes involve a bio-mechanical compromise of the articulations of our skeleton, principally our vertebral column (or spine). Misalignment of the spine directly affects the function of our body due to the spine's intimate relationship with the nervous system. Any factor that physically or bio-mechanically affects our spine will invariably affect its function. From our work posture to the effect of the impacts we absorb when we play sports. Whether it be the use of high heels, a low pillow, or a wallet in the back pocket of your trousers, numerous factors may alter normal spinal alignment, initiating the compromise in bio-mechanical function and nervous system integrity that will one day end up causing pain and other unpleasant symptoms.

Except for the acute pain felt after an obvious event such as a fall, impact, or accident, PHYSICAL causes are generally factors that are constantly present throughout our lives. Repeated over time, they provoke gradual loss of spinal function and as such may not always be easy to identify when pain and other symptoms appear.

CHEMICAL

As strange as this may seem, back pain may be stimulated by certain dietary habits, exposure to certain toxins, and inflammatory substances such as smoking and drinking alcohol. Many pathologies and resultant unpleasant symptoms that our body suffers originate from the toxins in our food or excessive sugar intake, including back pain. Many pharmaceutical drugs can cause back pain and muscle tightness and this fact is usually noted in the list of side effects that come with the purchase of any medication, however, very few people actually read this list. Any factor that affects the nutrition of the muscle can result in back pain. As 80% of our muscle's composition is water, inadequate hydration will understandably cause a reaction in the way the muscle functions and therefore the possibility of causing pain. Our body needs a sufficient amount of nutrients to be able to function correctly and will start to lose the health of any tissue if exposed to an excess of toxins. If you already suffer from a physical problem, this may be exacerbated if chemical factors are added to the mix. Many people have asymptomatic bio-mechanical problems for years until their internal bodily environment reaches a point of inflammation where the affected joints are inflamed to the point that they become symptomatic. For these people, true correction of their problem and consequent relief from suffering will only be met when both physical and chemical causes have been corrected.

EMOTIONAL

Many people find it difficult to accept that the cause of their pain and symptoms may be linked to stress or emotional issues. While we are understanding more and more about this connection, modern science still has not fully deciphered how emotional stress impacts our health so greatly. Our thoughts impact directly upon our state of 'stress' causing measurable hormonal changes. Elevated levels of hormones such as cortisol affect many physiological processes in our body, including the degree of inflammation. Increased blood pressure, heart rate, and muscle tone (caused by elevated levels of cortisol) can worsen the physical and chemical problems that we may already suffer from, taking previously bio-mechanical spinal dysfunction to a point where it becomes symptomatic. Have you ever noticed how happy people tend to get sick less frequently and suffer less when they do get sick than those of us who are less happy? Feel-good hormones such as serotonin are also pain-killing hormones. When deep emotional trauma has been suffered in the past, our pain can act as an amazing decoy from our subconscious mind to discourage us from thinking about this hurtful event. Emotional causes for back pain are real. Please don't disregard the role that they may be playing in your back pain.

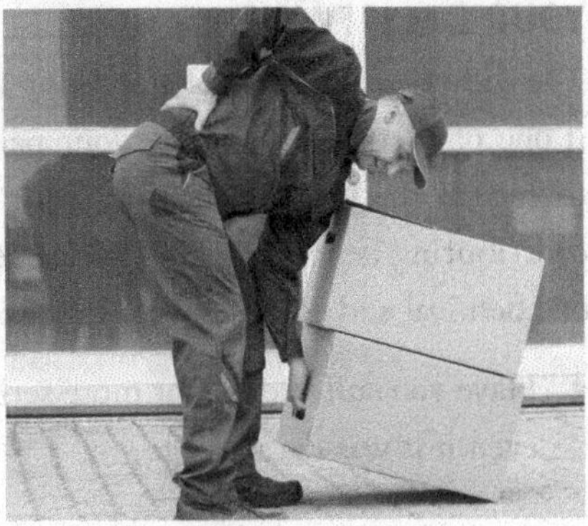

The following questionnaires will help you determine whether your problem is predominantly of a PHYSICAL, CHEMICAL or EMOTIONAL nature. More than likely, if you are

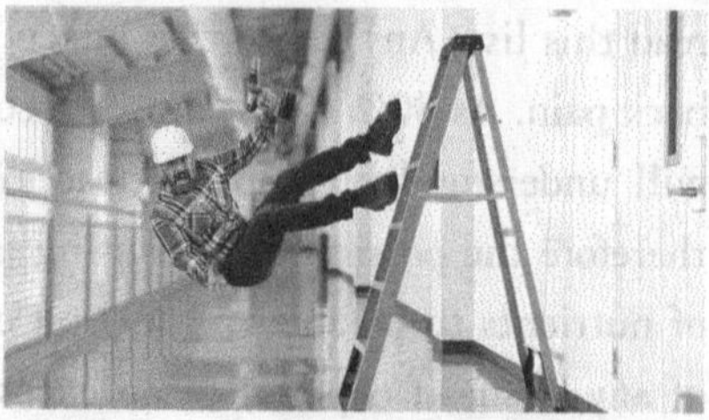

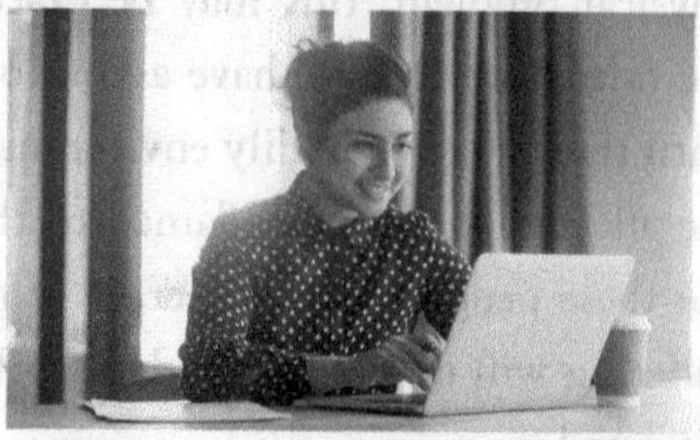

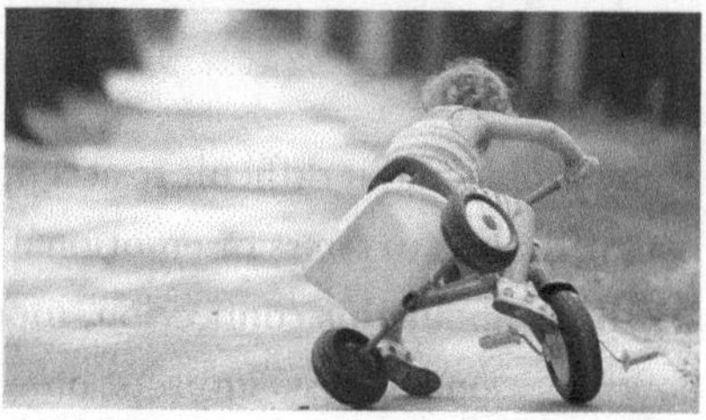

suffering pain and/or other obvious symptoms, the causes will be multi-factorial. We live in a modern world. One that is very different to the world that existed when the genetic make-up of out body was determined. It is extremely difficult to avoid the negative physical influences that our modern sedentary lifestyle promotes. At the same time, it is equally as difficult to avoid the normal falls, accidents, slips and tumbles that humans have experienced since the dawn of time. We now have thousands of chemicals that didn't exist as recently as a hundred years ago, foods and components of foods that are nothing like the nutrition that we were innately congruent with hundreds and thousands of years ago. Lastly, the stress that was once useful in defending ourselves from a dinosaur or to escape being eaten, has now turned chronic and continuous. Our sleep, moods, sensitivity to pain and so much more is detrimentally affected by these factors, principally because they are pro-inflammatory. This means that the inflammation traditionally caused by our day-to-day lives is now being frighteningly exacerbated by these other, more modern factors of life.

These questions serve to give you a general idea of where your inflammation and spinal problems may be coming from.

QUESTIONNAIRE – ARE PHYSICAL FACTORS CONTRIBUTING TO YOUR BACK PAIN?

The following is a list of questions that you may ask yourself to determine if one of the factors causing your pain is PHYSICAL. Remember, if you wish to correct the problem causing your pain you must identify and remove all contributing factors. As such, please review other possible causes in the section on chemical and emotional causes of back pain.

- Have you suffered one or more serious accidents or traumas in the past, even if it was decades ago?

- Do you maintain a fixed posture for extended periods of time (for example, in the garden or at work)?
- Is your mattress soft or older than 10 years?
- Do you sleep face down?
- Do you do exercise regularly?
- Do you sit for more than 4 hours a day?
- Do you feel pain relief when you walk? Is the pain worse when moving or sitting?
- Do you do anything in the gym or in your exercise routine that causes pain?
- Do you use a laptop?
- Does one of your shoes wear out faster than the other?
- Have you recently participated in a physical activity that you don't usually do?
- Do you travel long distances often?
- Is your life sedentary?
- Do you find it difficult to maintain yourself in good upright posture?
- Is one shoulder or hip lower than the other?
- Do you use high heels often?
- Do you play any musical instruments?
- Do you feel any pain when driving?
- Do you chew gum?

With the exception of the acute pain felt after an obvious event such as a fall, impact or accident, PHYSICAL problems are generally factors that are present constantly throughout our lives. Repeated over time, they provoke gradual loss of spinal function and as such may not always be easy to identify when pain and other symptoms appear.

QUESTIONNAIRE – ARE CHEMICAL FACTORS CONTRIBUTING TO YOUR BACK PAIN?

As strange as this may seem, back pain may be stimulated by certain dietary habits. Many pathologies and resultant unpleasant symptoms that our body suffers originate from the toxins in our food or excessive sugar intake, and so too can back pain. Many pharmaceutical drugs can cause back pain and muscle tightness and this fact is usually noted in the list of side effects that comes with the purchase of any medication. As 80% of our muscle's composition is water, inadequate hydration will understandably affect the way that the muscle functions and therefore increase the possibility of causing pain and other muscle related problems. Our body needs a sufficient amount of nutrients to be able to function correctly and will start to lose the health of any tissue if exposed to an excess of toxins. Any factor that affects the nutrition of the muscle can result in back pain, as resultant inflammation can compound with the inflammation caused in tissues suffering from bio-mechanical compromise (see the Chapter on Physical Causes of back pain). Many people have asymptomatic structural problems for years until their internal bodily environment reaches a point where chemical factors start to compromise the original structural problem even further. For these people, true correction of their problem and consequent relief from suffering will only be encountered when both structural and chemical causes have been corrected.

- Do you smoke?
- Do you suffer from constipation (fewer than 3 bowel movements a week)?
- Are you sensitive to many types of foods? Food sensitivity often results in diarrhoea.
- Do you suffer from flatulence?
- Do you suffer from indigestion, acid reflux, heartburn, or belching?
- Do you drink alcohol regularly or excessively when you do?
- Do you take medication or illicit drugs?
- Do you have a sweet tooth and consume many sugary foods?
- Do you drink more than 3 cups of coffee a day?
- Do you drink soft drinks/soda?
- Are you frequently thirsty during the day or night?
- Do you take vitamin supplements?
- Have you recently changed your diet or followed a special diet for a while?
- Are there any foods that cause headaches, insomnia, rashes, or other adverse reactions?

If the answer was yes to one or more of these questions, your body may be complaining about the type of 'fuel' that you are giving it, or the lack of nutrients that it may be receiving. Read on for the information in this chapter for a greater understanding of how these factors contribute to loss of health and subsequent back pain.

Have you ever had to perform or be on your best game only to fall short due to poor sleep the previous night? Does anything ever work out the way it should when we are stressed out or angry? These are two of the many emotional factors that can affect every cell of our body negatively. That includes our muscle and connective tissue cells and the cells of the nervous system and bones. When we add negative emotional input to a spine that is already less than optimal, we set ourselves up for even more pain, inflammation, and restriction.

In this chapter, *The Secret to a Healthy Spine* will guide you through fundamental knowledge regarding the emotional factors that affect all of us and empowers you to move to levels of function and performance that your spine may never have previously enjoyed.

QUESTIONNAIRE – ARE EMOTIONAL FACTORS CONTRIBUTING TO YOUR BACK PAIN?

Many people find it difficult to accept that the cause of their pain and symptoms may be linked to stress or emotional issues. Increased blood pressure, heart rate, and muscle tone can worsen the structural and chemical problems that we may already suffer from, taking the spinal dysfunction to a symptomatic level. Just as happy people tend to get sick and suffer less, those of us who are in less happy moments of our lives tend to fall sick more often and suffer from aches, pains, and other inconvenient symptoms. Sometimes our pain is an amazing decoy from our subconscious mind to discourage us from thinking about a hurtful or sad past event. Emotional causes for back pain are real and will be outlined later on in this book. Please don't disregard the role they may be playing in your back pain.

- Is the quality of your sleep compromised by insomnia, waking up frequently during the night, or sleeping lightly?
- Do you feel stressed?
- Do you work more than ten hours a day?
- Do you have financial problems?
- Are you nervous or anxious?
- Are you moody?
- Do you suffer or have suffered in the past from depression?
- Does your pain make you feel stressed or depressed?
- Do you have unresolved problems or emotional trauma?
- Is anyone in your family sick or has recently passed away?
- Do you feel happiest on the weekend or during the week?
- Are you unhappy in your relationship?
- Are you unhappy with your job?

THE COST OF PAIN TO OUR SOCIETY

Chronic pain is extremely common and generally preventable (when we learn how to prevent it). The high costs associated with a decrease in the productivity of employees, lost workdays and financial outlay from governments, private health insurance, and our own out-of-pocket payments could be substantially lowered if we as a society focused on the root cause of the problem instead of the resultant symptom/s. You will learn in the following chapters how our occupation, daily postures, lifestyle choices, and more, directly influence the function of our body and spine. We have control over those factors! We commonly ignore this fact until we 'feel' something. Sadly, for many people, by the time this happens, significant dysfunction or even degeneration has occurred, meaning that significant pain and suffering will be felt, as well as a considerable financial cost. The impact of chronic pain is expected to increase as obesity increases and the number of physical activities decreases. These factors are also expected to increase other conditions associated with chronic pain, such as other chronic, degenerative illnesses.

According to the 2020 study on 'The Cost of Pain in Australia' conducted by Pain Australia (painaustralia.org.au), 3.37 million Australians live with chronic pain. 53.8% (1.81 million) are women and 46.2% (1.56 million) are men. 68.3% are of working age. For the majority of Australians living with chronic pain, their pain restricts what activities they can undertake. In terms of financial costs, the total cost of chronic pain in Australia was estimated to be 144.10 billion Australian dollars. This equates to a cost of $22,790 per Australian in 2020! The World Health Organization estimates that osteoarthritis affects 10% of men and 18% of women aged 60 years old and over and lower back pain affects nearly everyone at some point in their lives and 33% of the population at any given moment. Not being confined to adults, 25% of children report having chronic pain and a third of them cite it as being severe. The economic impact of pain is profound since it affects absenteeism, reduces levels of productivity, and increases the risk of a person leaving the workforce. Chronic lumbar pain affects 1 in 5 Americans (approximately 50 million people) and costs the United States $635 billion annually, which is more than cancer, diabetes, and heart disease.

These figures and statistics are astounding. Similar percentages and dollar figures are observed in every country, from Sweden to Brazil, the United Kingdom to China. It seems that almost everybody, kids included, is damaging their health, and in particular their spinal health, through seemingly innocuous activities that they practice day after day, year after year. No, these activities will not

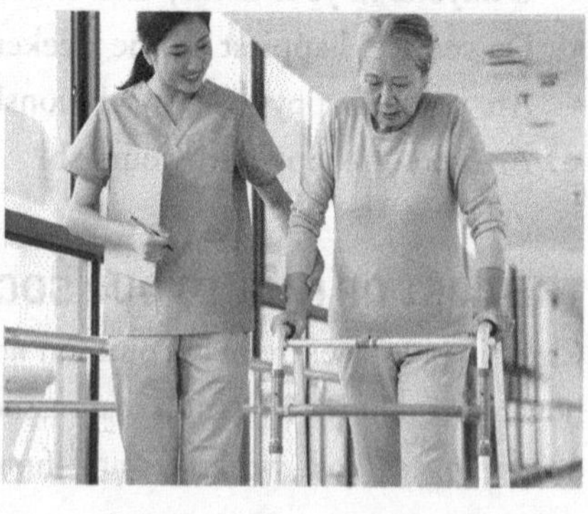

maim you today, but most of them, if not correctly executed, will maim you one day. At what cost will that pain, reduction in function, or incapacitation be? Even if somebody else foots the bill, no amount of money can reverse the intolerable pain that many chronic conditions cause. With such a high cost and a high probability of negatively impacting your life, wouldn't it be worthwhile learning what you are doing incorrectly today so that you can correct it and live pain-free tomorrow? You will not only be investing in your health and future pain state but also investing in your financial future, as paying for the cost of health problems is the number one cause of bankruptcy in the Western world. 66.5% of all bankruptcies in the United States in 2019 were due to medical-related problems such as the inability to work and the cost of treatment!

A huge percentage of the world's population suffers from severe pain that disables and prevents them from working and having a normal life. Most of these people are not aware of what it is that is causing their grief. The causes are so familiar to them that most don't even stop to consider them! Who would imagine, if they have used a chair their whole lives, worn high heels, or performed their job in a certain way, that certain articulations of their spine were being overloaded, and this could be the cause of their pain? Even less obvious would be the foods they have eaten or the stress they have suffered being inflammatory and increasing their pain sensitivity.

If you suffer from back pain, can you correlate the duration of your chronic pain with the persistence of an aggravating cause? It is time to understand what is behind your pain, and the pain of millions of others like you all around the world!

You are the only one who can dive deep and analyse what may be affecting your spine. If you're lucky, you will do this before your back starts to hurt and in turn become one of the few people who don't suffer from back pain. If you are already feeling the consequences of spinal dysfunction, take heart in knowing that you can, by recognizing what is causing it, turn your situation around and live a pain-free life. The combination of factors in your life that cause dysfunction is unique to you. By implementing the instructions contained in *The Secret to a Healthy Spine* into your life you will finally be making conscious steps towards correct function.

PHYSICAL CAUSES OF BACK PAIN

Any moving part, when intended to move in conjunction with another moving part, is prone to fall out of alignment. This occurs regularly in our lives with the simple machines that we depend upon, such as the wheels of our car or bicycle when they go over bumps or more complex machinery such as those used for construction or earth moving. Every object composed of moving parts will invariably need maintenance for this reason. This occurs due to factors such as gravity, bumps, and impacts that mechanically compromise surrounding structures whilst functioning. After compromise occurs, if these moving parts are not realigned back into harmony with those around them, they will start to wear and tear.

Our spine or vertebral column, as declared by Leonardo da Vinci, is one of the most amazing machines that humans have ever encountered. With 24 vertebrae all perfectly aligned one on top of the other, our spine can bend, flex, turn to the left and the right, and much more. It does all this while at the same time protecting the delicate and vital nervous communication structure held within it, the spinal cord. It's a tall order.

Every human being is exposed to influences that will invariably compromise the bio-mechanical function of their spine. From factors such as the 2,000 falls we suffer while learning to walk in our first years of life, to the posture a child assumes while studying at school, to the bumps and falls experienced during a normal childhood/adolescence. Less obvious factors such as having a wallet in the back pocket whilst sitting, using a chair that doesn't adequately support the lower back, a pillow or mattress that does not allow the neck or back to rest and recover while we sleep, and many more. We are exposed to multiple factors every day that compromise our spinal function and we must learn to recognize what they are if we are to avoid all of the pain and suffering that a degenerated spine will cause later in life.

Being aware of these factors and learning how to modify or avoid them is a critical strategy in guaranteeing a pain-free life. This book empowers you with the tools to help you return to a pain-free life, while accelerating healing and optimizing function. Focusing on the pain and how to relieve it has never gotten anybody anywhere. Using your pain and symptoms to identify the true cause of your problem provides you with strategies to rectify that course. This strategy simply makes sense as too many other interventions that have only focused on pain relief, and not the actual root cause of the problem, invariably leave the person with more pain, more restriction, and a lower quality of life for the future. The only way to continually enjoy a pain free life is to recognise causative factors and focus on removing them.

If you have suffered painful episodes or chronic pain that still hasn't resulted in the degeneration of your spinal function, consider yourself lucky. By following the pillars of spinal health outlined in this book you will not only be guided towards a pain-free life but at the same time achieve a level of function that you may have never enjoyed before.

In this section on the PHYSICAL causes of back pain, you will learn about the hidden risks behind such simple things as sitting, sleeping, the position of your car seat, the way that you should read or breastfeed, and how to execute chores around the house or garden without risking your spinal health. You will learn about the dangers of leaving an impact such as a fall or accident to progress to a degenerative state without being corrected soon after being caused.

GOOD AND BAD HABITS THAT LEAD TO GRIEF – LEARN HOW TO DO THEM CORRECTLY

SLEEP – EVERYTHING YOU NEED TO KNOW, POSTURE, MATTRESSES AND PILLOWS

Correct posture, whether we are standing or sitting, walking or lying down, is the position where the minimal load possible is placed on the muscles and ligaments of our body. In this particular position, the natural curves of the spine are preserved and its alignment is maintained (refer to previous sections on SPINAL ALIGNMENT and POSTURE). If we can manage to maintain our spine in its correct posture, gravitational forces are minimised thereby reducing wear and tear on our joints and also minimising the amount of energy our bodies use to hold that posture. Independently of what position we are in, whether it be while lying, sitting, driving, or working, correct posture will always have a positive influence on our body's health.

If we apply the rules of correct posture (previously discussed) to the position in which we sleep, we can quickly recognize that sleeping face down is most definitely the worst possible position for our spine. We should try and avoid sleeping on our front (prone position) unless there is a pathological reason that does not allow us to sleep in other positions. This is because it does not allow

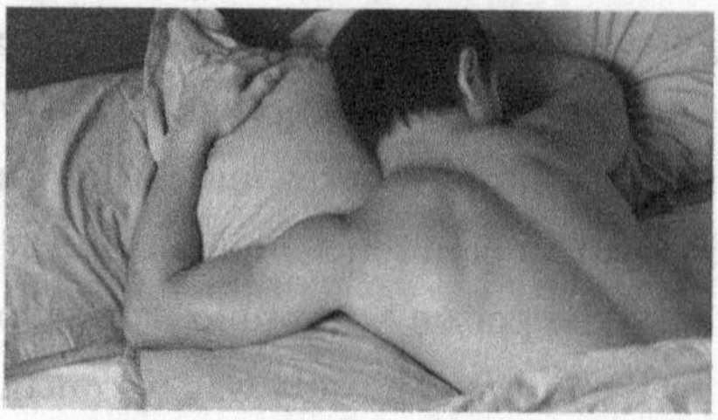

us to maintain our spine aligned, as we need to turn our head to one side or the other to be able to breathe, making it impossible to maintain the symmetry between the left and the right side of our upper back. Further, the curve of our lower back increases significantly in this position, which can jam up the facet joints and lead to muscle spasms and even nerve entrapment.

CASE STUDY

Danny came in complaining of intense headaches. They had progressively worsened over the years and now left him unable to work or leave his room when they were at their worst. Over the last ten years, he had been to many specialists and taken all types of medication. He had done a variety of diagnostic images from magnetic resonance imaging (MRI) of the brain, computerized tomography (CT), Doppler studies of the principal veins and arteries circulating blood to his head, and more. He had consulted neurologists, orthopaedic surgeons, and even psychiatrists and nobody was able to offer him a solution. He had taken all types of medication from simple pain killers, 'special' headache drugs to anti-depressants, all to no avail. Some of these interventions would relieve the symptoms for a while but the headaches would always return. By the time he came to see me he was extremely unmotivated and had accepted his 'fate' as being a future hampered by these incapacitating headaches. He had given up on many of the sports he loved and gained weight from the change in lifestyle that his continual pain had influenced.

When Danny first came in, we talked about times of the day that the pain was at its worst. He mentioned that it was far worse in the morning. I examined his neck and perceived that he showed a gross muscle imbalance between each side of his neck. His left trapezius muscle was fibrotic and sensitive to touch. When I palpated with an increased pressure a pain similar to the type of pain he felt in his head irradiated up over his cranium (skull). Eureka! As I always feel encouraged when I can reproduce the same pain a patient feels upon palpation of certain tissues, I was now sure that his pain was caused in the neck and not an actual 'problem' of the head. However, it was still necessary to find the cause and luckily this was found very easily with one simple question, remembering that his pain was worse after sleeping, "In what position do you sleep?" He told me that he slept face down, on his belly. I then asked if he was accustomed to sleep with his head turned to one particular side. He said "Yes" and I asked if it was the left side. He responded, "How do you know?" I knew because the resultant muscle contraction on the left side was glaringly obvious and much greater than the right. From my experience with many other patients like Danny, this could explain the asymmetry in muscle tension in his upper neck and the fact that his headaches were worse on one side and worse in the morning. Much to his surprise, his headaches progressively improved just by changing his sleeping posture (which isn't always easy) and one month of a combination of chiropractic adjustments and physiotherapy.

Additionally, people who sleep face down often complain of jaw pain as the pressure on the jaw in this position can jam compromise the function of the TMJ (temporomandibular joint). Other common symptoms of face down sleeping posture include bruxism (clenching/grinding of the teeth), tinnitus (ringing in the ears), vertigo (dizziness), stiffness, limited mobility of the neck and even radicular pain that irradiates down the arm to the hand and fingers. Always remember that these are healthy, normal warning signs advising you that something is compromising the correct function of your body and that your health may be jeopardized if not taken seriously. The warning signals are trying to direct your attention to the aggravating cause – your incorrect sleeping position.

Most people who sleep face down have a favourite side (either left or right) as muscles become chronically shortened and result in partially limiting full rotation of the neck. As a result, they tend to turn their head to the same side when they sleep as it is more comfortable, perpetuating the problem with time. People who sleep in this way will frequently (but not always) have symptoms on one side of their body only. I have no doubt at all in respect to the relationship between sleeping face down and the occurrence of the symptoms mentioned above, as thousands of patients over my career of 26 years have consistently proven this to me.

It may take up to several weeks to accustom yourself to not sleeping face down. Hang in there, you'll adapt! Just like any habit or attitude that we have developed over time, change isn't easy, but your health will thank you for it. If you are suffering symptoms as a result of sleeping face down, they will disappear quickly. If you haven't started feeling symptoms, you will not only avoid unnecessary suffering in the future, you will also reduce your chance of suffering from arthritis in the joints of the neck. If you haven't felt any symptoms yet, rest assured that spinal dysfunction is occurring.

If you wake up during the night on your stomach again, change position immediately. Little by little, you will rid yourself of this bad habit.

TIP – HOW TO MAKE THE TRANSITION TO A NEW SLEEPING POSTURE EASIER

As we tend to spread our legs when we lie face down some people have success with lightly and loosely tying their feet together with a stocking. Tie them a little above the ankles and make sure you don't tie them too tight. If and when you turn over onto your belly from a side or face-up position during the night, you will find it uncomfortable to stay in that position and not separate your feet. You will return to the side or face-up position, probably without fully waking in the same way that we move many times during the night without waking. If tying your feet together seems like it's too much of a task, try putting a squash ball inside a stocking and tying it at the level of the sternum (just under your chest). Similarly, the discomfort caused by the squash ball pressing into your bony sternum will remind you to roll out of that position. It understandably seems like great lengths to go to to be able to accustom yourself to sleeping in the correct posture, but believe me, it's worth it. Good luck!

If you have tried and simply cannot adapt to sleeping in another position and must continue to sleep face down to rest, make sure the pillow you use is low. Putting a pillow under your hips may help to minimise the extra load on the low back.

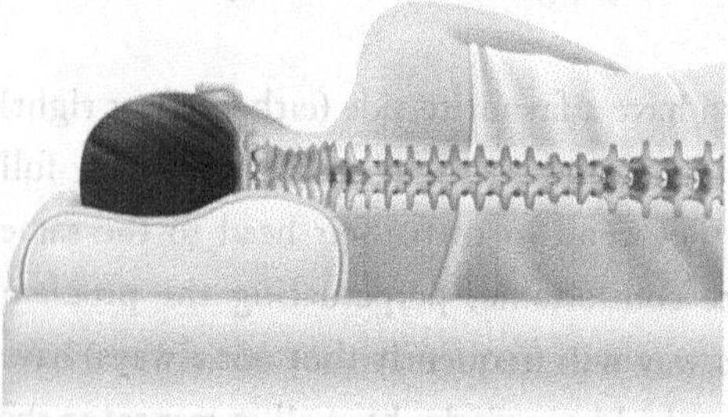

There are two options of sleeping positions that please the spine – on your back or on your side.

The degree of comfort you receive in each position will be determined by the firmness of your mattress and the height of your pillow. From my experience, a firm mattress is generally much better for the spine than a softer one, so start with the mattress. After that, look for a suitable pillow that will combine with the mattress. The purpose of a pillow is to support your neck, not your head. A firmer mattress will need a higher pillow when sleeping on your side. The same pillow when used in combination with a softer mattress may be very uncomfortable for your neck as it increases the lateral flexion (sideward bending) of the neck. Conversely, a firm mattress with a thinner

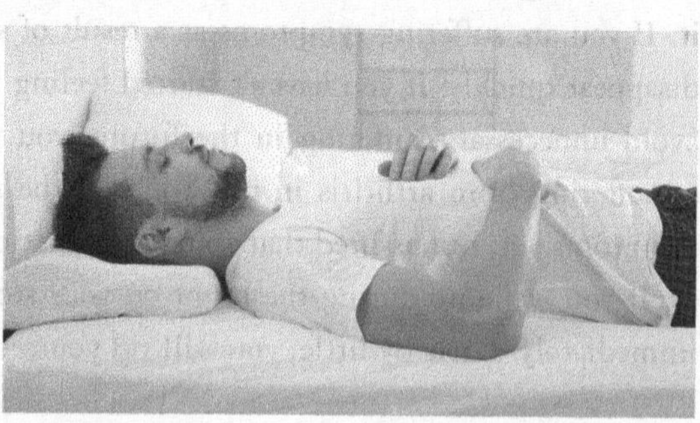

pillow whilst sleeping on your side is not recommended for the same reason, as it increases the lateral flexion of the neck. A softer mattress with a thinner pillow won't compromise the neck as much and therefore be a more comfortable option (until you change your mattress!).

If you are unsure of which position you sleep in at night (lucky you, because this probably means that you sleep deeply) confer which position you are in when you wake up. If you have a partner, ask them. Determining if this is the only position you sleep in will help considerably in the choice of your pillow, as pillows that are apt for side sleeping are considerably different from those that are more apt more sleeping on your back. Side sleeper pillows should be thicker and pillows for those who only sleep on their backs should be low. Interestingly, many people who try to sleep on their back due to the obvious benefits of this position fail because they use a pillow that is too high for them. As this type of pillow excessively flexes the neck whilst sleeping on the back, it becomes uncomfortable and the person has a natural propensity to turn on their side, where they head is better supported. Many people only sleep in one particular position the whole night. If there is doubt as to which position you favour try starting your sleep in one particular position for a few nights. If it feels natural and you don't move from that position more than likely this is your predominant position. Once this is decided you can then look for a pillow suitable for that particular position.

Of course, alternating between each position is fine and very common, as long as the neck is being adequately supported by the pillow. If you are using the correct pillow, there should be no space ever between your neck and the pillow.

Sleeping on your back has the added benefit of allowing you to have your airways more fully opened at night, especially if you are on a low pillow. It also gives your shoulders a break. Many shoulder problems that become symptomatic later in life can be contributed to the thousands of hours sleeping on our sides. When combined with a firm mattress, circulation to the shoulder muscles can be restricted. Muscle contraction, bursitis and cartilage damage can occur as a result. Most people would never imagine that the major contributing factor is their sleep position.

Side sleepers: if you can avoid sleeping with your knees excessively curled up (flexed) towards your belly, your low back and legs will thank you for it. This position unnecessarily flexes the spine promoting poor posture, loss of normal curvature, shortening of key postural muscles such as the ilio-psoas and even overloading the intervertebral discs of the low back. Who would imagine that a low back problem could be caused by simply sleeping on your side with the legs flexed? This position also allows the person to flex the neck for prolonged periods of time during the night, which can contribute to rectification and degeneration of the cervical spine. This is especially important if the person already spends their time during the day with their neck flexed and their head looking down at a computer or desk.

TIP

Side Sleepers! To increase comfort in this position, place a thin pillow between the knees. This avoids the bone-on-bone contact between the knees that can be quite uncomfortable. It also minimises excessive torsion of the low back.

HOW TO CHOOSE YOUR PERFECT PILLOW

Did you know that the quality of your sleep directly influences the quality of your day? This is why it is worth your while to take the time necessary to choose the most adequate pillow. A poorly chosen pillow can cause headaches, stiff neck, shoulder pain, numbness in the fingers and hands, and even insomnia. A pillow that has passed its 'use by date' is sure to contain fungus, dust mites, dead skin cells, and more which makes it heavier than what it was when you bought it! As surprising as it sounds, most people have never been informed how to correctly use or choose their pillow!

TIP FOR DETERMINING IF YOUR PILLOW HAS PASSED IT'S USED BY DATE

- If you are waking with a headache, pain in your neck, stiffness, pain in your shoulders or down your arms, or pins and needles in your fingers.
- If the pillow has lost its original shape, is lumpy or deformed. If it is more than one year old.
- If it has discoloured or has mould.
- If you are not sleeping well.

Considering that we spend between 25–30% of our lives in bed, sleeping with our 5kg head on top of a pillow, it is easy to understand how our pillow will wear out after a certain amount of time just as our shoes do. In the same way that worn-out running shoes can potentially damage feet, knees, and other joints of the spine if we continue to use them, so too can an inadequate, worn-out pillow. If you are starting to notice any of the above symptoms it's more than likely time to change your pillow. For most pillows, this is necessary after about a year of use.

In search of that magic pillow, many people end up buying a variety of pillows, which can be quite expensive. However, by understanding what pillow is most apt for you, you can minimise this unnecessary expenditure. Please don't choose a pillow due to its low cost. Even though many excellent pillows may be cheaper this doesn't mean that they will be necessarily apt for your body type, neck, and sleeping position. Don't be afraid to spend more if you feel that it would be more suitable. Think of how much time you spend sleeping and how much of an effect poor sleep has on the productivity of our day and the quality of our health. Based on a changeover of one year, even an expensive pillow (let's say around $200) ends up costing less than a dollar a night when calculated over a year. Having said that, please don't soldier on with an expensive pillow simply because it was expensive. Unsuitable is unsuitable, irrespective of whether it is cheap or expensive.

CHOOSING YOUR PILLOW

- Determine your sleeping posture – follow the steps previously mentioned to identify your predominant sleep position. Remember that your pillow must reflect this preferred position. Different positions require different pillow heights and degrees of density.
- Choosing a pillow is a process that is unique for each person. The human head weighs 5 kg and a pillow must not only be comfortable but must also provide support. It is not an easy task maintaining the head aligned with the neck and the rest of the spine while supporting the cervical (neck) curve and distributing the weight evenly between the neck and the head.
- BACK SLEEPERS – should use a pillow that supports the curve of the neck without excessively straightening it or worse still, bending it into flexion (see the section on Forward Head Carriage). A pillow that is too high will do this. Pillows with an 'anatomic' design that have a higher elevated side to support the neck and a lower portion to support the head are very popular with back sleepers. Alternatively, lower, thinner pillows prevent the cervical spine from losing its curve.
- SIDE SLEEPERS – as mentioned above, in this position a pillow that maintains the alignment between the neck and the spine is ideal. Latex, Polyurethane foam, and Down pillows are the most popular for their ability to support the weight of the head without deforming. From my experience, visco-elastic pillows generally do not have this ability and as they deform can compromise the spinal bio-mechanics of the neck.

FIRM OR SOFT PILLOW?

Your personal preference in respect to comfort should always guide you in respect to the correct choice of pillow. There's no sense in following the theory of what type of pillow composition is most suited to you if it simply isn't comfortable and doesn't allow a restful sleep. The higher the density of the pillow, the firmer it will be. Materials such as polyurethane foam, latex, and silicon fibre are generally firmer pillows and therefore more apt for side sleepers. Materials such as visco-elastic (memory foam), polyester, and low-fill down pillows are less dense, deform easier, and are therefore more suitable for back sleepers.

DUST MITES ABSOLUTELY LOVE PILLOWS!

Dust mites are micro-organisms that feed on fungus, bacteria, and skin cells that naturally peel off our bodies. They are prevalent in dark, humid environments such as sofas, cushions, carpets, and yes, pillows and mattresses! According to statistics from the World Health Organization, dust mites are a major contributing factor in respiratory illnesses. Considering that 30% of the world's population suffers from respiratory diseases it's worthwhile ensuring that your pillow isn't contributing to these statistics. Of all of the preferred places for dust mites to inhabit, the pillow comes in as the most worrying, as our faces are in direct contact with it and can therefore act as an easy entry for dust mites into your lungs. As your head moves over the pillow it can agitate the highly allergic and fine powder consisting of dead mites and their faeces, which ends up being inhaled.

TIP – Invest in a pillow cover. As well as protecting you from dust mites, it will increase the longevity of your pillow.

As basic as this may sound, regardless of the position you sleep in, your pillow should be under the head and not the shoulders. As mentioned above, there shouldn't be a space between the neck and the pillow, meaning that the neck is always supported. The thickness of the pillow should allow the head to remain aligned with the spine in both positions, whilst lying on the side or back, as it would be in a correct, upright standing position. In the lateral, side posture position, the pillow should be neither too high nor too low, as this leaves the head elevated or depressed, therefore misaligning it with the neck. This rule should also be maintained when lying on your back. A pillow that is too thick will leave the head elevated and the cervical spine (the neck) flexed, tensioning the muscles of the neck and promoting bio-mechanical dysfunction.

TIP FOR DETERMINING THE CORRECT PILLOW HEIGHT FOR SIDE SLEEPERS

If you buy your pillow from a store that also sells mattresses, test it out on one of their mattresses that is most similar to yours. Use your preferred sleep position to test it for the time necessary to know whether it is a suitable candidate or not. Now try others and eliminate those that are not supportive. If lying on a bed is not possible, find a wall, wedge the pillow between your head and the wall and test it for height and support. A rough guide would be that its thickness should be at least the same as the distance between the side of your head and the most lateral point of your shoulders.

EVERYTHING THAT YOU NEED TO KNOW ABOUT MATTRESSES

Have you ever stopped to think about how much time we spend in bed? If you sleep six to eight hours daily (the recommended amount), you spend between 25 and 30% of your life lying down! It is a long enough time to damage your spine if there is a compromising factor, such as an inadequate mattress. A large percentage of people who suffer back pain will say that it is worse when they wake. If this is your case, maybe your body is trying to tell your something.

Instead of listening to our body's signal, we usually get up, let the pain subside, and start another day of work and activities that distract us until the next day. If you do not suffer from back problems, you can help yourself to prevent them by using a proper mattress. Besides sleeping better, you will wake up with a good disposition, your life will be better, and your pain and muscle contractures will disappear. Good quality mattresses are not cheap, but they can last up to ten years and are an investment in your health.

To choose your mattress properly, here are some tips:

- Ask about the components of the mattress and the springs that support the spine; the number and configuration vary from one model to another. The pillow top (superior part of the mattress), is generally made out of memory (or visco-elastic) foam, is for comfort, and can have different thicknesses. In general, the height of the mattress varies between 16 and 40 cm. With these features, you'll have a product that provides the necessary support and comfort desired for a good night's sleep without compromising the posture and structure of your spine.
- There's no mattress that will please everyone, but if you prefer soft mattresses, consider that maybe over time that you have become accustomed to a softer mattress and that it will probably take a while to adapt to a firmer mattress. For people accustomed to sleeping on their backs a firmer mattress is indicated,

while people who sleep on their sides need a slightly less firm mattress to accommodate the fact that the pelvis and the shoulders sink into the mattress. Try a firm mattress (it can be a family member's mattress) to see how it feels, before you buy one.

- Know when the time comes to get a new mattress: if your mattress sinks in the middle and, of course, if you wake up with pain or stiffness (especially if the pain is in the lower back), it is time to replace your mattress! Putting a layer of wood under the mattress is just a palliative solution.
- Our body changes shape during our life for many reasons. Pregnancy, increases or decreases in body weight and certain injuries mean that we may require a new mattress to accommodate these changes.
- An expensive mattress is not a guarantee of good quality or that it is the most suitable mattress for you. Many patients, when talking about the quality of their mattresses, say it is good because it was expensive. Mattresses that have more springs and cushioning or coating, in general, have higher quality and therefore are more expensive, although the high price does not always guarantee that it is more comfortable or more supportive than a cheaper mattress. A good mattress should also give uniform support from head to toe. If there are 'spaces' in your mattress, you're not getting the support you need.
- Try out different mattresses before buying yours, for example, in a hotel or at a friend's house. When you're in the store, lay on the mattress for at least 10 minutes before deciding if it's good or not. If two people will be using the mattress, both should try it to make sure they have adequate space and that both consider it comfortable.
- Look for a mattress that does not move, deform or sink when your partner turns around and gets out of bed at night.
- Watch for the words 'orthopaedic' or 'semi orthopaedic'. There is no standard for testing the firmness of a mattress, which is why each mattress manufacturer adopts different parameters to classify firmness and comfort.
- Buy your mattress from a trustworthy business. If you know the brand and it has a good reputation, that is a start. Be sure to find out if you can exchange the product if you do not adapt to it.
- Take care of your new mattress! It is recommended that every six months, the mattress should be repositioned to ensure that the wear is uniform. Turn the side that has been slept on down and turn the mattress 180 degrees horizontally, i.e., where the head was before should now be for the feet. The weight must be distributed evenly across the mattress because the structures of a mattress are vulnerable to compression, just like your spine. For people who experience crises of acute back pain (lower back) and cannot afford to buy a new mattress

immediately (but recognize that theirs is too old/soft), there's a way to take care of that straight away: You can put several blankets on the floor with enough thickness to support the spine and still be comfortable. Your spine shouldn't touch the ground whilst lying on your back (supine). This will provide a fairly firm surface and the support needed to overcome the crisis. If sleeping on the floor in this fashion has you waking up without pain, the question has been answered: the mattress is not suitable for you and probably causing your back pain! Change it as soon as you can.

A third of our lives is a long time! That's exactly how long most of us spend in bed sleeping! Good sleep is essential for optimal health and as important as adequate hydration and a good diet. Proof of this is the fact that sleep deprivation can cause serious health problems in a very short amount of time, often in a few days. Sleep is a time for our body to regenerate and allow it to recuperate from the day's activities. A disrupted night's sleep results in a lowering of the body's immunity, difficulty concentrating, a reduction in the level of energy, all of which are essential for a productive day. When the disruption turns chronic (continuous) the consequences can be much more serious. There are many factors that we can't easily control, for example, external noise, temperature, the consumption of certain foods before bed, and the effect they have on our digestion. However, there are other factors frequently overlooked, such as mattress and pillow quality, that contribute to chronic sleep disorders. A comprehensive understanding of what constitutes a suitable mattress and how to choose is it is indispensable to be able to ensure a deep, normal, and reparative sleep. One that not only anatomically supports the spine but also promotes comfort. Through my work as a chiropractor, I have seen hundreds of cases of chronic pain due to inadequate mattresses. Funnily enough, although most of these people would wake up with back pain that they didn't feel before getting into bed, very few related their symptoms to their mattress. Most would use the same mattress for years or even decades, spending money on all types of medical intervention when they were lying on the real cause of the problem! A mattress becomes damaging to our health when it fails to provide adequate support to our spine when we are lying down. This support must be provided when we are sleeping on our side and our back. Mattresses that tend toward being too soft allow the area around the pelvis to sink into the mattress, overloading areas of the spine. The highest incidence of back pain from an inadequate mattress is most definitely in the lower back for this reason.

SLEEPING IN A BED THAT ISN'T YOURS

We can't always sleep in our own beds. Many people travel for work and holidays, sleeping in beds that aren't always suitable for their spines, especially when they have a pre-existing condition. To avoid unnecessary pain or an exacerbation of an existing back problem you must do your best to sleep on a mattress that is not going to compromise your spine. The majority of people that are suffering from low back problems will suffer more if they sleep on a mattress that is softer than their own.

When staying at a hotel, inquire before booking if they have firm mattresses. This is especially important if you plan to return frequently to the same hotel (for example on work trips) as a particular mattress that may suit your spine can be noted by the hotel and made available for future visits. If you have not inquired beforehand test the mattress as soon as you arrive. If you find it too soft, ask to change rooms. If this is not possible, ask the management to change your mattress for a firmer one. Don't be shy! Hotels usually have a variety of mattresses of different quality even though they may be the same brand as some may be newer than others.

Over the years I have received many patients, often in crisis, after sleeping on sofas and sofa beds, especially when these people already had a history of back pain. Exercise caution when sleeping on a sofa bed, as many have inadequate foam for spinal support. You may find more comfort from placing several blankets on the floor, to a thickness of 5–10 cm, and sleeping on them.

Some inflatable mattresses offer a surprising amount of support. If you buy one, make sure you test it out for one night before traveling, especially if you will spend a long time away from your bed. Inflatable mattresses do not provide the support of a normal mattress but are better than a couch or a hammock.

HOW TO GET IN AND OUT OF BED

Are you one of those people who 'bounce' out of bed in the morning? I certainly was. Until I suffered severe back pain and learned firsthand the importance of getting out of my bed correctly. By the time we get up in the morning, most of us have spent 6–8 hours lying down. While we may move a considerable amount during the day, at night we are predominately still, except for the minor adjustments made in changing position, etc. This period of inactivity can result in the shortening of important muscles, tendons, and ligaments. If we 'bounce' out of bed or even leave the bed in a way that overloads these shortened tissues, we may damage them. Worse still, as we depend on these structures to protect our spine and intervertebral discs from excessive load, certain movements may cause damage in these areas if our muscles, tendons, and ligaments haven't warmed up first. This is why it is so important to learn the correct way to get out of bed and repeat it every morning of our lives. For those people that live with back pain, are in crisis, or who suffer from bio-mechanical compromise, getting out of bed correctly will make a huge difference to the amount of pain they suffer and the rate at which their problem will degenerate or not. It is important to remember that any bio-mechanical activity incorrectly executed will accelerate joint and soft tissue degeneration, independently of what that activity is.

Turn sideways on the edge of the mattress facing the bedroom wall.

Bend both your legs slightly. Push yourself up to a sitting position using your superior arm. This should leave you sitting, probably with your feet touching the floor, ready to leave the bed. If you feel stiff or back pain, stay sitting in this position for as long as it takes to feel more comfortable, allowing the soft tissues of your spine and neck the time they need to adjust to the change.

Next step, engage your core muscles by activating your abdominal muscles and get up using both legs with equal force.

To lie down, repeat this process in reverse order.

HOW TO CARE FOR YOUR SPINE AT WORK

"People lose their health to earn money and then lose money to regain health. By thinking anxiously about the future, forgetting the present, for not living in the present nor future, they live life like they will never die and die as though they have never lived."

BUDDHA

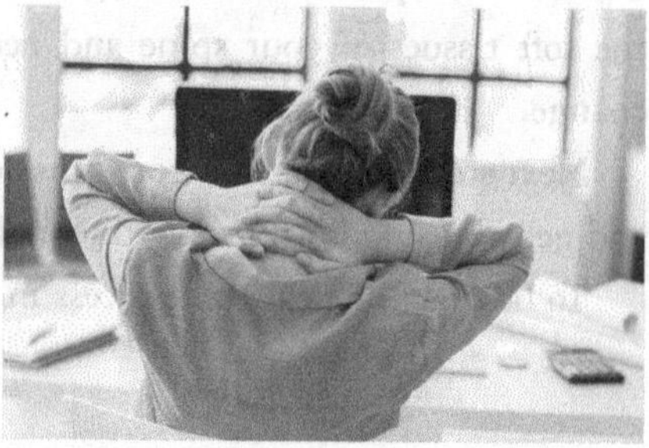

To the untrained eye, your workspace may seem harmless, however, it possesses many hidden potential dangers that can cause serious problems to your spine. Based on my experience, I would say that at least 50% of my patients present with bio-mechanical problems caused by their work posture or work-related activities. If we stop to think of a few professions and the postures that they require their professionals to maintain during the day, it is quite easy to understand how the intricate bio-mechanics and function of the vertebral column can be compromised without the professional being aware of what is happening.

Picture a dentist who is seated most of the time with their head looking down into a patient's mouth, and worse still, rotated to the same side every day! Wow! This poor professional has lost the ability to maintain spinal symmetry, as well as being obliged to pass hours and hours with a forward head carriage, straightening of the neck curve (rectification), and last but not least, load on the lumbar spine from sitting excessively. As dentists get accustomed to their work posture from the very first day they start work, most will pass their careers without feeling pain until a certain moment when the body simply can't adapt anymore.

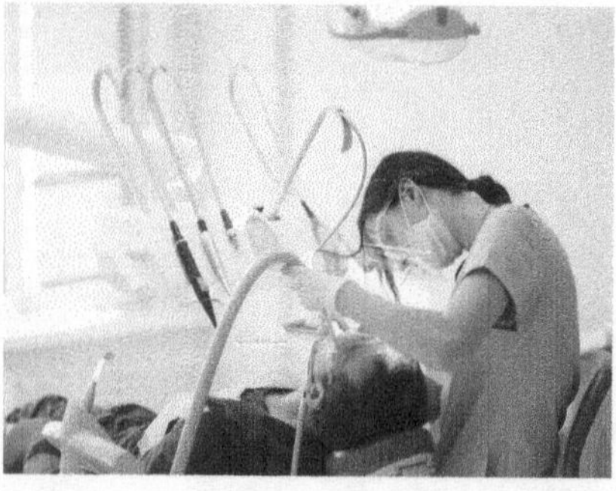

At this time a crisis of neck pain or stiffness can and often does uncover years and years of osteoarthritic degeneration in the form of bone spurs or vertebral disc wear and tear. While I won't discuss specific preventative measures here, I will highlight the necessity for dentists and all other professionals that receive continual asymmetrical load on their spines to implement specific stretching and strengthening measures throughout their whole career. In reality, these preventative measures should be taught while they are studying. Being a chiropractor, I can relate to the effects that my work posture and repetitive movements have had on my own spinal health and wish that I had have been taught how to care for my spine earlier, before spinal surgery obliged me to. I have examined literally thousands of patients throughout my career that sadly showed avoidable spinal degeneration, simply because they worked and sustained postures that were causing harm while the professional was oblivious to the damage being caused and the necessity to counteract it.

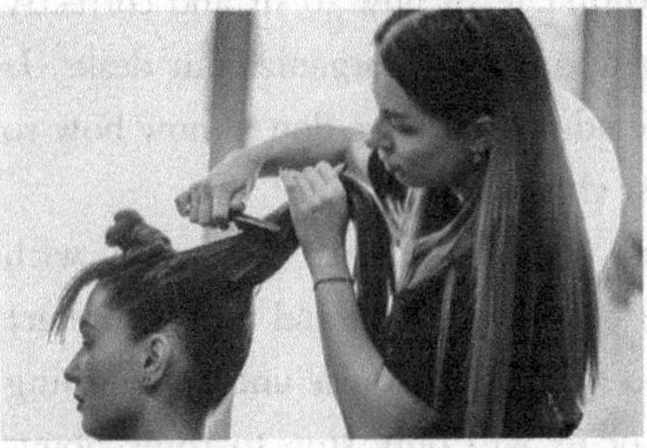

Consider hairdressers, architects, writers, secretaries, and lawyers who work with similar postures to the dentists or builders, electricians, and plumbers who have jobs that are more active but place a bio-mechanical load on the spine in a different way. People who lift weights, perform repetitive movements, or work asymmetrically overload certain articulations and tissues much more than others and as a result speed up the degenerative process.

If we classify patients according to sedentary or non-sedentary professions, based on my experience, the sedentary jobs pose far more risk to the health of the spine than the non-sedentary ones. This fact surprises most people as they forget just how dangerous lack of movement is for our mobile, articulating vertebral column. Imagine leaving a bicycle without being ridden or a door handle without being opened. With time they both seize due to lack of movement. Lack of function. It must be remembered that the spine, like the bicycle and the door handle, is a machine composed of movable components and if it is not functioning and fulfilling its purpose as long as possible during the conscious hours of our life, will slowly lose its function. How this happens has already been discussed in previous sections. This gradual loss of function and subsequent irreversible degeneration usually happens without obvious signs and symptoms. Those who pass 8–10 hours a day sitting, must understand that the function of their spine will invariably be affected. Physical activity outside of those hours is obviously vital to compensate (to a certain degree) for this time of inactivity. Understanding the correct way to sit, how to use a computer or smartphone correctly, how to choose a suitable chair, or adjust a computer monitor to the correct height is vital if we are to avoid the unnecessary suffering that comes from avoidable spinal degeneration caused by our professions. As discussed earlier in 'Forward head carriage', even a 1–2 cm forward shift in head position whilst using a computer can overload the joints of the neck by 5–10 kilograms! As these and other effects are cumulative, repeated day after day for the duration of somebody's professional life, we must learn the basic rules and apply them to our work posture. The way we write an email or send a text message and other routine tasks that we perform many times a day during our adult lives can all be detrimental if done incorrectly. Remember that as kids we didn't learn how to sit and correctly position ourselves when we read and write or how to organize our desks. Is there any wonder then, when we become adults, why we don't know how to set up our workstations or choose the best chair for our spine?

Ergonomics, (*Webster* definition – an applied science concerned with designing and arranging things people use so that people and things interact most efficiently and safely) isn't given too much importance until 'something has already happened'. In reality, most of us will only stop to think about ergonomics when we are already suffering headaches from incorrect work posture, a sore low back from an inadequate office chair or pins and needles in the fingers from having our keyboard too far forward or too high. It is important to highlight that by the time symptoms appear to advise that a position or posture may be detrimental to us, irreversible degeneration has often already occurred.

SITTING YOUR LIFE AWAY?

Our spine was never intended to pass prolonged periods of time in a sitting position. Even if your chair is the most modern, most expensive chair on the market, no degree of technology or expense will successfully negate all of the

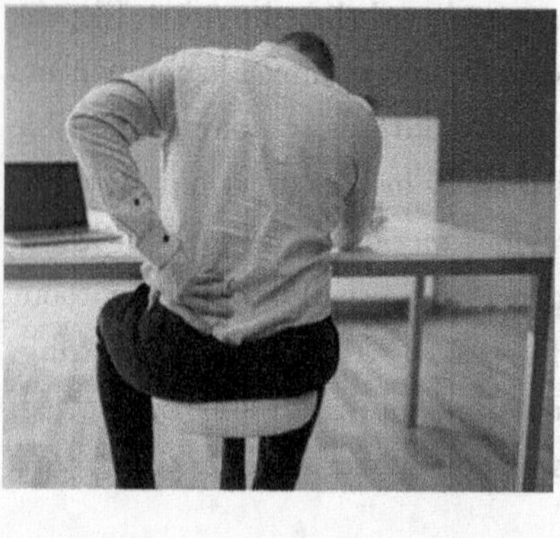

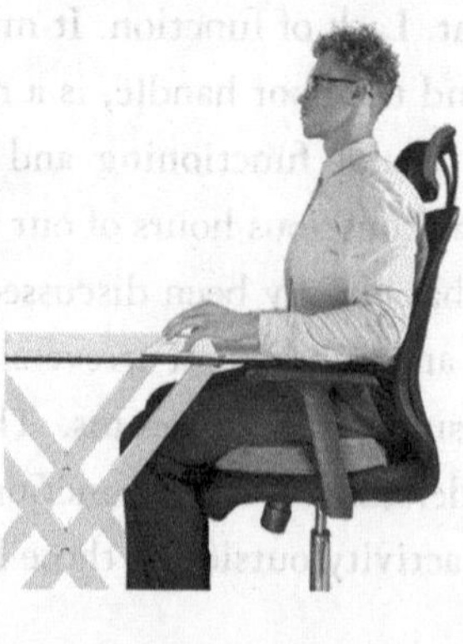

excessive load that gravity exerts on our spine whilst sitting. That said, a good quality chair can drastically reduce the amount of load that your lumbar spine receives whilst sitting and is a worthy investment. Poor quality chairs and stools simply cannot provide the support necessary to comfort the spine whilst working.

Our distant ancestors didn't work sitting. They were predominantly active and the times that they were stationary it is believed that they did so squatting. Many cultures still adopt a squatting stance whilst eating or doing routine tasks, especially indigenous ones.

Correct posture whilst sitting keeps the spinal curves preserved, especially the lumbar curve, also maintaining the body's centre of gravity and therefore minimising the effects of gravity upon the spine.

HOW TO SIT ON A CHAIR CORRECTLY

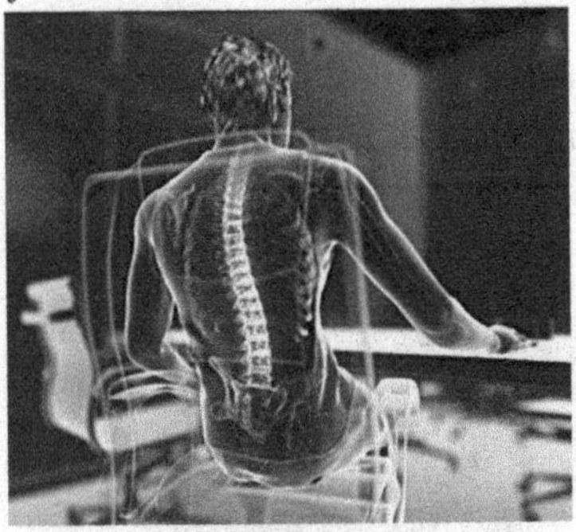

If you have to sit, sit correctly! A correct posture for sitting can be achieved by lowering yourself slowly onto the chair, allowing the buttocks to slide down the lower part of the vertical back support. This will position the buttocks at the base of the chair, allowing the rest of the spine to be well supported against the vertical part. Our challenge is to not slide forward with time, whether it be due to the effects of gravity or because we are simply more accustomed to slouching in the chair. Chairs made of slippery plastic or wood can also encourage the buttocks to slide forward, making it difficult to maintain a correct sitting posture. As this happens, frequent adjustments must be made to reposition the buttocks. It is estimated that this type of postural adjustment should occur every 15 minutes to compensate for this forward movement. Those who slump and pass hours incorrectly positioned with the buttocks well forward and the resultant increase in thoracic curve, frequently relate low back pain, thoracic stiffness, pain in the neck, and permanent postural changes leaving them 'hunched' over. Passing enough time in this position actually changes the permanent posture of these people, causing them to be stuck with this hunched posture permanently.

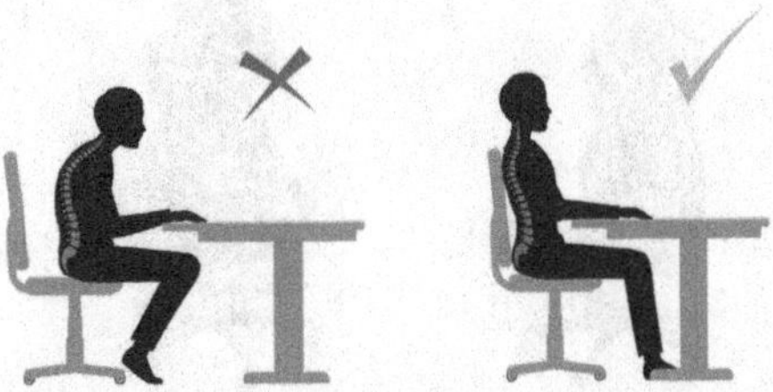

When the buttocks and base of the spine are correctly positioned in the chair the rest of the thoracic and cervical spine will follow into correct alignment. The spine will consequently be kept in it's correct anatomical position.

CASE STUDY

Sarah was a writer who came in with marked stiffness, loss of low back mobility and strong low back pain of only a month's duration. When we talked about traumas that may have happened around the time of the onset of her pain, she couldn't recall anything specific that may have influenced the state she was now in. When I asked her if anything had changed in the last month (for example a new exercise routine, new bed, or a new chair), she told me that she had renovated her home and had been writing on a bench from her outdoor dining setting instead of her normal chair. After treating her once I asked her to go home and dust off her normal chair. On her second visit a week later, she was feeling 100% pain-free.

Sitting on a bench or slouched in a chair causes the spine to lose its normal lumbar curve, as the support necessary to keep the low back curve preserved isn't being provided.

MYTH – Curves are not normal!

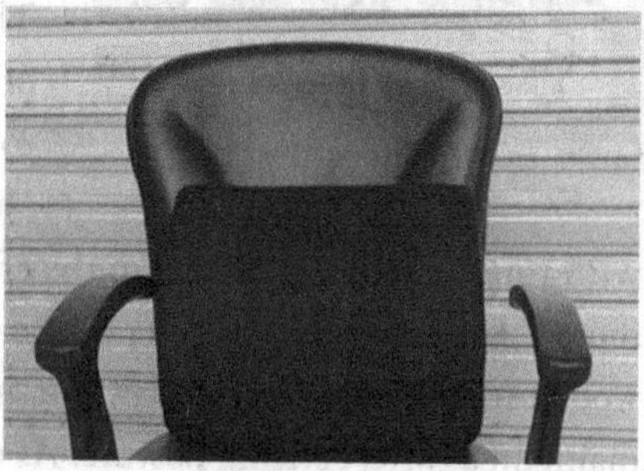

Actually, curves are essential for normal movement (compare the neck of a giraffe with no spinal curves and consequently no spinal mobility, to the neck of a flamingo that has two curves and as a result can turn 360 degrees!) An ergonomically sound chair will always have some type of support for the lumbar spine. As benches do not have this support, they are unable to maintain the anatomical curves of the spine and are therefore terrible for passing long periods of time on.

For the correct posture whilst sitting, get the right support!

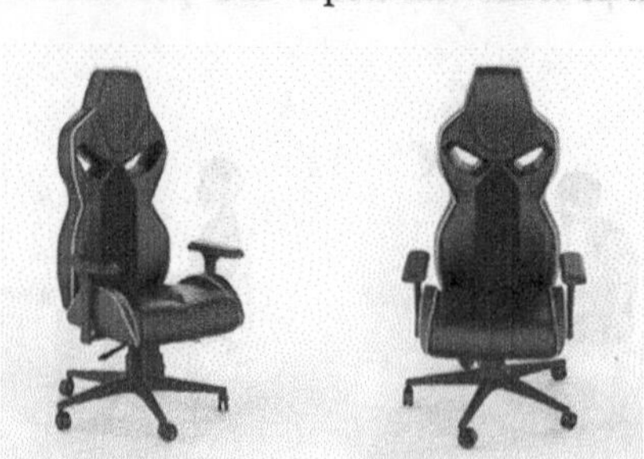

Ergonomic chairs are an excellent option for office workers or those who have to pass many hours a day sitting. Their structure provides the correct support for the spinal curves and minimises the effects of gravity on the back. If one of these chairs is out of your budget, look for a chair that adequately supports the lumbar spine, preferably with a curve at the base that encases the lumbar spine. Foam and visco-elastic lumbar supports are also excellent and cheap options for improving the support given by a normal chair.

A suitable chair will also have an armrest, that helps prevent slouching in the chair and helps the person sitting in it to maintain their torso erect. Armrests also allow the person sitting in the chair to support their forearms on them while they type. Another advantage of ergonomic chairs is that they can rotate. This is important because it means you are not constantly causing unnecessary rotation to pick up documents or when you move to meet a client or answer the telephone. Remember that rotation combined with flexion is one of the worst things for your spine, so do not rotate your back whilst seated.

A footrest can also help, as keeping the feet slightly elevated redistributes some of the weight, even if it is for a short time. Two other chairs are becoming popular – the kneeling chair, and the Swiss ball.

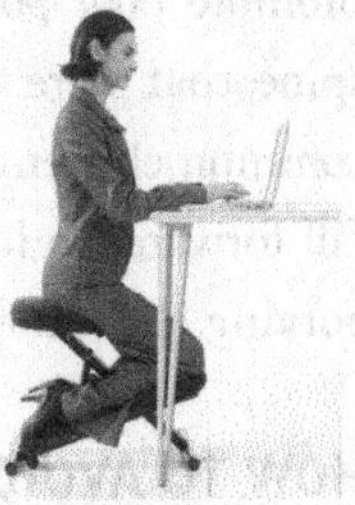

The KNEELING CHAIR can be very beneficial as it puts most of the weight on the knees and not on the lumbar spine. These seats are tilted forward with a platform to support the knees. It may take a while to get used to, however, they can really help because they keep you from sitting crouched or bent forward. As this model has no back support, it obligates the person to sit up straight and contract their abdominal muscles to maintain good posture. However, as there is no support for the arms, the knees can get a little tired, which is why I suggest alternating the use of this one with another ergonomic chair with lumbar and arm support.

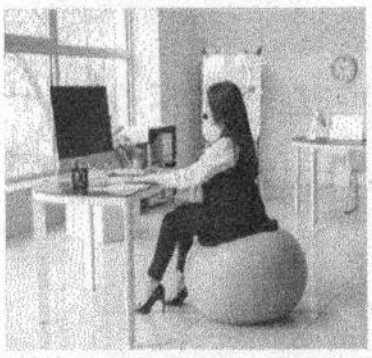

SWISS BALLS oblige the person sitting on them to maintain their core activated. You can also move your pelvis and lower back when you work. This can be done by moving your buttock forward and back and in a clockwise and anti-clockwise motion. The abdominal muscles should be activated and the legs contracted to stay upright and balanced. Some people grow tired of it because they have no lumbar or arm support, but others speak very well of this way of sitting. You can also kneel on it to vary the position and load that your spine is taking. Kneeling can activate the proprioceptive nerve receptors in the lower back which govern the level of muscle contraction in the lower back. This subsequently strengthens the lower back. Working may not be avoidable however back pain certainly is with these options and with possessing a knowledge of the correct way to use a chair.

Why not try these chairs and see which one is better for you?

Try not to cross the legs whilst sitting because it puts an uneven load on the spine and pelvis. overloading certain muscles, ligaments, and joints and interfering with the normal movement of the lower back. If you really need to cross your legs, switch between the two sides and cross them at the level of the feet and not the knees.

Remember that your spine was not meant to sit eight hours daily. Get up a minimum of every 50 minutes (ideally every 20 minutes) to walk and stretch for at least five minutes.

COMPUTERS

In today's society, it is impossible to imagine our lives without a computer. While being revolutionary and contributing enormously to productivity, it comes with a huge toll. Besides promoting a sedentary lifestyle, the use of computers, whether they be desktops, laptops, or smartphone technology, also promote poor posture, placing excessive loads on certain articulations of our spine that were never intended to be overloaded in this manner. The most common challenge for computer users is to resist the tendency for the head to fall forward, to look down, or to slouch in the chair that they are working in, curving the spine even more.

HOW TO AVOID COMPUTER BACK

The computer must be directly in front of you and not at your side.

The centre of the screen has to be at eye level.

The keyboard should be at the level of the elbows and, if possible, tilted slightly upward. Leave enough space between you and the keyboard to support the wrists while typing.

Try not to use the mouse more than necessary. Use the keyboard most of the time because when we favour one side, we create uneven loads, causing certain muscles to contract and become dysfunctional.

Place the mouse as close to your body as possible.

Your feet must be flat on the floor and legs bent at an angle of 90°.

Maintain your spinal curves (with ears, shoulders, and hips aligned – see 'anatomical centre of gravity line'), because only then are we evenly distributing the load and forces of gravity without overloading any particular region of the spine.

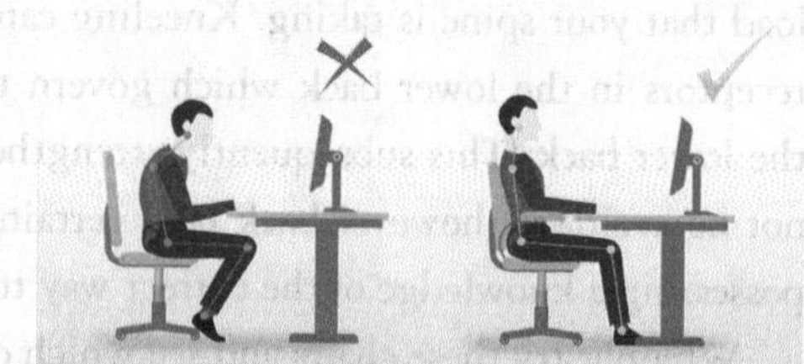

You can also use a lumbar support to maintain good posture because it enables one to sustain an upright posture longer with less energy expenditure.

Unfortunately when the computer was developed it didn't come with an instruction manual on how to correctly use it without compromising spinal health.

It is important to be your own doctor and recognize the pain that may occur from an incorrect sitting posture while at a desk, for example, when the computer is positioned to the side of the keyboard and not directly in front of the person using it.

If we calculate a working week of 8 hours a day, five days per week 48 weeks per year (subtracting four weeks of annual leave), in an average career of 40 years (8 x 5 x 48 x 40), we spend at least 76,800 hours of our lives at work! Now imagine how incorrect postures and repetitive movements etc. at work can overload certain joints, muscles, tendons and ligaments. For many people who are using their technology and other instruments incorrectly, this wear and tear could have been avoided or at least minimised by simply stopping to adjust the computer screen, adjusting the height of the chair, learning to elevate your mobile phone whilst texting, and checking the height of the keyboard, etc. This can make an enormous difference over time. Do not let the configuration of your computer and workstation be another detrimental factor to your health, beyond those of everyday life that we cannot control as easily.

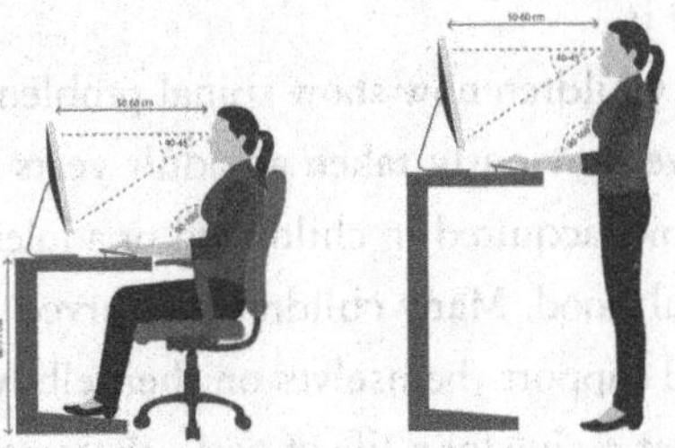

It is important to have your screen at the correct height! If the screen is too low, the head needs to be tilted down, flexing the cervical spine and rectifying it's curve. Remember that for every 1 cm of forward head movement, the neck and its articulations receive an increase of 5 kg of load! This increase in load falls even greater at the base of the neck and this is why people complain of more tension between their shoulder blades, over their trapezius muscles, and at the base of the neck. The head is kept in a position where it doesn't add excessive load to the neck when the ears are exactly in line with and above the shoulders as previously explained, the head is kept in a position where it doesn't add excessive load to the neck.

You can correctly position the screen by placing a box under it. Alternatively, if your chair is adjustable, it can be adjusted to a height that leaves your eyes in line with the computer screen. It is also important to remember that the desk needs to be at elbow level.

LAPTOPS and iPADS

Intended for portable use, laptops are extremely convenient and enable us to work from practically anywhere. Airports, coffee shops, bus stops, and trains can now literally be offices away from the office. However, this convenience comes at a cost and the aches and pains of those who regularly use laptops are the proof.

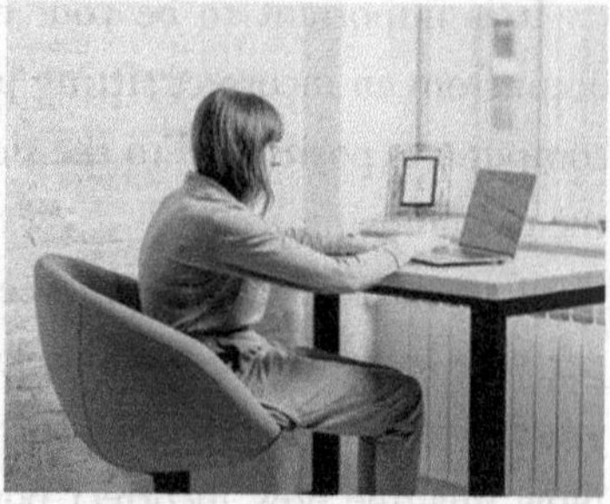

There is no way to maintain correct posture when using a laptop on your lap! The only way to use it properly is to have it propped up and make sure the screen is high enough to be level with the eyes. Likewise, if the keyboard is in line with the height of the elbows, the head is obliged to look down at it, setting up the problems described previously.

We must remember that a laptop was designed to be used for only short periods of time, and not permanently. Try alternating between your desktop computer and laptop/iPad as much as possible to mix the loads on your spine up a little.

Before purchasing a laptop, consider how much time you will actually use it.

Children now show spinal problems from the use of tablets etc. that would have previously taken an adult years or decades to develop. Furthermore, the habits acquired in childhood or adolescence are very difficult to be changed in adulthood. Many children sit curved in a chair looking down or lie face down and support themselves on their elbows to use the iPad, and that is certainly a great recipe for a life of neck, thoracic, and lumbar pain. The children of today will be the workers of tomorrow, and they are already showing bio-mechanical problems long before they reach their work age.

FOR OCCASIONAL LAPTOP USE

Use a comfortable chair that allows you to recline it slightly backward.

Place the laptop on your lap until you find the most neutral posture possible for the wrists, with a minimum of extension or flexion – as straight and aligned with the forearm as possible.

Tilt the screen to minimise flexion of the neck with the head forward.

FOR MORE CONTINUAL USE

Place the laptop on the desk in a position that allows you to see the screen without bending the neck forward. To do this, you may have to raise it by using a stable support (a book, box, or a block of wood or a support specially made for laptops). It is also a good idea to use the keyboard and mouse separately.

Many laptops offer a large screen (15 inches), but you should ask yourself if you really need it, because they are more difficult to manage in places like airplanes and automobiles. Currently, there are several smaller portable laptops, but you have to consider the screen size and resolution. With small laptops, the keyboard is small and it is very difficult to keep your hands in a good position.

The weight of the laptop is very important if you are a professional who works in the street and often uses the laptop. Also consider the total weight of all accessories (battery, desktop drive, wires). If everything weighs 4 kg or more, you should consider loading them into a suitcase with wheels. If you prefer a smaller bag, a shoulder bag, ergonomically sound, could also be used.

LIFTING LOADS AT WORK (AND AT HOME)

Learning correct ways to carry excess weight is important even from an early age. One of the most common ways to damage the spine is to carry heavy weight incorrectly, and for many people, this starts in childhood when kids overload their backpack.

Later on in life, the load continues! Everything from carrying groceries to the car or luggage when you travel, to lifting the kids, picking up a weight in the gym, organizing the garden shed, to picking up a piece of clothing off the floor. Correctly lifting any object can minimise the chance of injury as well as minimise unnecessary wear and tear on your joints.

Think before your lift!

Steps to correctly carry an object:

Plan how you will carry a certain object before and visualize your movements prior.

If you are not confident that you can safely carry an object, do not lift it. There will always be another way to move it without overloading your spine. Even if the object being carried doesn't seem heavy there is still a risk of getting injured from lifting light objects, such as carrying groceries to the car or picking up a trash can. There is a correct method to lifting and carrying heavy objects, which protects the spine, and should also be applied to the times that we are lifting lighter objects.

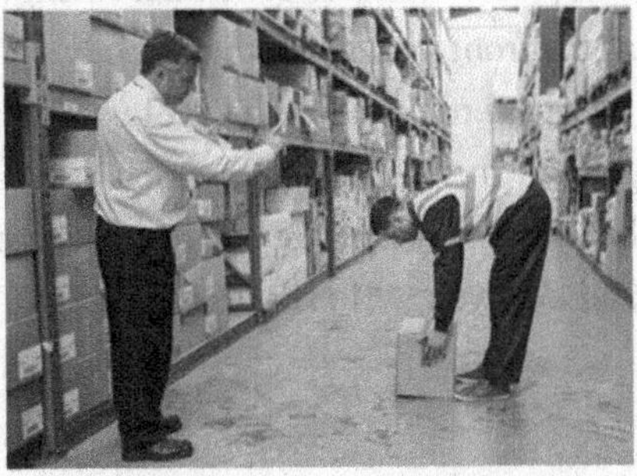

When you pick up an object off the floor, never bend at the waist.

Lower yourself by flexing the legs and hips, keeping your back as upright as possible. It helps to look to the front and not down to the floor where the object that you will carry is.

If you can, place the heavy object between your feet, which should be separated the same width as the hips.

Hold the object as close to your body as possible when lifting it off the ground, ideally having it against your body.

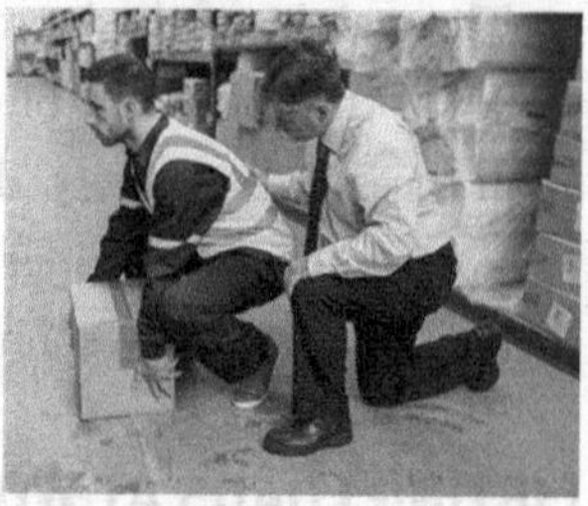

Breathe in deeply, contracting the abdominal muscles while you grab the object.

When you exhale, breathe out slowly to maintain the support for the spine whilst lifting.

Leave your elbows as close to your torso as possible. Raise yourself using the muscles of the leg and buttock, making sure to avoid rotation.

Another point to note, when practical, is to avoid carrying weight with only one hand. This will create an imbalance that may jam articulations of the spine and lead to reflex muscle guarding of support muscles and soft tissues.

If the object you are wanting to carry is too heavy, ask for help. Coordinate your lifting plan with the person helping you. If you cannot lift the weight alone or with assistance, arrange for machinery that can assist – It's simply not worth hurting yourself doing something that you could have done in a safer way.

When you lift a load, your intervertebral discs also absorb some of the load. This is generally not a problem if you do it whilst maintaining the natural curves of the spine. But if your spine is bent forward or sideways, or worse still, twisted, the unbalanced load is concentrated in one specific spot rather than being distributed throughout the entire disc. Similarly, ligaments and intrinsic muscles around the disc and vertebral segment can be strained. Negative consequences may occur from one single event in which we lift an excessively heavy load or it may occur in a cumulative manner over time with repetition.

Developing and using your core strength will not only assist you whilst lifting but will also protect your spine. This will be extremely helpful if your occupation involves continual lifting. A strong core means that both muscles at the front and back of your body are sharing the load.

These rules should be applied when picking up anything from a shoe on the ground to heavier objects such as a heavy box in the garage. Every time you bend down for any reason, take a second and think about what you're doing, and how you will execute the process. And remember, bend the knees!

SPINAL CARE AT HOME

"The future is formed by our daily decisions, inconstant and changing, every event affects all the others."

ALVIN TOFFLER

PETS

Who would have thought that even our pets could harm our spine? In fact, having a pet can attribute to exacerbating pre-existing spinal problems and causing new ones. Like any other daily habit, repeated day after day, we should stop to access what movements and postures are involved in interacting with our pets and change or modify them (the habits) if they are detrimental.

When walking your dog, you need to be the one who is in control, as many owners allow their dogs to walk them. If you have a larger, stronger dog or one that continually pulls you along, you are subject to forces that can biomechanically compromise the spine every time you walk. Besides straining the muscles of the arms and shoulders, the sudden change in direction and excessive force can also overload your neck and spine.

TIP

Consider working with a dog trainer if your dog needs to learn who is boss. Well trained dogs pose little or no threat to their owners spinal health whilst on a lead.

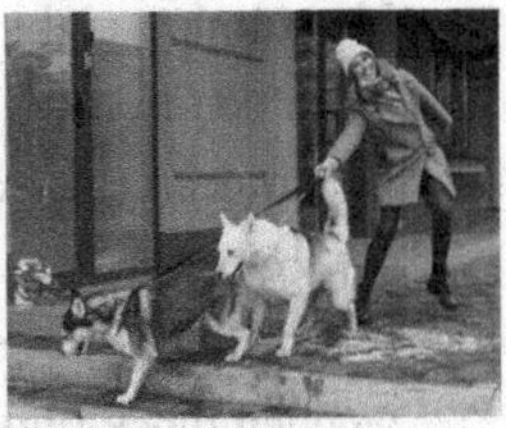

Be mindful to avoid bending your spine when leaning over to put food or water in your pet's bowl. Keep your spine straight, bend with your knees, place the food on the floor and stand up, maintaining the spine straight. If you are in pain, you can also kneel, or bring the bowl to the table to fill it.

Be especially careful when you bathe your dog, especially when carrying it in and out of a tub!

HOUSEHOLD CHORES

Housework is never-ending. Clean clothes will get dirty, dishes will need to be washed (again), beds need to be made, groceries need to be bought and carried to the car. The lawn will need to be mowed, the garden hedged, the car washed and the list goes on.

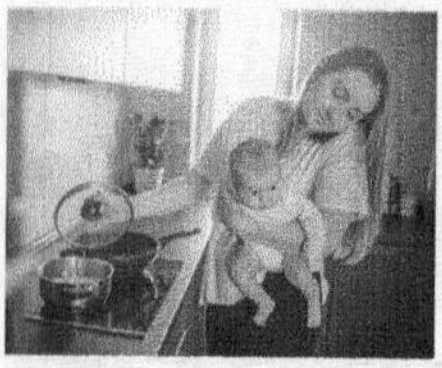

These tasks are recurrent and really need to be performed correctly, as an activity incorrectly repeated over and over, will have a much more damaging effect on the spine. As these activities have to be done daily, it's worth learning how to perform them in a way that will minimally load the spine. This is especially important if we are to avoid the degenerative problems that appear as we get older.

Over many years, I have seen many women and men suffer from avoidable problems caused by incorrectly executed daily activities such as ironing, washing, shopping, etc. Even though it is very difficult to remove the entire load that each activity produces on your spine, there are ways to minimise the damage. Here are some examples of how to practice these daily activities safely:

IRONING

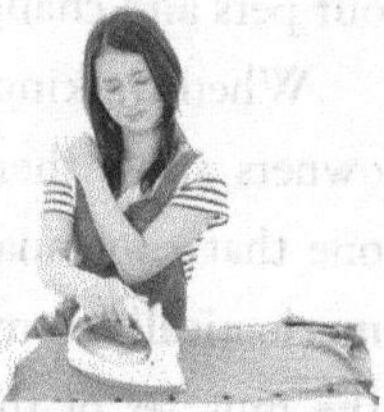

- Start with an adjustable ironing board! Adjust the ironing board to the correct height for you and, if it is not adjustable, consider buying one that is. The higher the ironing board, the less you need to look down and this will minimise neck flexion and the consequent straightening of the cervical spine and its tendency to encourage the shoulders to fall forward.
- Keep your bodyweight equally distributed on both legs so you maintain an even load between left and right.
- Use a lightweight steam iron so you can apply less pressure on the clothes when you iron.
- Do not iron the clothes all at once. Multiple shorter bouts (half an hour or so) are better than one marathon session.
- If you have pain or problems in your lower back, place a phone book or a wooden block under one of your feet, leaving the knee slightly bent. That takes some of the load off your spine.

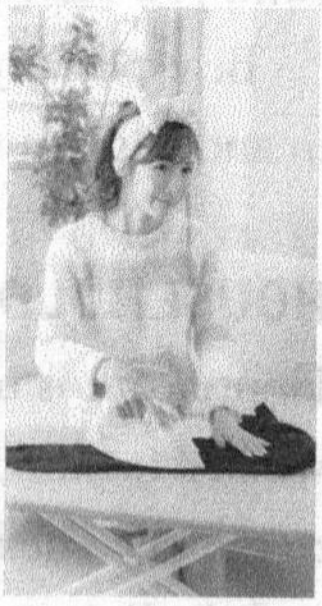

Warning! If you suffer from dizziness or headaches, and they worsen as you iron, please listen to your body and stop! This is a signal from your body that a tissue, muscle or neurological structure is being adversely affected due to poor posture. These symptoms are a serious warning that you should find the root cause of your problem.

You can actually sit while ironing if this makes it easier for your neck, however if this increases low back pain, try sitting on a firm surface and mix the standing/sitting combo up a little. Follow the rules detailed above to minimise the load on the other areas of your spine and shoulders.

WASHING THE DISHES

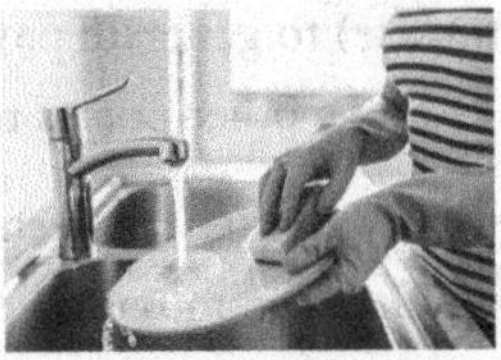

Washing dishes requires us to look down for a long period of time. This is made even more difficult if your sink is too low. As it's not always easy to install a new, higher sink, you will more than likely need to adapt to the one you have.

Here are a few things you can do to minimise the impact that this activity has on your spine:

- If there is a cupboard under the sink, you can open the door and put one foot on the bottom shelf. This will keep your spine straight and prevent you from leaning forward while doing the dishes. As little as 5 degrees of lumbar flexion whilst standing considerably overloads your spine, so do your best to keep it upright.
- If there is no cupboard, use a phone book or a stool to support the foot; this will have the same effect.
- Be careful when lifting something or bending over (for example to get dishwashing liquid out of the cupboard below the sink), especially if your spine is not straight. Check first and then lift the object. Remember to follow the simple rules previously discussed explaining how to lift loads or pick objects up.
- If you are in pain, ask for help! Delegate people you live with to do the tasks that threaten your spinal health.
- We need to be aware that the everyday tasks such as washing dishes, can be contributing factors to several spinal problems that can take years or decades to appear either in the form of pain or other obvious symptoms. Do not wait for these signs from the body, start carrying out these daily activities with the lowest possible impact on your spine.

SWEEPING AND VACUUMING

These activities pose a risk to normal spinal bio-mechanics function because many people bend over whilst doing them. In addition, these activities are asymmetrical, in other words, we use one side of our body more than the other. To counteract this, the best thing we can do to protect our spine is to alternate between the two sides. For example, sweep one minute with the broom on your left side followed by a minute with it on the right side, and so on. You could even set an alarm to remind you to switch sides – this may even make the time doing a mundane job more interesting and challenging!

To minimise harmful effects on your spine, keep your back as straight as possible. You can bend your knees slightly and use your quadriceps (thigh muscle) to generate power instead of using the spine.

Some other points to remember:

- Try to vary between push and pull, between movements to and fro.
- Get help moving heavy furniture such as beds when you need to sweep under them.

Remember the most important rule is that your spine needs to be as straight as possible.

- Keep your shoulders relaxed and make sure that they are in this position and not high, to avoid locking the neck.
- When purchasing a vacuum cleaner, try to buy one that has a long hose and consider choosing one that is upright to prevent you from bending over.

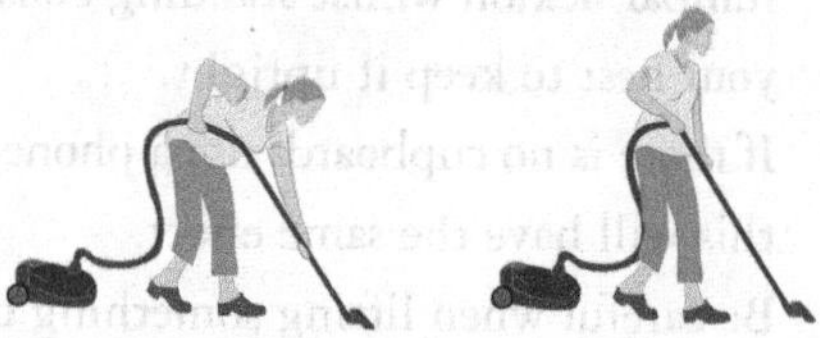

incorrect posture   correct posture

- If you do not have someone to help lift the large pieces of furniture, try cleaning underneath them by kneeling. This will put less load on your spine.

GROCERY SHOPPING

My number-one tip is to swap a basket for a shopping trolley! Using a basket can cause unnecessary strain and we tend to favour one side (usually our strongest side) when carrying a basket. This tip is especially important if you are already in pain.

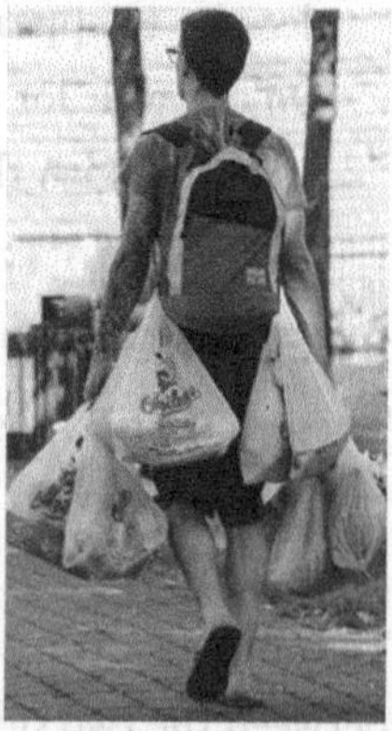

A trolley needs to be treated with caution too! When using a trolley – do not overload it as it will become difficult to push. Also, avoid using a trolley that has broken or stuck wheels – these may stop or change direction suddenly, straining your spine.

- While buying in bulk may save you some money it may not save your back! Even though we could save money by buying food or cleaning products in large packages, it might be better to choose smaller, lighter packaging so you can carry them more easily.

- Be careful of how you are choosing your groceries at the shops. If you reach for a product that is on a shelf close to the ground, squat down and bend your the knees, then lift yourself back up again with the product as close to your body as possible. Don't be afraid to ask someone at the supermarket to assist you if you need a heavier product, such as a big bag of dog food. If you can't find anybody to help you and decide to get it yourself, bend your knees and remember to do the same when you transfer the products to the car or when you get home.
- If you do not find a shopping cart, you can use two baskets to balance the weight between both sides, putting them on the floor when you get a product off the shelf.
- It is also important to balance the weight of your shopping bags when carrying them back to the car and once home, from the car to your house. Call for some help from friends or family to help you unpack.

MAKING YOUR HOME SPINE SAFE

Falls and accidents at home can injure you, sometimes seriously, even fatally. We are all guilty of doing things in a rush and without taking due caution at certain times whilst at home. Unfortunately a large proportion of serious accidents happen at home, and in most cases could be prevented by going slower and thinking about what we are doing before we do it.

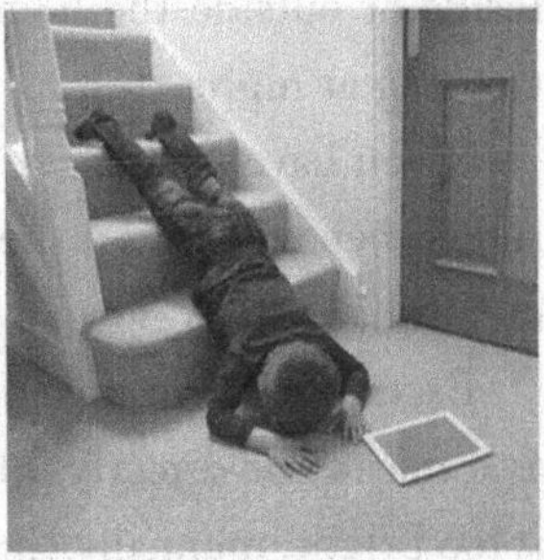

Your home could endanger your life and that of others. It is important to recognize any risk before it causes a seriously inconvenient and possibly painful or fatal accident.

- Walk around your house and identify anything that could cause injury in each room, in the yard, and garage. Look for loose rugs that you could slip on. If in doubt about a rug or something else on the floor, remove it and leave the floor bare. Many unnecessary falls occur due to people tripping on the corner of a rug or sliding on a rug that is not fixed to the floor.
- Be cautious with toys or objects left on the floor also. Cultivate the habit of removing them as soon as you see them. Better still, teach your children to put them away themselves, as they can also trip on them and begin a process of wear and tear in their spine.

- Most serious injuries in the home tend to occur to older people and those suffering from osteoporosis. They are at greater risk, since the chance of fractures is high, especially in the hip if they suffer a fall. Refer to the section on the Elderly.

STAIRS

Many serious accidents occur on the stairs of our home, but we rarely examine them to pin point possible risks. It may sound obvious, but check to see if the handrail is fixed firmly on the wall. A loose handrail at a moment where you may be off balance can mean the difference between a fall or torsion of the spine or an easy descent of your stairs. Can you pull the rail using your whole body weight without it moving? If not, call a tradesperson to secure it.

If you don't have handrails, you may need to have them installed, especially if there is a possibility of elderly family members or guests using it.

If the stairs are exposed to the weather, they can become slippery very fast. Cover the surface with a non-slip tape or paint.

LIGHTING

As obvious as it sounds, good lighting is imperative but is often overlooked when moving into a new home if the home doesn't already have ideal lighting. We often become accustomed to it instead of replacing the lights with stronger lighting. If your home is well lit, you're less likely to stumble on objects left inside or outside the home, as well as being able to fully see where you are treading at night.

If you have sensors, be mindful of the fact that a light sensor may turn off right when you need it the most, for example when you're about to step into an unfamiliar area or down a stair.

Excessively bright or direct lighting can also be a problem for some people as it may shine directly into their eyes, blinding them temporarily. If the light is too bright, manually change the direction that it is pointing so that it shines towards the ground.

STORAGE SAFETY

Avoid storing heavy objects on the ground or in places that are hard to reach as you will need to overload your spine when you need to use them. If they are at levels that make access difficult, remember to keep your spine as straight as possible and think about squatting. Squatting once or twice does not pose a problem, but these activities when repeated several times a day generate a cumulative effect on the spine, hips and knees. Lack of organization, for someone who suffers spinal problems, can be their worst enemy, so get on top of this by installing shelves at different heights in your closet or garage, to be able to keep heavy, cumbersome objects at waste to shoulder level!

Many injuries are caused when we stretch out excessively to reach objects in cupboards. Beware! Often these objects are heavier than you think and, may cause you to lose balance and fall, or strain areas of your spine that are bio-mechanically compromised, whether you know it or not. Your safest bet is to ask for help to do this activity if there's any chance of risking your spinal health.

To lighten the load of a garbage bin or bags, garbage can be deposited into smaller containers for easy transport. This rule is also valid for boxes used for storing clothes, books, and other items. Get a garbage bin with wheels and leave it by the door near the kitchen or backyard so that you do not have to carry it for any great distance.

MOVING HOUSE

Moving can not only be emotional stressful, but it can also result in physical pain if not planned well, so why take your chances? If you are going to move houses, you should plan it in advance so that you do not damage your spine.

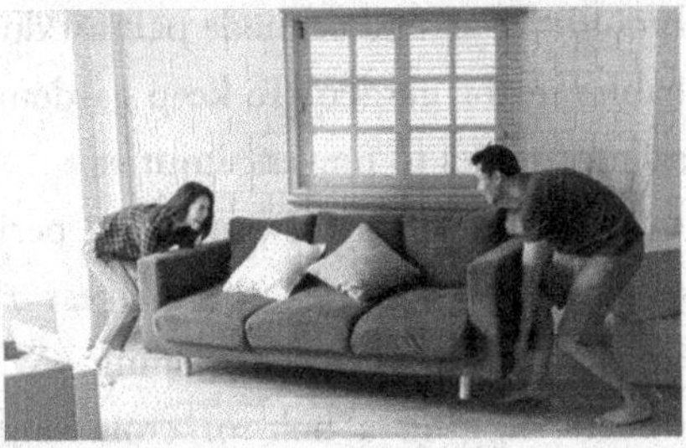

Hiring a professional moving service should be considered, especially if you already suffer back pain, or have an excessive number of heavy objects to deal with. You will still need to put your belongings into boxes, and this alone can exacerbate any pre-existing spinal problems. So if you are suffering, ask for help or start well in advance, avoiding the inconvenience of an injury that may make moving houses even more difficult and stressful.

When moving, you will carry all kinds of objects with different shapes and weights. It is important to stop and think before lifting or moving any heavy object. Think about where your centre of gravity is and only then position yourself in a way that allows you to raise the object whilst holding it as close to your body as possible.

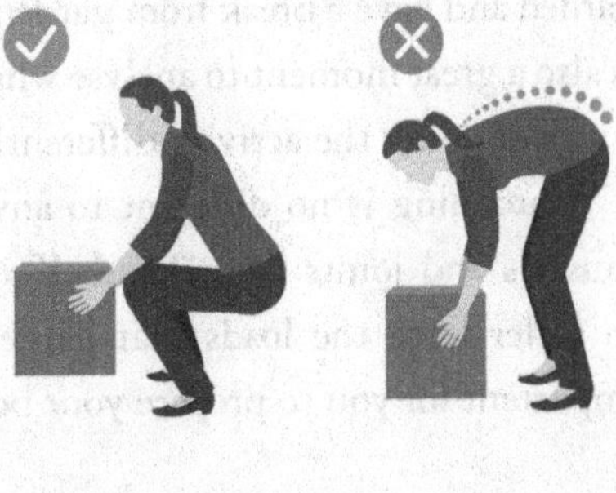

Lift with your legs and not your spine when picking up any object from the floor, activating your core when you do. Do not look down. Look forward when you are lifting. By looking down, you tend to carry the weight using your spine and not your core. If possible, use a cart that can be manoeuvred with ease, to carry heavy furniture.

TIP

Place both lighter and heavier objects in the same box to lighten the load. If this is not possible, write on the outside of the box if it is heavy, or very heavy to warn anyone now or in the future that will lift the box. Remember that these boxes can be stored for years, especially if your new home is smaller than the previous one. Years from now when you lift that box again your spine may not be as healthy as it is today, and you will appreciate the fact that the label on the box may have saved you from avoidable grief.

When moving furniture down the stairs, use pillows, rugs, and ropes to pull them whenever possible.

Use gravity to your advantage whenever you can.

IN THE GARDEN

Spending time in the garden brings joy to so many gardeners. This joy is often brought to an end or made painful due to basic postural errors and poor spinal habits in the garden. To keep gardening pleasurable, it is important to adopt safe strategies to prevent injuries.

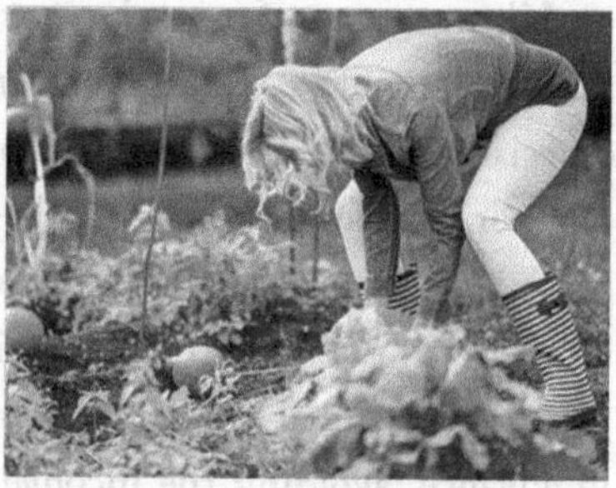

Bending down for prolonged periods of time poses one of the biggest risks to the spine whilst gardening. When we are digging a hole or crouching to remove weeds, our spine's normal curves are compromised. They can remain this way for extended periods of time and, commonly, pain isn't felt at the time because we are distracted by the activity that we are doing. However, stiffness and pain are often felt when we stand. When this happens, listen to your body and stop. Go for a walk around the garden and have a break from gardening before you go back and continue. This is also a great moment to analyse why your body caused that symptom and plan a way of doing the activity differently, in a way that is kinder to your spine.

Gardening is no different to any exercise in regards to warming up your muscles and joints beforehand. If your life is sedentary, you are more prone to suffer from the loads that gardening places upon it and it is even more important for you to prepare your body for gardening.

TIP

One of the best ways to do this is to walk at least 30 minutes or start gardening a little later on in the day, after your body has had enough time to move, circulate the blood and loosen your joints and muscles. Preparing your body via stretches and warmups for any exercise is essential. Why would gardening be any different?

Another way to avoid the muscles being contracted for long periods of time is to start the activity and stop every 30 minutes to walk for at least five minutes. This will help maintain the mobility of your spine and minimise the risk of it locking up. As a general rule, it is advisable to dig for 20 minutes at any one time.

When doing any action that requires force, do it with your knees and hips, using arm and shoulder strength as well to reduce the load on your spine.

When possible, place a pillow or blanket under your knees to make kneeling more comfortable. I have treated numerous avid gardeners over the years with advanced arthritis in their knees that they attributed to the time they spent kneeling in the garden.

Keep yourself as close as possible to the tree or shrub that you are working on to avoid unnecessary effort. Avoid rotating the spine when pulling any plant, as the force combined with rotation will be more detrimental to your spine.

Choose the right tools for the job!

Use a wheelbarrow to carry heavy plants, dirt, or sand around the garden and from the car!

Always keep the space where you keep your garden tools tidy to avoid tripping over the mess. This will also help you avoid stretching out when reaching for them. Using adapted gardening tools with long handles, such as forks and tools with extensions means less stretching and you can adapt them to your body as well.

Invest in a good hose, which is easy to pull, avoiding the need to carry buckets or watering cans of water. Think about installing an irrigation system to minimise the effort involved with watering.

Yes, an aesthetically pleasing yard is important, however, it should be easy to maintain and care for. The little details can make a massive difference in the long run. Plants can be arranged on an elevated level to avoid having to bend down to take care of them. Favour plants that do not need to be changed every year or watered regularly, even in the summer – which also prevent water wastage. Make flower beds narrow to work on them without stretching yourself too far. Avoid bare patches as this encourages weeds to grow (and removing them can add load to your spine).

Planting slow-growing shrubs that do not require heavy maintenance can also save your spine from additional wear and tear with time.

BATHROOM

The bathroom can be one of the most dangerous rooms of your house. It poses a series of threats to your spine, not only because of the obvious risk of a fall on a slippery floor, but also other infrequently considered factors.

This section covers the areas that pose the greatest risks.

DRYING AND STYLING YOUR HAIR

Drying and styling hair can place unusually heavy loads on the head while it is in positions that it is not adequately supported in. When done consistently and incorrectly over time, this can cause neck and spine issues or exacerbation of pre-existing ones.

TIPS

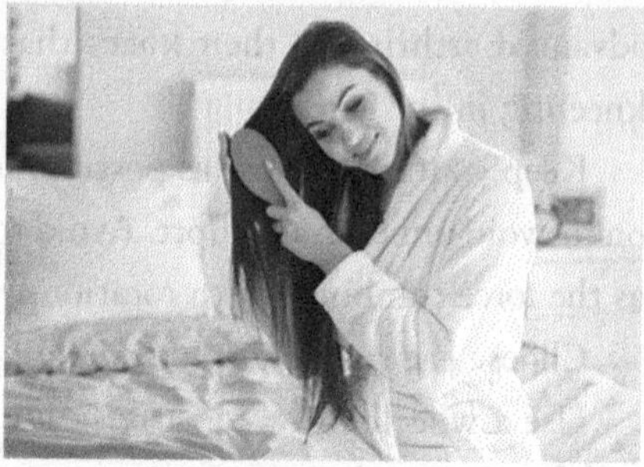

- Comb your hair without tilting your head.
- When you find a knot, use the strength of your arm to try to slowly work it out in several attempts, not just in one, with the use of force.
- Parents should adopt this same procedure when combing their children's hair. The child's neck is much more delicate and pulling a child's neck at this age can result in spinal bio-mechanical dysfunction and consequences that may only be felt in the future.
- When most people use their hairdryer, they usually tend to bend or rotate their heads to dry hair evenly and quickly. This becomes even worse when you have the dryer in one hand and comb the hair with the other as it can overload the shoulders and the base of the neck.
- Dry your hair first, keeping your head aligned with the body and spine, and then brush it, keeping the correct position of the head in relation to the spine. Avoid doing both at the same time.

DRYING YOURSELF WITH A TOWEL

Even a seemingly basic and routine act of drying the body with a towel can overload certain joints of the spine and the body. We can balance on one leg while lifting the other one up, pivot on a foot to bend down to dry a calf and so on. For people who are physically prepared for this and flexible, their bodies are totally prepared for the extra loads that certain positions can place on their joints. However, for those who have spinal problems such as arthritis, previous surgery or even plain old stiffness from lack of exercise, this everyday act can end up being the straw that breaks the camel's back.

TIPS

- Be careful when drying your feet; crouch down, bend your legs and not the spine, dry your feet and lift yourself back up again.
- If you have good flexibility and sufficient strength to support yourself on one leg, resting one foot on an elevated object such as a stool or the edge of the bathtub can help you avoid unnecessarily bending over.
- If the two tips presented above are simply too demanding, leave a stool or bench in the bathroom that allows you to sit down and dry the rest of your body whilst sitting.
- If you suffer from neck problems, when drying the head and neck, do not tilt your head, keep it straight.
- Using a longer towel will enable you to dry both sides of your body (each with one hand). Like this you'll be able to dry your back and your head without bending or leaning.

BRUSHING TEETH AND SHAVING

People with low back problems such as osteoarthritis or intervertebral disc degeneration often report feeling pain and/or crisis when doing simple hygienic tasks, such as shaving or brushing teeth, even though they are not 'apparently' overloading their spines. This is due to the fact that forward inclination of the body, with slight flexion of the lumbar spine (required when bending over a sink to reach the tap or the sink) significantly increases the load on this area of the spine. If you suffer from spinal problems in the lower back region, do all you can to avoid this slight forward inclination until you have heeled. This is often made worse when the sink is too far from the edge of the vanity. Only 5% of flexion (forward inclination) is required to overload the discs of the spinal column up to five times more than normal.

To minimise this is, stay as close as possible to the mirror and avoid leaning forward while brushing your teeth or shaving. When it is necessary to lean, bend your legs a little, activating the core first.

BATHROOM CABINETS

Bathroom cabinets placed too close to the floor require us to continually bend over to reach their contents. The only safe way to use these cupboards over time is to bend your legs and squat down without bending the spine. This is OK for somebody with a healthy back, however for those who don't, it can be a real challenge.

TIPS

- Place the items used most often in the front of the cabinet and as high as possible for easy reach. This will reduce the time your posture is compromised if you need to access them.
- If you are lucky enough to design your bathroom, put the cabinets at an appropriate height for you (preferably at arms or eyes height). It will be worth the effort as you may live in the house for a long period of time and be using the bathroom for many years! Alternatively, consider installing a cupboard on the wall which will keep the most used items at eye level.

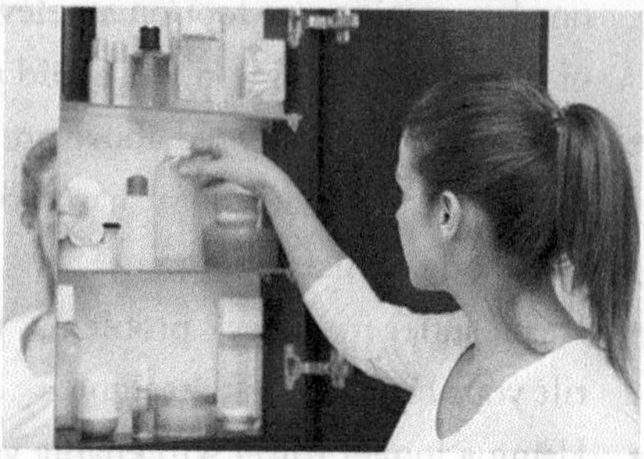

SHOWER AND BATH

Regardless of your age or your health, the possibility of a fall in the shower is higher than in other areas of your home. Most of the serious falls that occur in the home occur in the bathroom. Cranial traumas, fractures, and even death are common. Bathrooms need special attention for this reason alone and if you suffer from any type of back problem, you have one more good reason to give your bathroom the attention its needs.

TIPS

- Avoid leaving shampoo or soap on the bottom of the tub or shower after using it as it can remain there and cause a slip or fall the next time you use it. Always wash the surface down and remove any excess product, using your feet if that is easier.
- Use good quality rubber bath mats in these areas as well as on the bathroom floor. The bottom of the mat must have suction cups to prevent them from slipping while you are standing on them.

- Using a handheld shower head can help you avoid angling yourself in awkward positions to expose difficult areas of your body to the water stream coming out of a mounted shower head, especially if it is weak.
- Special chairs and stools for bathtubs and showers can dramatically reduce the risk of falls and increase comfort for elderly people or those who have lost flexibility through their spinal problems.

  They are easy to use, effective and greatly lower the chance of a fall.
- Install handrails in the bathroom and the shower box, placed strategically to support you. Such bars are very important in elderly people's bathrooms, whose strength and balance are already compromised, and this helps to avoid preventable falls. Many people live in their homes for decades and as they age understandably accept the structure and layout of the home as it has always been. As humans, we lose bio-mechanical function of the spine gradually so the necessity to make changes such as installing handrails is not always obvious. If your parents are elderly, check the safety of their bathroom. It may just save their life.

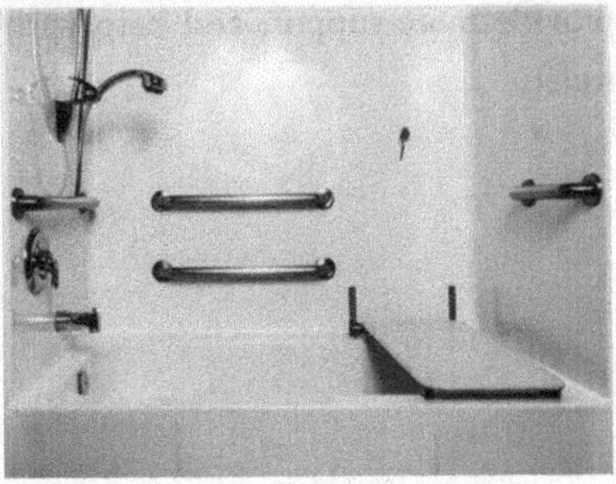

Two types of bars are recommended for an elderly person's bathroom:

- To enter or leave the bathroom in an orthostatic position (standing);
- Next to the toilet bowl to support themselves when lowering or raising themselves.

The installation of diagonal handrails is not recommended because the hand can slip, and if the feet are not firmly supported, there is a greater likelihood of falls.

SITTING ON A TOILET SEAT

Many toilet seats are too low. Often people only realise this when they are suffering a crisis of low back pain. If you've ever suffered severe low back pain you'll appreciate this fact. Imagine those who live with it day after day! Raising the height of the toilet can greatly relieve the pain associated with getting on and off the toilet.

TIPS

The toilet can be raised 7–14 cm by placing a special extension or seat, which can be removable or permanent, that helps to significantly minimise the effort of sitting down, reducing the load on the spine.

A bench to elevate your feet can allow you to slightly flex your hips and reduce some load from the low back. This tip won't help everybody but it will be a salvation for others.

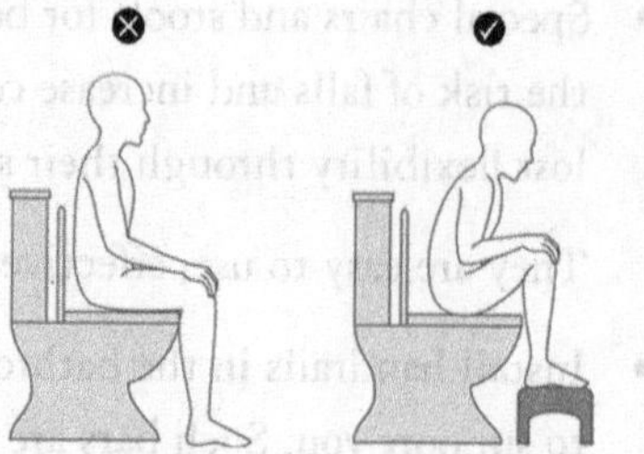

If you're building a new bathroom or have a chance to change your toilet now, consider installing a unit with a seat attached to the wall, so that you can adjust it to a more appropriate height.

Rails or safety bars can also be placed on the wall next to the toilet to provide more support and help with lowering and raising yourself from the toilet.

TRANSPORTATION – A COMMON CAUSE OF BACK PAIN

DRIVING IN A CAR

There is no one particular model of car that has seats and internal spaces that are suitable for everyone. This is why taking time to ergonomically scrutinize your future car before buying it is so important. Your car has to match your height and body type, as you spend a large percentage of your life driving to work, dropping the kids off at school or traveling around town.

ADJUSTING THE SEAT OF YOUR CAR

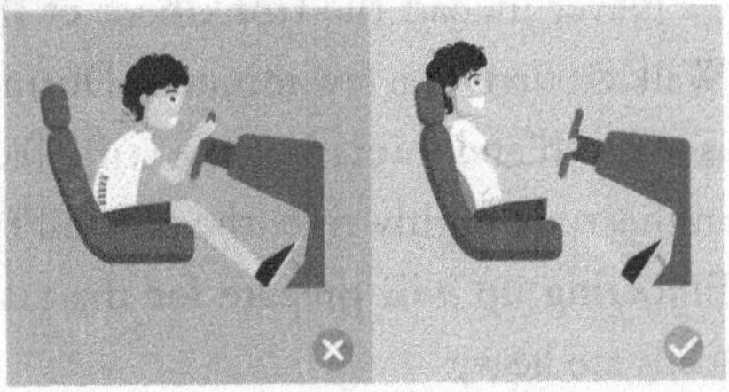

The car seat should be adjusted according to your body type. It should slide back far enough to allow your legs and arms to be relaxed and slightly bent whilst driving and at the same time provide support to your upper and lower back.

The seat should be wider than your hips, and be high enough to support your shoulders. The ideal model should have an adjustment for height and angle of inclination of the back support.

Make sure that the angle of the steering wheel can be altered.

LUMBAR SUPPORTS FOR CAR SEATS

If your seat does not have decent lumbar support, consider using one. They are an excellent way of compensating for any support that the seat may be lacking. They keep your spine supported and aligned as it is maintained in its correct anatomical posture. If your lower back is correctly aligned and supported, your neck will sit comfortably above your shoulders, minimising the extra load that a forward head posture causes. Many motorists drive with their head way too far forward, caused by the excessive inclination of the car seat or inadequate lumbar support. This consequently fatigues the neck and upper back.

Correct posture whilst driving will also ensure that your shoulders aren't unnecessarily elevated, which causes contracture of the trapezius muscle.

GETTING IN AND OUT OF THE CAR

Getting in and out of the car places a surprisingly large amount of load on the lower back. Anyone who has ever done this during a painful crisis will attest to this. It can be absolute agony. During these times of increased sensitivity we can actually appreciate the considerable amount of force that the spine sustains whilst doing this routine task, helping us to recognize how this can affect any spine, whether it is in a symptomatic state or not. This is one of those activities that we repeat thousands of times during our lives. If done forcibly or fast, as it is done by many of us when we are in a hurry without consciously positioning our body, certain ligaments and muscles overload articulations of our lower back.

The correct way to do this is to move your whole body towards the door, keeping your thighs together. Turn your body 90 degrees to put your feet on the ground, and only then get up and stand, using your activated core to do so when you do.

Never unload the trunk/boot of the car immediately after a long journey. Walk around for a few minutes. During long trips muscles contract, blood flow is reduced and joints become stiff. Tackling heavy loads while your tissues are in this state highly risks the possibility of injuring them. Walking around and limbering up will prepare for the task at hand, especially when some of the loads are heavy.

When you bend over or squat, activate your core and hold the weight as close to your body as possible to lift it. Lower yourself at the same level of the load you will be lifting, facing it front on, and then looking toward the place where you will take the object to.

When you are in the front seat and want to retrieve small objects such as purses from the back seat, do not twist your body to do so. Get out of the car, open the rear door and remove them. Many people only find out that they have a spinal problem when they actually 'tweak' it when they stretch out in positions like this.

Many people recovering from an acute back pain crisis take a turn for the worse after sitting for prolonged periods of time.

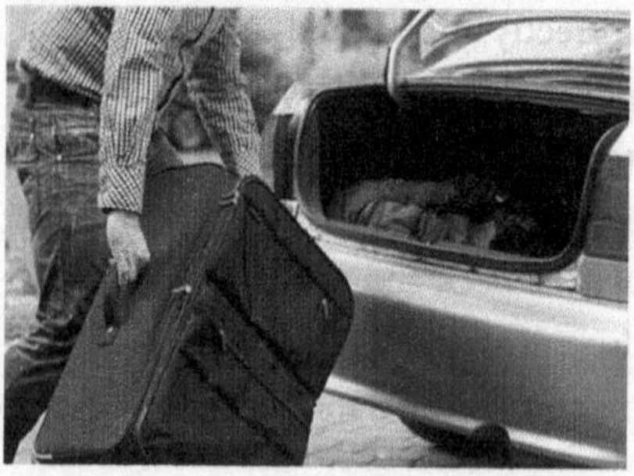

Prolonged sitting is one of the most detrimental factors to worsen a spine that is already inflamed. When sitting in a car at these times is unavoidable, stop for a break and walk around for at least 10 minutes every hour during the trip. These regular breaks allow the spine to decompress the tissues, promote blood circulation and help the joints from 'stiffening up'. Walk around, lifting your knees as high as possible to introduce movement into the pelvis. Do some stretches if possible.

MOTORCYCLE

It is understandable why motorcycle riders commonly suffer back problems, as the body is flexed forward in order to ride, making it difficult to sustain correct posture.

From my time working on social projects in South America in areas such as Iquitos in the Amazon, where the majority of the population rode motorbikes, I noticed that many patients suffered pain and postural problems in specific areas of the spine due to this mode of transport. I noticed that many of them had hyper-kyphosis of the thoracic spine (increased thoracic curve or hunchback) and/or a lump on the base of the neck, meaning that the normal function of these regions was compromised by bending forward.

Furthermore, consider the higher percentage of falls and accidents that affect motorcyclists, and that any trauma on the body (e.g., arm or shoulder) is also absorbed by the spine. If you do fall from a bike, always get your spine checked by a good chiropractor, physiotherapist or osteopath as soon as possible to correct any possible bio-mechanical dysfunctions that developed after the fall. This is important even if you never felt any apparent symptoms after it.

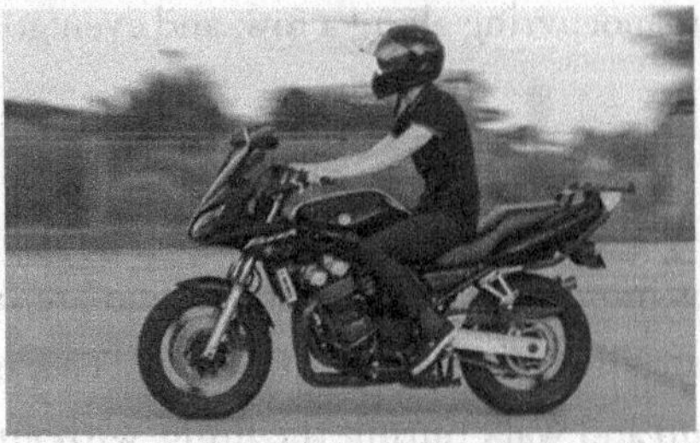

Sitting for prolonged periods of time without lumbar support limits normal range of motion and consequently causes low back pain or sciatica/numbness of the legs and toes for many riders. Interestingly many don't join the dots and identify the motorbike as a source of suffering.

When we sit on the motorcycle, it is practically impossible to sustain both the cervical (neck) curves and lumbar curves because the handlebars are generally low and forward (except in a few cases such as the Harley Davison), there is generally no lumbar support and we have to arch the spine forward, rounding the shoulders to reach them. Over time, this increases the tension on the cervical and lumbar muscles and causes chronic fibrosis of the surrounding muscle tissue. Motorbike enthusiasts need to do some type of compensatory exercise or stretching routine to minimise the risk of their riding posture causing chronic spinal problems.

TIPS

When riding, do your best to maintain the most upright posture possible and if you already suffer from back problems, find a model of motorbike appropriate for your spine. One that makes it easier to maintain a posture as close to optimal as possible. A racing bike requires much more bending than the 'chopper' or 'custom' models, which allow the rider to maintain a more erect position.

Use full helmets with protection under the jaw that will protect your neck in case of an accident. Do exercises for your core to increase your abdominal strength and protect your spine.

PLANES

Travelling on a plane can challenge even the most asymptomatic spines, especially during longer flights. As it is widely known, the limited space of an economy class seat on an airplane is not very comfortable. On long haul flights, the spine is incredibly restricted, with the confined space complicating movement and the ability to sustain good posture. If you've ever travelled with back pain, you'll understand just how much getting in and out of a seat, manoeuvring along a row, and even going to the toilet can be utterly agonizing.

TIP

At the time of check-in try to reserve a seat near the emergency exit where there is more space. Only people who are free of pain or other physical restrictions are allowed to request this area. This means that you will then be able to stand up and walk during the flight without disturbing the passengers seated beside you. If you are debilitated and therefore unable to sit in this area, request a seat on the aisle which will allow you to stand up and walk around whenever you need to.

Moving and stretching also helps you avoid the fluid retention that accumulates around the base of your ankles and in the body and also minimises the risk of thrombosis.

Another good idea is to do some stretching before boarding, during a stopover, and even on the plane near the emergency exit when the plane is in the air. Walk as much as you can before you get on the flight to loosen the tissues and promote blood flow before your body is obliged to be in a position that will promote the opposite.

If you decide to read to pass the time, keep the book at eye level. Many people get off the plane with a stiff neck and even numbness in their shoulders, arms, or fingers because they spent too much time looking down during the flight. The same approach should be taken when using laptops. In this case, it

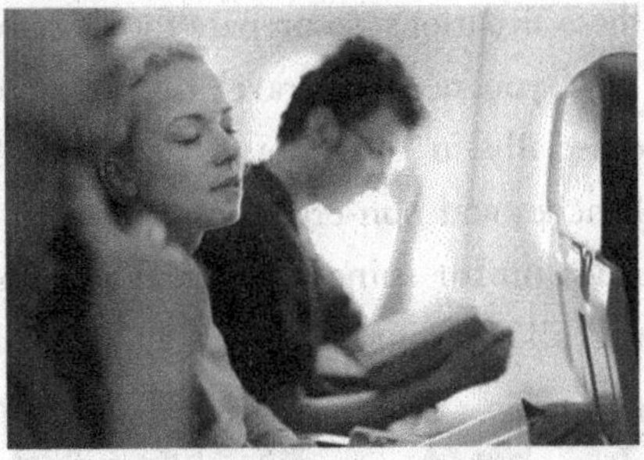

may be more difficult to leave it at eye level, so compensate for this fact by doing some neck extension stretches (looking back) when you take a break.

Long trips can also cause sleepiness, which leads many people to be careless about the position of their head and neck when they sleep. Try to sleep with the head well supported and maintain its normal alignment. Do not lean your head on the window. Place a roll in the curve of the neck, recline, and sleep peacefully. The blanket offered by the airline is more effective than the pillow as it nestles perfectly between the neck and the top of the seat. Don't forget to carry an extra sweater to keep warm (as you won't have the blanket).

Use the pillow that the airline provides to support the curve of the lumbar spine while you are seated. Keeping this lumbar curve supported and not allowing it to flatten out is crucial if you wish to leave the plane pain-free. It is amazing how fast a low back can seize up when it is deprived of it's curve.

When watching movies, keep your head resting on your chair, which will allow the neck muscles to remain relaxed.

There is a certain tendency for dehydration during long-distance travel, increasing the risk of cramps and consequently the intensification of any pre-existing pain. Drink plenty of water and avoid alcohol consumption (which promotes dehydration). Of course, this will make you want to go to the bathroom – a good excuse to get up and stretch out!

Most people carry an excessive amount of luggage when traveling, which invariably increases the load on the spine, especially the low back and shoulders. As difficult as it may be, try to pack only what is necessary instead of an entire wardrobe. Leaving your bag lighter will have your spine thanking you!

When choosing a suitcase, opt for models with wheels, including carry-on luggage, and try to keep yourself straight when you are pulling it. Bon voyage!

PUBLIC TRANSPORTATION

Getting on the bus or the train often sees us rushing to enter before it embarks. Sometimes, these moments can lead to impacts on the spine such as a stumble, a shoulder impacting against the door, or a sudden movement that could aggravate an already sore back.

You should always stand near a bar or rail and hold on tightly as these modes of transportation can be jerky. Your body often absorbs the forces in these situations, so prepare for those bumps and sudden stops.

If you need to travel by bus or train/metro/subway daily or frequently, especially in busy hours, and have back problems, try to soften the hard benches and non-ergonomic seats by rolling your blouse or jacket and using it as lumbar spine support. This allows you to be more upright in position and allows your head to stay aligned with your shoulders. If you're sitting by the window, take great care when getting off because other passenger's feet and bags etc. can trip you causing a stumble or fall. And lastly, don't use the window for head support if you want to sleep. You will wake up with a stiff neck and maybe miss your stop!

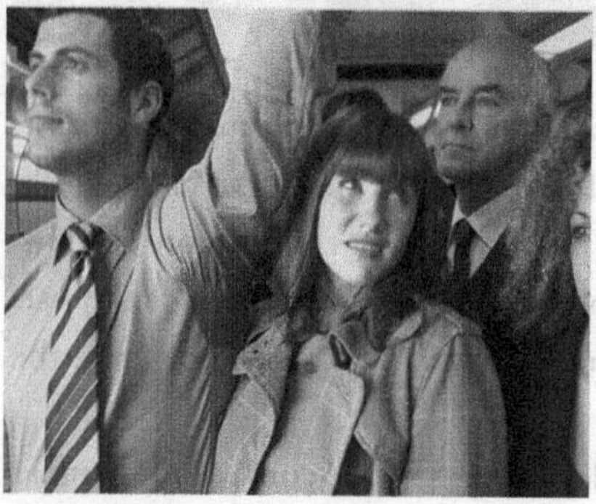

If you are on a bus, avoid sitting on the seats located over the wheels because the impact is greater, particularly as the vehicle passes over speed bumps. The rear seat should be avoided at all costs, especially for those who are suffering acute back pain or have a history of back problems. Hitting a speed hump at speed may throw the body of the passenger up in the air and when 'landing' can cause a compressive force on the lumbar spine. Ouch!

WOMEN AND THEIR SPECIAL SPINAL NEEDS

There are a series of influences specific to women that need to be focused on separately. Major events in women's lives such as pregnancy, giving birth, raising children and even menstruation put additional loads on a woman's body and her spine. While many of these things cannot be avoided, it is worth learning the technicalities of such events so that the loads may be minimised, and the resultant impact on the spine reduced.

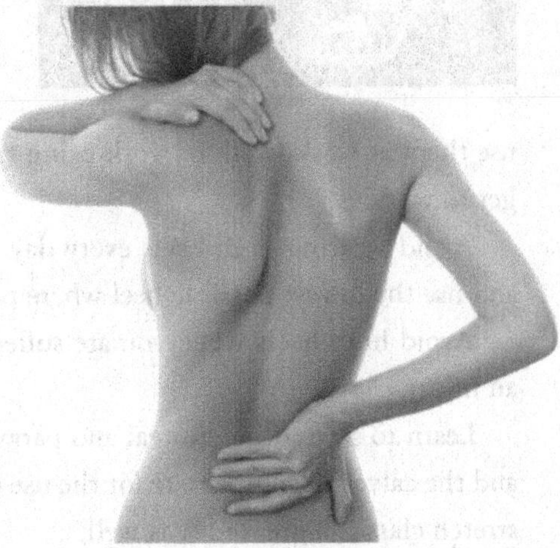

Accessories such as handbags and high heels also negatively affect the bio-mechanical function of a woman's spine. Read on and learn about ways that you can lessen your chances of developing degenerative problems in the future.

HIGH HEELS

High heels drastically modify the normal function of the spine and other joints. Our centre of gravity should fall in a line that connects the ears, shoulders, hips (femoral heads), knees, and ankles. When we elevate our heels with high heels, the body alters its natural position to accommodate and stay balanced. When the centre of gravity moves forward, the curves of the spine accentuate, from the lumbar curvature (causing hyper-lordosis) to the thoracic spine to compensate for the imbalance. This is similar to what we see when we observe the spine of a woman in late-term pregnancy. The lumbar curve increases to a lordotic state to compensate for the forward shift of weight. The thoracic and cervical curves react accordingly. High heels cause the muscles and tendons of the legs and gluteal muscles to become chronically shortened, which complicates the bio-mechanical function of multiple joints in the body.

TIPS

Restrict the use of high heels for special occasions such as parties, weddings, etc., especially if you are in a crisis of low back pain.

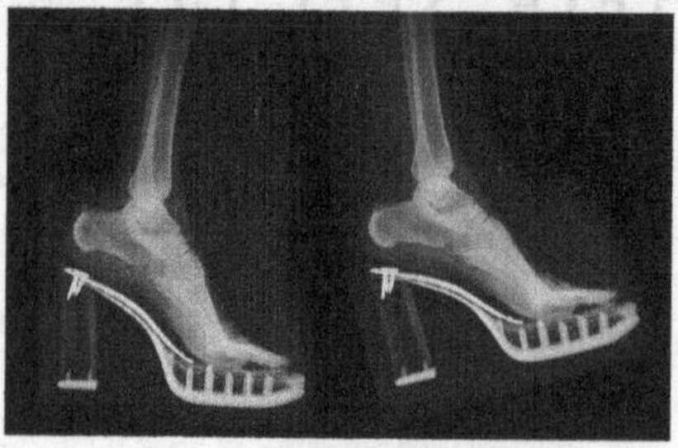

Stretch your calves.

Put a ball under the arch of your foot and then roll it back and forth, as this also helps stretch the muscles of the arch under the foot that are shortened by the use of high heels.

On days that you need to wear high heels, walk beforehand. If you use them at work, walk to work using trainers and put the heels on when you get to work.

Avoid wearing high heels every day. Try to vary the height of your shoes, and use the lowest possible heel where possible or practical.

Avoid high heels when you are suffering back pain or are recovering from an injury.

Learn to stretch the gluteal and paravertebral muscles of the lumbar spine, and the calves to compensate for the use of high heels. Doing yoga, Pilates or a stretch class is a great idea as well.

It is interesting to note that many women cannot tolerate using sneakers, low heel shoes, or walk barefoot after using high heels continuously, since their lower limb has adapted to high heels. For this reason, it is vital for the health of your feet and spine that you continue to use flat shoes or walk in bare feet, even if you initially feel pain. At this time, a good massage therapist will help to work the contracted muscles of the calves to allow them to relax and facilitate walking without heels. Don't give up! Give your body and feet time to re-adjust, and return to the correct function.

PREGNANCY

Nine months is a long time, especially if a woman is suffering back pain that has appeared during her pregnancy. This beautiful time in a woman's life must be as peaceful an experience as possible.

During pregnancy, a woman's body is going through many changes. These include hormonal fluctuations influenced by hormones that have not previously influenced her health, bio-mechanical adaptions with her spine, and effects in almost every system of her body, from cardiac and respiratory systems to digestion. Many women who have never experienced pain or other health problems before pregnancy often do, and those already suffering before falling pregnant often see their problems accentuate during pregnancy.

You can do a lot to minimise and prevent back pain due to the harmful effects caused by pregnancy. Some of the effects can manifest themselves many years after the birth of the baby. During pregnancy, the female body goes through many changes. Bodyweight increases (in some cases up to 25%), requiring significant adaptions in other areas of the woman's body to compensate for the extra weight and how that weight is concentrated around the abdomen. With so many changes occurring at the same time, it is easy to understand why a female body that is physically well prepared for this time undoubtedly better deals with this new state.

Preparing your body for pregnancy by strengthening the spine and making it stronger and more flexible before conception will help it not only during pregnancy but also after the birth of your child, when new activities such as breastfeeding and putting your baby into a crib etc. will occur. Regular physical activity improves aerobic capacity. Specific stretching (such as yoga or Pilates) prepares muscles for the changes that altered spinal bio-mechanics will have on them. Strength training prepares muscles for the loads that new activities will place on them. Exercise should be multi-faceted, including an emphasis on aerobic, strengthening and flexibility. If you are accustomed to a certain type of exercise you can continue practicing it throughout your pregnancy, however it is not advisable to start certain, more strenuous activities during pregnancy if you have never done them before. Always consult with your specialist before starting something new.

When you're pregnant, the ligaments of the spine become lax due to the increase in circulating levels of a hormone called Relaxin, which allows the pelvis to expand and accommodate the passage of the baby through the birth canal during childbirth. However, this hormone can unfortunately also leave the articulations of the spine and the pelvis unstable. Laxity of these ligaments, and consequent pelvic instability, may continue for many months or even years after birth, so it is advisable to avoid overloading the spine at this time. Daily activities such as housework, lifting bassinets or shopping bags, etc. should be done more cautiously than normal.

The abdominal muscles are stretched progressively during pregnancy as the baby grows. During this time, the rectus abdominis (which descends in the anterior part of the abdomen), separates to allow the uterus to expand. It is, for this reason, gentle exercises of these abdominal muscles such as swimming, yoga, or Pilates are recommended, especially in the first trimester.

As the breasts increase in size the centre of gravity can also be influenced causing the shoulders to fall forward, resulting in the rectification of the neck curve and an accentuation of the thoracic curve (kyphosis). This is one of the most common reasons for pain during pregnancy, with symptoms such as headache, neck ache, neck stiffness, tingling/pins and needles in the hands or fingers, and tenderness around the shoulders being the most frequent complaints. Be conscious of what an ideal posture (refer to earlier texts on Posture) is and do your best to maintain it at all times, especially when standing or sitting. It is also beneficial to invest in a bra that adequately supports the breasts and allows the shoulders to be properly supported, facilitating alignment with the ears. If this still isn't effective in helping you achieve and maintain correct posture, use a posture corrector for a few weeks until it becomes easier to maintain an erect posture.

Muscles of the pelvic floor, that span the bottom of the pelvis, provide important stability to the pelvis and support pelvic organs such as the bowel, bladder, and uterus. These muscles frequently lose tone during pregnancy. It is for this reason that it's essential to begin pelvic floor strengthening exercises as soon as possible after the birth of the baby.

TIP

When they become weak, symptoms such as urinary incontinence, where urine can leak whilst coughing, sneezing, laughing, or running, can occur. Women who suffer this also report failing to reach the toilet in time, reduced vaginal sensation, and difficulty retaining a tampon as other tell-tale signs. To help combat or rectify this problem, you can do a simple exercise that can be done anywhere. Whilst sitting, comfortably squeeze/contract these muscles for 15 seconds. If you are unsure as to whether you are doing this correctly, insert your thumb into the vagina whilst squeezing. You should be able to feel this squeeze is contracting the vagina. Repeat at least 10 times each session, 5 times a day.

Returning to regular physical activity such as walking, swimming, yoga, and resistance training with weights as soon as possible after childbirth will greatly assist you in your return to normal life and prepare your body to be physically prepared for all that life as a new mother will demand of you and your spine.

AFTER THE BIRTH

Maternal life is a new reality for your spine. New movements and positions combined with the continually increasing weight of the baby put surprisingly large loads on your spine. For these reasons, physical activity and increased attention to your health are even more important at this moment in your life. Keeping up with regular spinal maintenance with your chiropractor, osteopath,

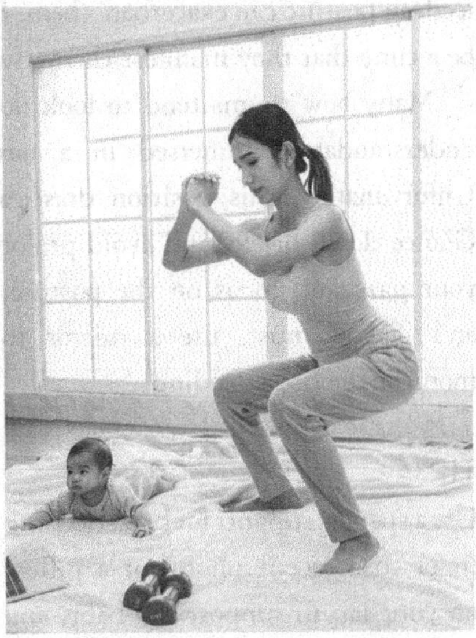

physiotherapist or massage therapist will help compensate for the harmful effects that these activities have on your spine.

It is very easy to forget to take care of yourself after the birth of the baby. You're busy, your sleep is compromised and life has been turned upside down. It's really easy to forget yourself. As a result, a new mother's health often suffers. You need to do your best to keep yourself and your health a priority, because if you aren't your best, how are you going to adequately take care of your child or children? Simply do your best. Do what you can in the home, in the backyard, or wherever you may be to make it easier on yourself and your back. Read about exercises that resonate with you, sign up for an online yoga, Pilates, or high-intensity interval training course. You can squeeze 10–20 minutes in front of the TV or a lap top while your baby is sleeping. Even though there'll be times you are exhausted you'll soon see your body's strength and resistance improving. You'll have more energy! And with a higher level of health, everything will flow more smoothly for you.

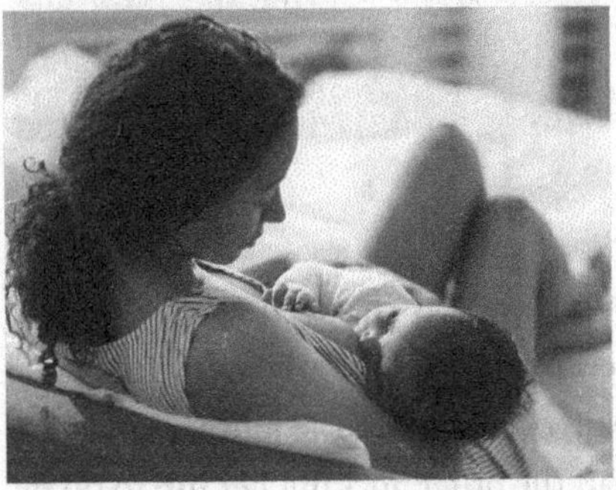

TIP

No time to do any of the above? Simply jog on the spot or walk for 20 minutes inside your own home. Movement is everything for you right now and your body will thank you for it. If exercising is new for you start walking and gradually increase the speed or time devoted to this activity.

BREASTFEEDING

Maintaining a correct posture is crucial whilst breastfeeding. Remember just how many hours you will be doing it in the first 12–24 months of your new child's life. If there are already problems in your neck or upper back poor breast feeding posture can exacerbate them. If you've never had problems this can also be a time that they manifest themselves, so take care.

Many new mums tend to look down at their baby when they breastfeed, understandably immersed in a new and beautiful time of their lives. Unfortunately, this position drastically overloads the neck and shoulders. Glance down briefly and avoid prolonged periods of time looking down. Lift your gaze and focus on the posture, and if you must, use a mirror to monitor the breastfeeding.

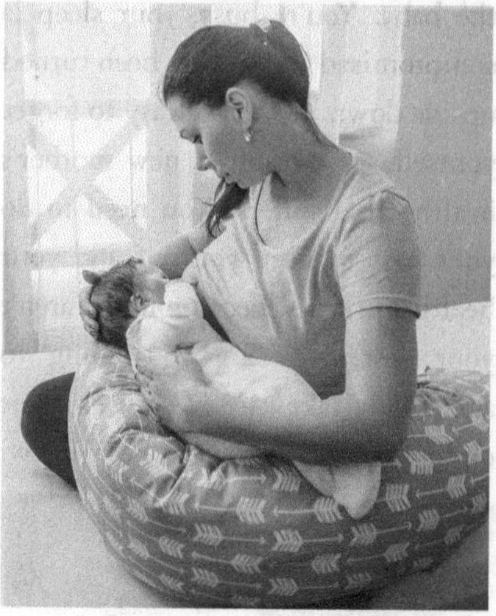

TIP

Use a specific support for breastfeeding (refer to adjacent photo) or a pillow on your lap to support the baby, and raising him/her close to the breast for feeding. This will help avoid the harmful stooped posture that can lock the cervical joints and tighten the neck muscles.

CARRYING YOUR BABY

Your baby's weight is no different to any other load that you carry, so apply the rules previously discussed on how to correctly lift load when carrying your baby. A very common cause of low back pain occurs when the mother holds the baby on one side that she favours more than the other, locking her hip to do so, This causes an imbalance as the weight is placed asymmetrically on the spine and pelvis, causing lumbar or sacroiliac joint dysfunction. Remember that the levels of Relaxin are still high and that the pelvis isn't as prepared for uneven loads as it usually would be. Holding your baby consistently on one side will increase the chance of subluxating the sacroiliac joints.

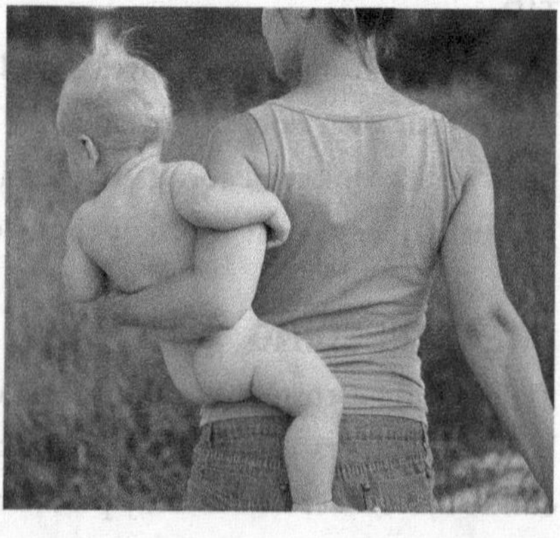

The resulting subluxations can cause inflammation of the low back or sciatic pain, pain in the buttocks, or even pain radiating to the inguinal region (groin). If you can, keep the baby's weight very close to the centre of your body. If this is not possible, alternate between both sides.

The weight of your baby is constantly increasing. This phase of life requires significant physical exertion. If a new mother has back pain, she can find it hard to give it the rest it requires and avoiding the daily chores is often not possible.

When squatting to pick up your baby, do so with the legs bent. Don't bend your spine. When moving the baby, it is important to get as close to where he/she is as possible because this will minimise the load that goes through the lumbar spine. At times like these, the more strength in the abdominal muscles and elasticity of the lumbar spine, the fewer problems the mother will have. Strong abdominal muscles allow loads to be lifted without using the muscles of the lumbar spine, hence protecting it from strain. Always activate the abdominal muscles before lifting a baby.

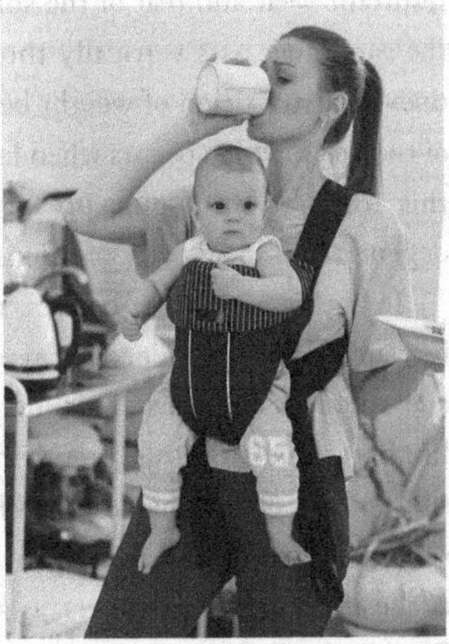

A stroller is the safest way to carry your baby. Besides saving your spine from carrying the weight of your baby, you can hang a purse or shopping bag on the handles to lighten the load as well. They offer a great opportunity to get out and about, exercising your body and strengthening your spine in a way that doesn't feel tedious.

Another option that you may consider is a front pouch or sling. These are excellent to use while a baby's weight is still light. They are positioned in the front of the body and are great because they keep you and your baby very close, while at the same time leaving your arms free to do other tasks or carry other objects.

Important note: Front pouches are great for newborns, but when the baby gains weight, it can make the weight considerably harmful to the lower back, neck, and shoulders. It is only recommended for use if the mother has strong abdominal muscles and not for extended periods of time, since the compression of the spine and intervertebral discs is inevitable. If you find that your baby is becoming too heavy, stop using it and go for a stroller!

Slings have been used by women for centuries and are very efficient. Be cautious if the child's head is loose and if they are sleeping, because the movements caused during the walk will be absorbed by their delicate neck.

As your child gets older and is learning to walk, resist their constant requests to be picked up. In the beginning, it will be difficult, but be firm to keep your back in good condition and better prepared for the coming years. Opt for a cuddle on the couch instead.

WELL-ENDOWED WOMEN

For women with small breasts, it is difficult to imagine that having large breasts could be in some way negative. Any woman who has larger than average breasts may not find them as desirable, especially when they can suffer the deleterious effects that larger breasts pose for their posture. When this occurs, increased loads on the spine compromise not only the cervical spine but also the dorsal and lumbar spines.

As explained in previous sections, an ideal posture should be maintained as much as possible during life to minimise bio-mechanical dysfunction and its resultant wear and tear of the spine. The centre of gravity that passes through the ears must pass vertically through the shoulder, hip, knee, and ankle. The uneven distribution of weight between the anterior (front) and posterior(back) of the body, which occurs when larger breasts, pregnancy, and obesity, interrupt this line, sets the spine up for uneven distribution of loads and resultant degeneration in the way of osteoarthritis and degenerative disc disease.

In the case of larger breasts, the centre of gravity line frequently falls way forward of the shoulders because the weight of the breasts can pull the head and shoulders forward. This increases the dorsal curvature (kyphosis) and the lumbar curve (lordosis), resulting in dysfunction of the spine, accelerating the process of degeneration. When the body uses symptoms to advise that something isn't quite right, pain at the base of the neck, numbness or tingling of the arms, hands, or fingers, as well as headaches, dizziness are most common. Restriction in breathing (due to difficulties expanding the thoracic cage) and other physical and emotional symptoms can also occur.

Specific exercises and stretches can be extremely beneficial in compensating for the unequal distribution of load that larger breasts can cause. While exercises such as swimming, resistance training with weights, and high-intensity interval training can promote and restore the range of motion of joints negatively affected by postural changes, specific stretches, yoga and Pilates lengthen muscle fibres that may have been chronically shortened by postural compensations.

Swimming is a more suitable alternative than running or aerobic exercises that increase the impact caused by the additional weight of the breasts on the spine. Obviously, the effects of gravity in the water are reduced and the spine can move without suffering the influence of the breasts' excess weight. Swimming has the added benefit that it can be done with the neck extended which is excellent compensating for the curved, forward flexed, posture.

TIP

Look for a bra that can distribute the weight of the breasts over a larger area, which reduces the amount of force that the muscles need to exert to support larger breasts supported by less suitable bras. These bras are especially important in women with a smaller stature, as their larger breasts concentrate a heavier load over a smaller area.

HANDBAGS

Fashion has influenced the growth in the size of popular handbags to a point where the women carrying them put their spinal health in jeopardy. The ideal way to carry any bag is to share the load between both sides of the body. This is possible in bags such as backpacks, where straps over each shoulder, distribute the weight of the bag in a manner that has all joints equally contributing to support the bag. Handbags don't allow for this luxury, worse still when they are the in-fashion larger ones capable of accommodating everything but the kitchen sink!

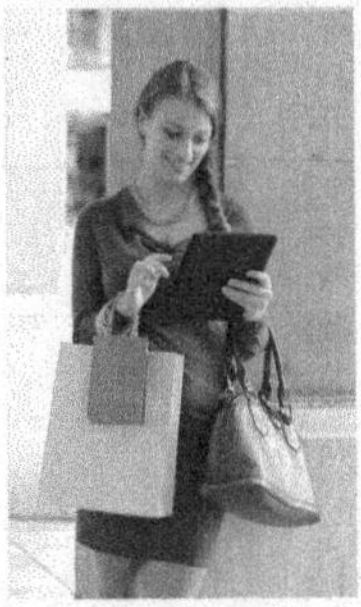

When the bag is being carried on one shoulder, it results in the body leaning in the opposite direction to maintain balance, interfering with the alignment of the spine and consequently affecting the normal bio-mechanical function of the upper and lower body. Some women prefer to carry the handbag over their forearm, which tends to overload the elbow and shoulder on that side, eventually straining the muscles of the neck as well.

Pain in the lumbar spine is not unusual, especially when a woman has scoliosis or a pre-existing bio-mechanical dysfunction in the lower back. Other common symptoms of problems caused by heavy handbags include pins and needles in the wrists or fingers, tendinitis over the elbow and even head aches.

TIPS

Periodically remove everything from your handbag and start again, returning only essential objects. Over time all sorts of unimportant and occasionally used objects find their way into a woman's handbag, increasing its weight and resultant load on the spine.

Alternate the shoulder that you use to carry your handbag, especially if walking long distances or standing for too long on the bus or in the subway.

Choose a bag with a long or adjustable strap. It should be long enough to go over your head onto one shoulder and cross your body diagonally, helping distribute the load more evenly.

Put frequently used objects such as your purse and cell phone in the front pockets (if your bag has them), as reaching out to pull items out can result in straining muscles in the neck or back.

If you travel with your laptop, try putting it in a backpack to avoid overloading your spine.

Consider using a fashionable, smaller handbag-sized bag that can be worn over both shoulders. They look great and pose very little threat to the health of your spine.

KIDS HAVE SPINAL PROBLEMS TOO – FIND OUT WHY

The future depends on what we do in the present."

MAHATMA GANDHI

Adults are not the only ones who develop back problems from daily activities. Children are exposed to the same risks as adults however their spines are delicate and malleable, making them even more susceptible than an adults spine.

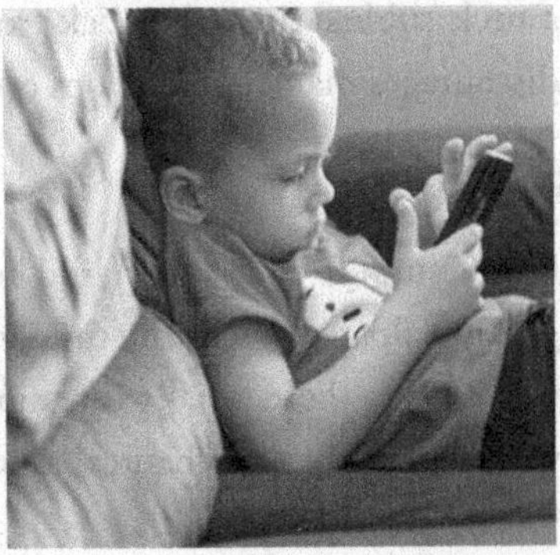

Unlike adults, when children suffer impacts that cause spinal problems and misalignments they rarely manifest as pain or other symptoms. This makes problems in the spine and neck of a child difficult to diagnose. Remember that babies and young children cannot communicate verbally. If problems occur at this time of life, the child may have no reference of what 'normal' is, which would otherwise allow them to compare a certain pain state to how they feel before the pain started and communicate it to their parents (if they were older). Spinal problems need to be detected in childhood as they will worsen with time and can progress asymptomatically for years until the day that pain or symptom advises that advanced spinal has already occurred.

BIRTH

"The disease must be fought at birth."

AULUS PERSIUS

Trauma sustained by the spine, particularly in the neck, during child birth is sufficient to provoke misalignments and bio-mechanical dysfunction of the spinal articulations. Childbirth involves forces such as pulling the baby by the neck, twisting the thorax, and rotational movements that bending the cervical spine. While these forces are often unavoidable as the doctor is understandably focusing on the wellbeing of the baby and the mother, it is undeniable that the delicate spinal column of many babies can be in injured on their very first day of life. When you consider that studies show that birth fracture of the clavicle occurs in 0.4–10% of babies, it is totally viable to recognise that the force exerted by the vagina during childbirth could misalign a newborn's spine.

Subluxations resulting from these misalignments can lay dormant for years or the body may use symptoms to communicate that something isn't quite right. Symptoms such as poor appetite, regurgitation, and difficulty sleeping can be some of the ways the brain tries to call attention to the problem. Babies with irregularities during breastfeeding (such as those that favour one particular breast) may have some joint restriction (subluxation) due to spinal misalignment. Another common sign is a baby preferring to drag itself along the floor in a sitting type position as opposed to crawling. If the baby has a neck subluxation, the neck extension required to crawl is painful and this discourages many babies from even trying.

TIP

If you suspect that your child may have a spinal misalignment in the neck gently palpate (touch) the muscles under the base of the skull. If they do they will change their facial expression while you do it. If this is the case consult with a spinal bio-mechanical specialist on how to correct it.

FALLS

Between the stages of crawling and walking with confidence, falls are very common. It is estimated that by the time child has reached five years of age, it has had approximately two thousand falls. Falls such as falling out of bed, off the changing table or chair, out of the stroller, whilst learning to walk and of course the numerous falls that occur when they are confident on their feet and running around.

For parents, it is often unclear whether the fall caused a serious problem or not as the child may cry for a while and when it stops a parent can understandably think that everything is OK. Even a seemingly light impact can cause misalignment of the vertebrae, which can interfere with the function of the nervous system from the time of the impact onwards or contribute to early arthritic degeneration, visible on an x-ray as soon as a decade or two later on. Parents should always be alert and consult a spinal practitioner who is specialised in restoring any bio-mechanical

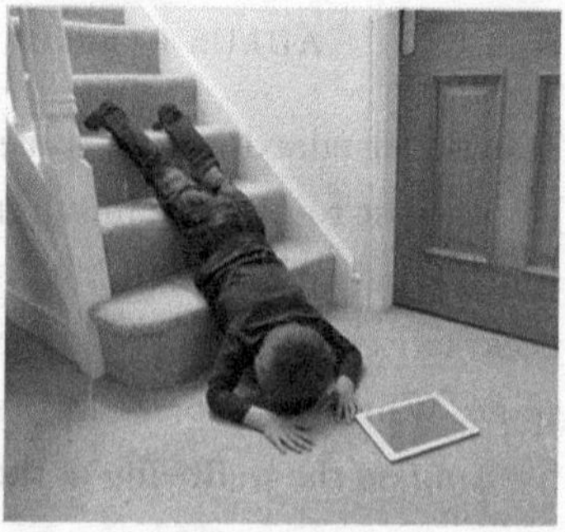

compromise that may have occurred due to the fall or impact.

Older children (five to nine years old) usually fall at parks and playgrounds, and the severity of the fall is often directly related to the height of the fall and the area where they fell.

Falls are scary for parents and it is important to remain calm. Here are some tips on helping you decide the best course of action.

AFTER A FALL:

- Examine the limbs, head, and body to check for any signs of bruises, inflammation (red areas), swelling, or deformities. If there are no such signs, there is probably no significant injury.

You should take your child to the doctor or emergency room if:

- you observe inflammation or deformity in the extremities (arms or legs) or that they are limping for more than two hours;
- they do not stop crying;
- they are sleepy and having trouble waking up;
- they vomit more than two or three times;
- they complain that the pain is increasing;
- they have difficulty focusing their eyes on objects;
- they show changes in behaviour.

Do not remove your child from the fall site and call the ambulance if they:

- are unconscious or were temporarily unconscious;
- have seriously injured the head, neck, or spine;
- are having difficulty breathing;
- have clear fluid or blood coming out of the nose, ears, or mouth.

If you think it is safe to move the child:

- hold and support them until they stop crying;
- use ice on any surface damage or bruising;
- watch for 24 hours following the fall, noting any unusual occurrence.

Always get them checked by a chiropractor, physiotherapist or osteopath who specialises in children after you are sure that nothing serious happened.

AT HOME

Your home may seem safe however it is full of traps for children. Here are some specific things to look out for around the home that may increase the chance of a child suffering from a serious falls:

Furniture

- Do not leave babies alone on the bed, couch, or changing table.
- When the child is sitting in high chairs, use a belt to secure them.
- The crib should have a distance of 60 cm between the mattress (top) and the upper part of the crib (sidebars). The space between the mattress and the bars should be no greater than 10 mm. The crib bars should have a separation of 50 to 80 mm.

Stroller

- Do not leave children unattended on balconies or stairs. Remember that children love to play on stairs.
- Remember that the baby carriage may tip if we carry shopping bags on the side. Get a stroller with a shopping basket to carry the bags.

Windows

- Windows must remain closed and locked when there are children around. Never leave a child alone in a room with the windows open. When you open a window for ventilation, open only those that the child cannot reach.
- Provide special protection (such as safety nets or bars) for the windows that will prevent the child from falling.
- Do not leave chairs, cribs, beds, and other furniture close to the windows.

Stairs

- Use safety gates at the top and bottom of the stairs, especially if you have small children. The stairs should be well illuminated. Remember that children love to go up and down the stairs. The stairs are responsible for a high percentage of falls.

On the Floor

- Secure rugs and pillows, especially on wooden, ceramic, or plastic floors. Foam under the carpet also helps prevent slipping.
- Walkers are not recommended, because many children are injured while using them. Allow your child to walk when they are ready (approximately thirteen months of age).

Car

The family car can cause numerous problems for the child's spine. When accommodating them in the back seat do not use the car seatbelts, as their specifications are only suitable for adults.

- Use the regulation car seat for children until your child is older and big enough to sit in the back seat with the appropriate support.
- When we put a baby in a car seat, the body is easily protected and supported, but the head is free and can suffer forces from the motion of the car, during curves, sudden braking, and lane changes. Sudden movements produce a large load on the baby's delicate neck.
- Drive slowly and leave home early to avoid speeding with your baby on board. Avoid changing lanes abruptly and braking violently. Support the baby's head in the best way possible to avoid unnecessary movements.

Automobile accidents, in general, affect the whole family. It is very common after an accident that the parents and older siblings go through proper medical examinations due to the ease of communicating with the doctor. Very young children who show apparent symptoms may be released without adequate testing when in reality they require even greater attention.

The child's spine is very flexible and, therefore, the impact and force of the accident can affect the spinal cord even more than adults.

SLEEP

A baby's spine is constantly evolving, and they spend a lot of time sleeping. Therefore, they must have a good quality mattress that will provide adequate support.

- Ideally, use a firm mattress and provide a proper pillow for your child. Pillows made for adults do not have the appropriate measurements and may deform the curves and the normal alignment of the child's spine and neck.
- Look for a pillow suitable for your child's age. Change it when necessary, according to the child's development.

BACKPACK

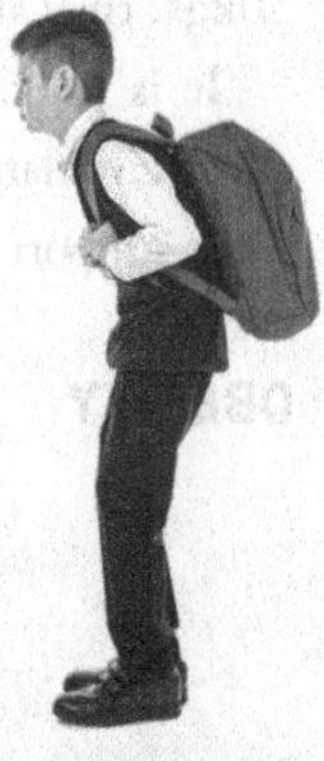

For young people, a backpack is more appropriate than a bag or purse, especially if it has to be used for a long period of time. If used correctly, the stronger muscles of the spine and abdomen (which work together to stabilize the midsection and keep our body in postural alignment) help to carry it, distributing its weight evenly. However, if used incorrectly, it can cause problems in the low back, shoulders, and neck, as well as causing headaches and even scoliosis.

If your child complains of the above symptoms, take note of the following:

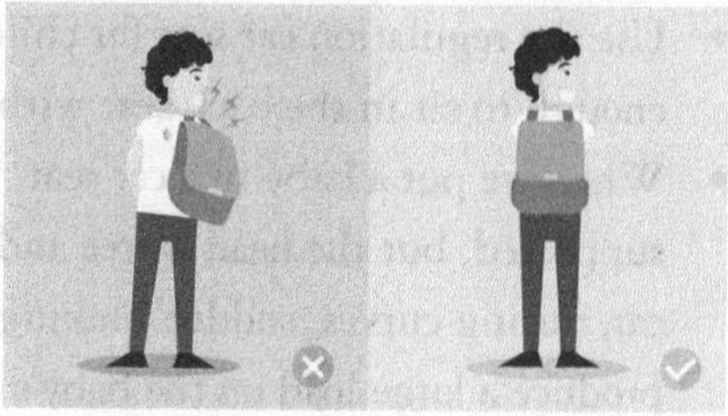

- Do they have to change their normal posture to compensate for the load they carry?
- Do they complain of numbness or tingling in the arms?
- Do they carry more than 10% of their body weight in the backpack?

Support the backpack on both shoulders because if you hold it on just one shoulder, you will overload that side to offset the imbalance, bending the spine and causing subluxations.

With time, this speeds up the process of joint degeneration, and eventually symptoms such as pain in the cervical (neck), upper, or lower back, headaches, and even functional scoliosis (lateral curvature of the spine). Remember that the consequences and especially the symptoms appear much later on in life, which is why you should teach your child from the start.

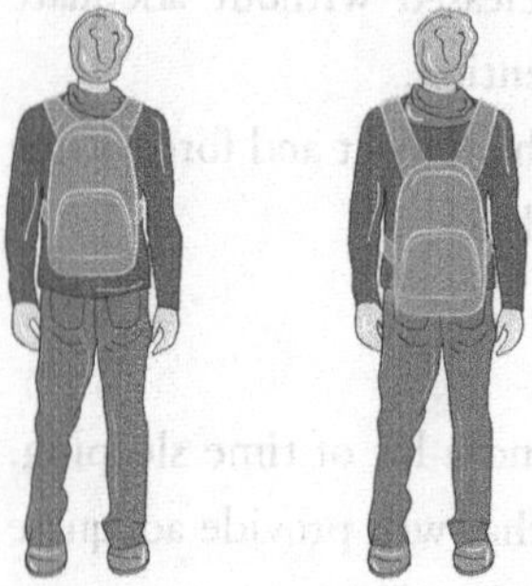

correct incorrect

Limit the weight your child carries. Students of all ages often unnecessarily fill their backpacks (excess books, clothes, or shoes for after-school activities, etc.). If you notice that your child has to lean forward to maintain balance, their backpack is too heavy and can cause loss of the natural spinal curves, leading to cervical and lumbar compensation and increasing the load on the intervertebral disks. 10% of your child's body weight is the maximum load that should be carried in the backpack. So if your child weighs 50kgs, they shouldn't carry more than 5kg.

It is important to buy backpacks with wide straps, as narrow straps can affect circulation, causing numbness or tingling in the arms. Backpacks with waist support are better still because they assist in evenly distributing the load.

OBESITY

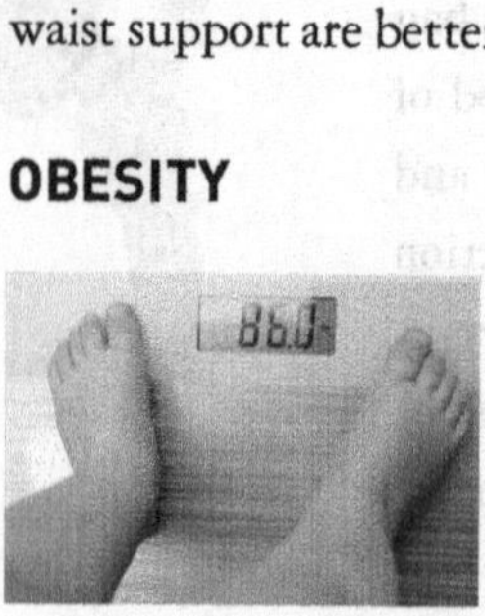

Children, in general, are now more likely than ever to be carrying excess weight. Being overweight impairs health, affecting the normal function of the spine as well as a myriad of other consequences. An obese child has a high probability of becoming an obese adult. In the past obesity in childhood was rare, however, universally it is now one of the most serious medical problems, especially in developed societies such as Australia, the United Kingdom, Canada and the United States.

According to the World Health Organization (WHO), there are 22 million obese children in the world under the age of five years old. In the U.S., 30.3% of children (between six and eleven years old) are overweight and 15.3% are obese. In adolescents, the rate is almost the same: 33.4% overweight and 15.5% obese (according to data from the American Obesity Association)

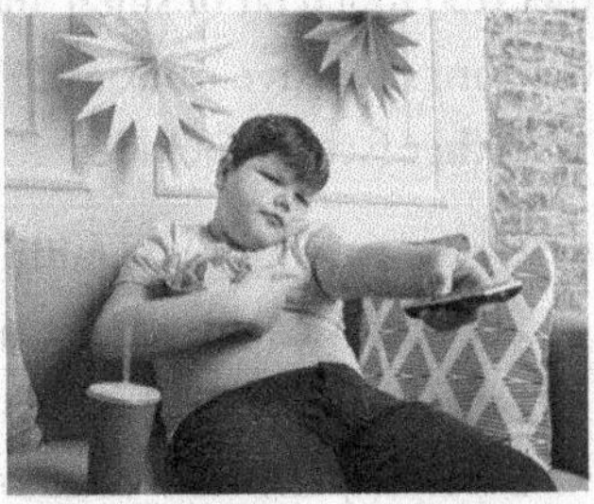

Obese children carry more weight, suffer from reduced mobility, and have greater difficulty maintaining a correct posture necessary for the normal functioning of the spine. Furthermore, they may suffer from slipped femoral epiphysis (a hip problem related to growth) and genu valgus (bow legged) or other serious problems of the legs that invariably end up affecting the spine. Let's not forget the effect on the bones of the feet, because weight gain can lead to structural abnormalities in this region as well.

Other serious health problems caused by obesity in childhood include:

- type 2 diabetes (suffered only in adults until a few years ago and currently having a very high incidence in children);
- high blood pressure (hypertension);
- liver problems;
- fatigue;
- respiratory problems;
- diseases of the heart, bladder, and ovaries (polycystic ovary syndrome).

As for the psychological consequences, being an obese child is the trigger for a series of damaging factors that, unfortunately, similar to an addiction, accompany the child throughout their lifetime.

In most cases, being obese means that the child may not be able to practice physical exercise or join sporting teams. This has social and physiological impacts.

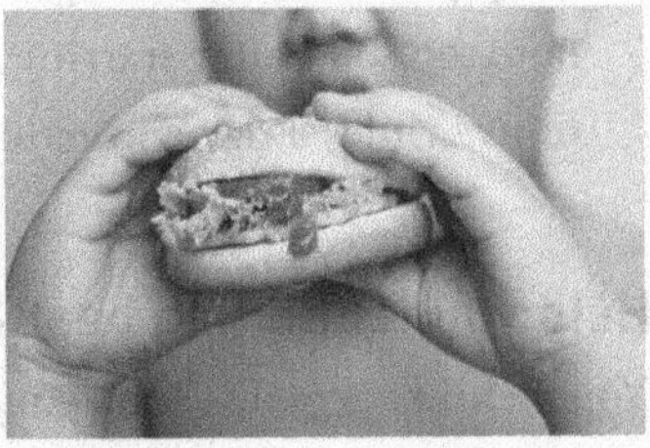

A sedentary lifestyle impedes the spine from the movement that it requires to maintain or achieve health and normal function. Exercise and proper diet are vital to avoid the 'extra pounds' that overload the discs, dehydrating them and making them more prone to degeneration with time. Bony degeneration or osteoarthritis can be accelerated due to an overloading on the joints and lack of normal function.

CAUSES

Obesity in childhood is caused predominately by two main factors: incorrect diet (too much fat or sugar and eating adult's sized portions) and lack of exercise (to burn excessive calories).

Other factors include:

- Obese parents – the family's incorrect eating habits contribute to a child's obesity. A balanced diet not only keeps the child at an ideal body weight but also helps maintain their health and consequent resistance to sickness.
- Sedentary habits – technological advances also mean that our children have more distractions and entertainment that do not require physical exercise. TV, video games, and computers are sedentary pastimes that are replacing physical activities such as soccer, volleyball, basketball, cycling, outdoor games, walks in parks, etc.
- Genetics – some genetic disorders cause severe obesity in children or adolescents, as well as hypothyroidism and Cushing's syndrome. In these cases, parents have to be even more conscientious and choose healthy foods for the whole family. Obesity caused by these causes is rare compared to obesity caused by the factors cited above.

SOLUTION – Help your child to get to a healthy weight!

- Obesity is diagnosed by body mass index (BMI). This is calculated by dividing the child's weight by the square of their height. This index should be evaluated according to age and should not be compared to those of adults.
- If your child is overweight, consult a dietician or nutritionist. Do not submit the child to an aggressive diet as this may have its own dangers. Make healthy eating choices and long-term subtle changes for the whole family.
- Help your child find a sport they like, a physical activity that they will not stop soon after starting. Increase consumption of fruits and vegetables to five times a day and reduce fats and sugars.

Help your child find healthy and tasty snacks.

Your child depends on you to lose weight. Obesity affects the child psychologically, their confidence, and their relationship with their classmates. Obese teenagers are more likely to have low self-esteem, which can influence the establishment of friendships and school performance. Your child depends on you to make responsible and healthy decisions that can have positive consequences for the rest of their life.

SEDENTARY LIFESTYLE

Sedentary lifestyle in children is a serious problem. Between the ages of eight and 18 years, children spend more time (44.5 hours/week) in front of the computer, television, and video games than doing any other activity (this is without counting the time they spend asleep) according to research from the Kaiser Family Foundation. These stats are worsening every year and some kids don't even do exercise at school any more.

Childhood is a remarkable stage of life and physical activity is vital for muscle development, cardiovascular health and healthy bone mass. A study of preschool girls revealed that the girls who watched most television have a lower hip bone density.

A comparative study done on obese and non-obese children, between eight and twelve years of age, correlating time spent in front of the TV and their metabolic rate, showed that the metabolic rate was significantly lower in the obese group while they were sedentary in front of the television. Lack of movement effects a child's concentration, focus and brain function, their hormonal balance and even their self-esteem. Physical activity costs nothing and besides a healthy diet, can be one of the most cost-effective investments that you can give a child in regards to his/her future health.

WHAT IS THE SOLUTION?

Respect your child's body and encourage your kids to exercise; their little bodies were never intended to be left long periods of time without moving.

Among other benefits, physical activity helps build bones, muscles, and joints and a healthy musculoskeletal system; it increases and maintains strength and endurance, controls body weight, and reduces fat. It also reduces anxiety and stress, increasing self-esteem and overall energy levels, and may improve blood pressure and cholesterol levels, preventing disease and promoting health.

HOW YOU CAN HELP

- Reduce the time that your child stays on the computer and television, and keep both items out of their bedroom.

- Encourage them to find an exercise or sport that they like. Exercise with your child. Be a role model for them.
- Motivate your child to take regular breaks to stretch and walk while doing homework, because sitting for too long fatigues the muscles of the spine. Obese kids suffer from back pain significantly more than kids who have a normal weight.
- Do not be a bad example for your child. If they see you leading a life of little physical activity, they will have no motivation to listen to your advice and exercise, because the advice is contradictory.

YOUR CHILD NEEDS YOU

Children, like adults, develop spinal problems.

The simple fact that your child does not feel pain does not mean they do not have problems in the spine. Spinal problems may be the cause of several common childhood complaints, seemingly unrelated to the spine such as headaches, cramps, asthma, and enuresis (bedwetting), among others. These effects can occur because of the intimate relationship between the spine and nervous system. Organs can be affected when there is an interference in nervous communication at the level of the spinal nerves, due to spinal bio-mechanical dysfunction.

STUDY TIME!

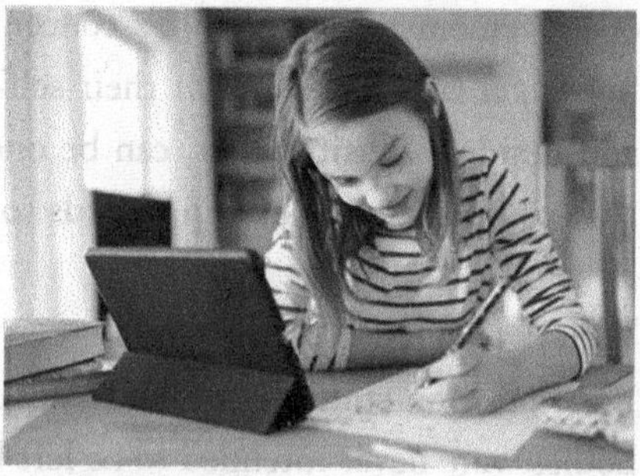

Studying for exams at school or university is stressful for a child or young adult. Spending hours in front of a computer, with the head forward and shoulders slumped causes poor posture and consequent subluxations in the neck and the spine.

The influx of young patients at the chiropractic/physiotherapy or osteopathic clinic greatly increases in the months before final school or university exams. The most common symptoms include headaches and stiff necks and shoulders and even symptoms such as insomnia, dizziness, numbness and tingling in the fingers, irritability, and anxiety.

At this phase of a student's life, physical activities are usually put aside and forgotten when, in reality, it is one of the most important times in for kids and young adults to be active. Physical activity stimulates brain function, improving memory and retention, focus and concentration. It also greatly contributes to maintaining important physiological functions such as immunity, gastrointestinal function, mobility and flexibility etc. at healthy levels, which can easily be compromised by the prolonged periods of time that a student is sedentary whilst studying. Students who continue with exercise and sports at these times are typically those who suffer less muscle aches and pains, meaning that they are less likely to have their concentration affected by avoidable muscle-skeletal symptoms or the adverse reactions to medication that may be taken to calm those aches and pains.

Sitting down for hours and staring at a book or computer screen most definitely does not please our spine. It needs to be kept mobile and when we have a sedentary lifestyle and poor posture, pain is the best way to emphasise this necessity to us. Exercise promotes spinal mobility and it is congruent with health, boosting various bodily processes. The body responds accordingly by decreasing pain and symptoms.

While studying, many students spend hours looking down and sitting in positions that are terrible for the spine, many of which increase the dorsal curve and the load on the lumbar spine. Follow the rules for correct posture already discussed and sit up straight, adjust the position of the book or computer and study hard.

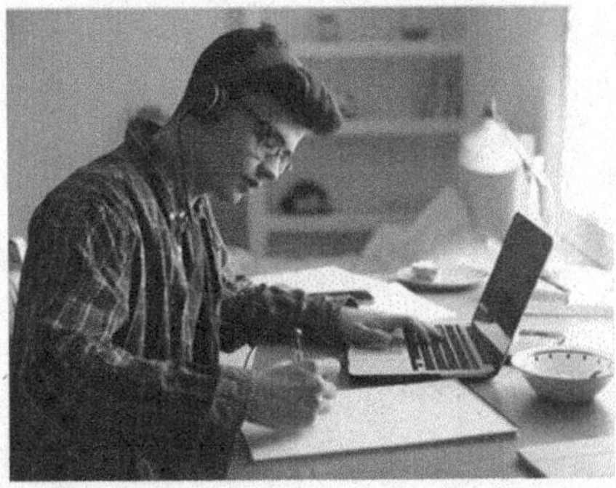

Spinal alignment can also be gradually lost with time when writing or working at the computer, as gravity is constant and our muscles gradually fatigue. It is important to constantly check in with your posture and adjust it accordingly as we relax towards more detrimental positions. Many students also lean their heads to the side when they write or leave the computer off centre to one side or the other, which contracts (shortens) certain muscles and can negatively impact upon normal neck function.

Unfortunately during exam time there is no way to avoid the hours and hours of preparation required for exams. Many students leave their study to the last minute, cramming as much as they can into the time they have. This is why many students only really find relief from the pain and symptoms that studying causes after they finish their exams. If this description fits your study style, do your best, follow the rules and rest assured that you'll be able to focus on your spine and give it the attention it needs on the other side.

Here are some tips to start preparing your body well before the tests, just as you prepare your brain:

- Get up every 30 minutes to walk or stretch;
- Do not change your exercise routine – you may exercise less, but try not to give it up, decrease the time spent rather than the frequency;
- Learn exercises and stretches that can be done at home or your place of study;
- To assist in minimising neck flexion while writing, place a few text books under the opposite elbow to the writing arm. This will help to keep the trunk straighter and avoid slumping;
- Keep the screen in front of your eyes (refer to the tips on safe computer use in the previous section 'How to care for your spine at work') and also be careful with the use of a laptop – prop it up to eye level!

THE ELDERLY – MAKING LIFE PAIN FREE

"Few people know how to get older."

FRANÇOIS DE LA ROCHEFOUCAULD

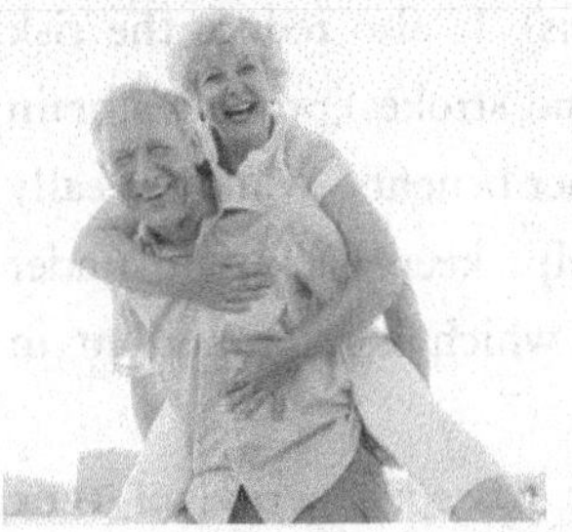

Every day, the ratio of elderly people in the population increases worldwide. Average life expectation is increasing, due to changes in lifestyle and advances in medicine. Incorrect choices often lead to early chronic and degenerative joint disease, while correct choices result in longevity and health. Healthy habits adopted in childhood, including those directed towards respecting proper posture and the correct way of using your body, can result in an elderly spine that works as well as a young adult's spine, with minimal wear and tear. If you are in your senior years and have never suffered spinal problems due to the healthy spinal practices that you have maintained throughout your life, please continue doing what you are doing. If you are in your senior years and being bothered by aches and pains that you never felt before, please don't accept that this a normal facet of ageing. It isn't. While it may be common it definitely isn't normal. Work with someone who specialises in restoring spinal bio-mechanical function, such as a chiropractor, physiotherapist or osteopath who focuses on treating the cause and not simply relieving you of its symptoms. When you are once again asymptomatic, continue on with all of the healthy practices that you have learned about in this book.

EXERCISE

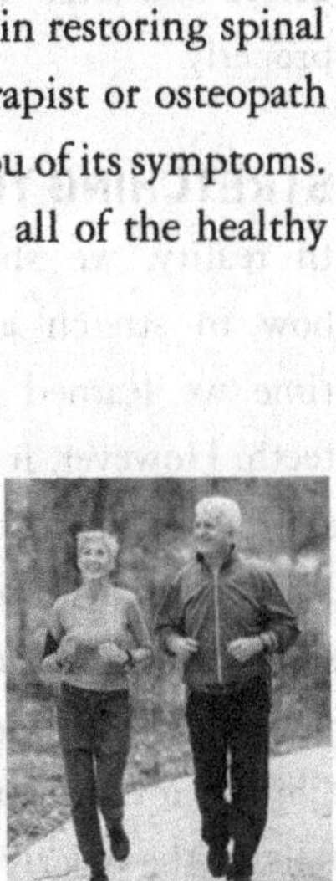

The most debilitating thing for our ageing health is a sedentary lifestyle. Exercise in this phase of life is as important as a proper diet and regular sleep. Movement guarantees improved circulation and the demands that our muscles place on our body during exercise ensures this. Weak muscles decrease joint function, accelerating bony degeneration such as osteoarthritis and also the degeneration of intervertebral discs. Exercise helps maintain digestive function, hormone levels, brain function and minimise the chance of suffering from anxiety and depression. It is simply too valuable not to do.

> *"A sedentary and consequently rigid thirty-year-old is old, while a flexible eighty year old is young."*
>
> JASON GILBERT

WALKING

Walking is a simple activity for the elderly that provides endless benefits for their health. Walking significantly helps in maintaining normal bone density levels (lowering the chances of osteoporosis). It also reducs the risk of cardiovascular disease (including heart attacks and strokes),promotes brain fuction, regulates digestion, and offers countless other benefits. Walking really is a perfect physical activity for the elderly. It helps keep back pain under control, keeps limbs agile and muscles activated, which is so important in maintaining balance and avoiding falls.

If you have been suffering from back pain or passed a period of time convalescing, start slowly by walking as little as five minutes in one direction and five minutes back. If you need help, because you do not have the confidence to walk alone, ask someone to accompany you. Add five minutes per week until reaching a minimum of thirty minutes each time you walk. Do not be alarmed if during these first weeks the lumbar spine and legs ache a little, especially if you are not accustomed to physical activity. They key is to keep going gently and increase the time gradually! Make sure that you drink sufficient water before and after the walk to give your muscles what they need to function properly.

STRETCHING YOUR MUSCLES

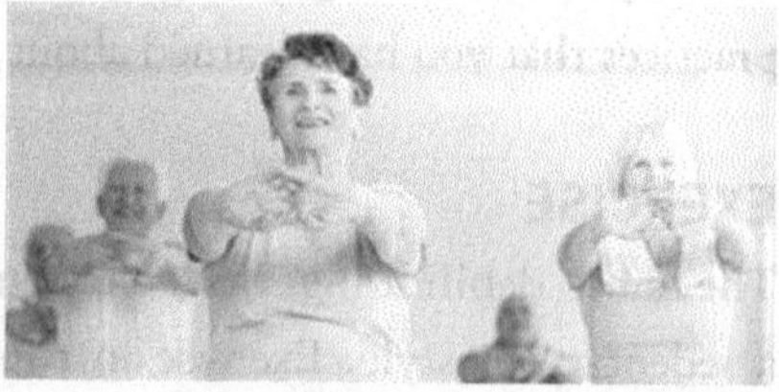

In reality, we should have learned how to stretch at about the same time we learned how to brush our teeth. However, it is never too late to start and a good stretching routine is important to prevent chronic muscle shortening also decreasing the possibility of spinal problems. In a study published in the *Journal of Advanced Nursing,* the effectiveness of Tai Chi (the Chinese martial art that improves flexibility and balance) on the incidence of falls in the elderly population was investigated. During three months, those who practiced Tai Chi three times a week presented significant improvement in knee and ankle strength and more flexibility and mobility than the control group. The people who practiced Tai Chi were also two times less likely to suffer a fall. Similar results would be expected if the group practiced yoga or any type of standing stretching routine.

FALLS

If you have suffered a fall, you'd understand how some people can be seriously injured or even lose their life. As we age, our ability to maintain balance and equilibrium, coordination and correct posture worsens. Our vision and hearing often degenerate, further affecting our balance and coordination and consequently the risk of suffering a fall. Our reflexes become slower, reducing our reaction speed in threatening situations such as avoiding a bicycle on a footpath or staying upright on a wet floor. Loss of muscle strength and flexibility may interfere with our ability to get up or remain standing, also increasing the likelihood of falls. Once you have suffered a fall it may affect your confidence and cause concern that it will happen again and encourage a more sedentary lifestyle, perpetuating all of the factors mentioned above. Many falls result in a person deciding to never walk again or use a walker or mobility scooter.

THERE ARE SEVERAL FACTORS THAT MAY INCREASE THE CHANCE OF SUFFERING A FALL:

MEDICATION

Certain medications can increase the risk of suffering a fall. Common medications used by elderly people can have side effects that could affect brain function, causing vertigo and decreased coordination.

Taking multiple medications such as antidepressants and antihistamines increases the risk of falls, and taking them with alcohol complicates the situation even further and should also be avoided.

Have your doctor review your medications and if possible, discuss the possibility of decreasing the dosage of those that may increase the risk of falling. Consider using a cane for support while taking these medicines which will give have more confidence and security when walking.

Many elderly people who rely on painkillers for many years or even decades also suffer serious side effects in other organs like the stomach, kidneys, and liver. The use of these drugs for pain control, as well as their side effects, can be reduced and even avoided if the person follows healthy habits, such as maintaining good posture and minimising sedentary time as well as nourishing the body with a nutritious diet and good quality sleep.

OSTEOPOROSIS

Osteoporosis is a major cause of fractures in the elderly, particularly in women. The word means 'porous bones' and the disease occurs when bone density deteriorates until it can no longer bear the weight of the body. Hormonal changes, calcium and vitamin D deficiency, and reduced physical activity are the most common causes.

Please refer to more information about Osteoporosis and how to deal with it in 'Chemical Causes of Back Pain'.

POOR VISION

The risk of falling also increases as vision worsens with age. Eye diseases related to ageing, such as cataracts and glaucoma, may alter the perceived distance of objects, the brightness of light and visual acuity, impairing locomotion. Get your eye sight examined regularly to ensure that your spectacles are apt for your level of visual acuity. Also, keep your glasses clean for better visibility.

HIDDEN DANGERS IN THE HOUSE

At least one third of falls occur at home, mostly caused by objects on the floor. Check to see if your home has hidden dangers. Refer to the section on the home previously discussed in this chapter.

DEPRESSION AND CHRONIC PAIN

> *'Unhappiness makes people age faster'*
> HESIOD

Depression is the most common emotion associated with chronic pain, up to four times more common in this group than in the rest of the population. Many of the factors that increase the effects of depression are reported by the elderly, such as insomnia, inability to do normal activities of daily living, the need to depend on someone for even the simplest of tasks, and of course the underlying problems of the spine that cause pain. This begins a vicious cycle in which pain is the trigger for depression, which frequently results in an increase of pain. Many elderly people, particularly those suffering from chronic pain and depression, are confined to a bed or couch obliged to a sedentary lifestyle which directly leads to a reduction in brain function and mental health.

Signs of clinical depression persist for two weeks or more and include many of the following factors:

- feelings of sadness, despair, and moments of crying for no apparent reason;

- decreased concentration and memory;
- loss of interest or pleasure in normal activities;
- low self-esteem or guilt;
- lack of appetite;
- sudden increase or loss of weight;
- insomnia;
- tiredness/fatigue.

WHAT TO DO

The first step is to identify the cause and not let the pain be the focus of your life. Try to maintain normal activities and start an activity you enjoy if your life is very sedentary.

Tell your family how you feel. Ask for help. Whether it be from a professional therapist or psychologist, or someone to simply walk with you.

Distract yourself from the pain by changing environments and keeping yourself busy. (See 'Depression and its effects,' in the chapter 'Emotional causes of Back pain', to understand more about this problem and tips on how to fix it.)

EXERCISE – FUNDAMENTAL FOR SPINAL HEALTH

"Overcoming laziness is the first thing that a person should do if he/she wants to own his/her future."

THOMAS ATKINSON

According to the World Health Organization (WHO), "physical inactivity has been increasing alarmingly throughout the world, no longer a purely aesthetic problem to become a serious public health problem in a global epidemic." Yet according to data from WHO, "70% of people worldwide are sedentary, leaving them predisposed to developing heart disease, diabetes and obesity. Lack of physical activity has been cited as contributing to 54% of deaths from heart attack, stroke by 50% and 37% by cancer".

People who lead predominantly sedentary lifestyles are at greater risk of suffering when they are in situations that are 'outside' of their normal routine, such as doing activities like digging in the garden, pushing a car that does not start, or even cleaning the house, simply because their body is not used to exertion.

They are more prone to injury due to the lack of preparation and the fact that soft tissues such as muscles and tendons are simply not prepared, sometimes leaving the spine sore and stiff for weeks and contributing to absences from work and other modifications in their daily activities due to the pain. Many of these 'flare ups' or simple injuries result in discomfort that can last for weeks afterwards or even exacerbate pre-existing problems, perpetuating a non-active lifestyle and often promoting an even more sedentary lifestyle.

People who work in office jobs or professions that oblige them to be seated are surprisingly much more prone to suffering spinal problems when compared to those whose employment requires physical activity.

"Laziness hinders, while activity facilitates everything."

MARQUÊS DE MARICÁ

If we calculated the time that our spine is inactive in any given week we would be surprised! We sleep an average of 6–8 hours a day (approximately a quarter to a third of our life), we sit at desks working or studying or at tables for meals and there's the time spent commuting on cars, buses, trains etc., to school, university or work. Let's assume that this represents a minimum of 18 hours each day. In those 6 hours what are you doing? Is your spine getting the movement that it needs to function correctly? Or is it sedentary while watching TV, using your smart phone or computer or lounging on the couch? If we don't allow our spine the opportunity to function it will actually stop functioning correctly. As the human body is resilient this could occur without any 'obvious' signs from the body until the 2nd, 3rd or maybe 4th decade of life, however in this time you can rest assured that it is slowly degenerating and that your health and the quality of your life is no where near the potential that it could be. Movement stimulates the cerebellum, which is the homeostatic (control) centre of the brain. The cerebellum relies on movement to be able to coordinate all of the functions that it must coordinate. Even the amount of pain you feel will be regulated by the amount of movement occurring at a segmental level of the vertebral column. Movement is quite simply the most important nutrient for our body (after sleep) and is grossly ignored in our modern society by a large sector of the population.

Many people say that they simply do not have time for exercise during the week. That is understandable. Sometimes family, work and other commitments have to be juggled in a busy week and exercise is overlooked, especially if somebody is asymptomatic. This priority often changes when back pain rears it's ugly head, as people learn first-hand what must be done to provide the spine and the body with what it needs. Other people leave exercise to the weekend, when their schedule permits. While any exercise is obviously better than none at all, it is advisable to simply move more during the week if you can't find time to go to a gym, park or other area where you usually exercise. Move more at work, in the home, or even commuting to work. Anything you do will make a huge difference in the long run.

Our body actually tries to guide us towards exercising. An interesting example of how it does this is seen when patients, during their first consultation, relate that their complaint worsened after they stop exercising. I have heard this literally thousands of times in my career! Many of these people, upon feeling pain, stop exercising because they think it worsens or actually causes their problem or because someone (often their doctor) advised them to stop. Instead of looking at the cause and considering whether a certain exercise or aspect of it was excessive, they often refrain from every form of physical activity. This can be devastating for their spine and their overall health and wellbeing! Perhaps a simple and temporary change to another type of exercise, a lighter weight or the treatment of a pre-existing problem was all that was needed.

LACK OF TIME

If my clients say that they don't have time to exercise it really means that they don't understand the importance of exercise for good health or their health is not a priority. This of course is common when we have never been taught about spinal care and the intimate relationship between the spine and the health of our body. Imagine telling a dentist that you don't have time to brush your teeth. The dentist would quickly be able to join the dots and recognise how devastating that would be for your dental health. Interestingly, many people would dedicate more time to caring for their teeth than their spines. Brushing teeth is not a source of joy for millions of people, but they do it every day, liking it or not, because they know the consequences if they do not brush them. If exercises could be done in three minutes, three times a day, I wonder if more people would exercise? Teeth are important but the spine is undeniably much more important. Please don't wait until you are suffering, possibly from an irreversible degenerative condition to start to prioritise your spine. Exercising is free and it is vital for the maintenance of our health, which is our best investment to avoid multiple degenerative diseases that would otherwise end or shorten our life span.

There is no doubt that doing exercise involves an investment of your time, in the same way that work or sleep occupy our time. They are both however, important aspects of life. We do not complain of the time taken to earn money or the time invested in a good sleep to rest and recover the body. Investing sufficient time to exercise is as essential as these two examples.

Every day, there are many opportunities to exercise our bodies. All we need is to change little habits such as using the stairs instead of taking the elevator or walking or riding to work, moving whenever we get a chance. Walk instead of using your car or public transportation if you have to go somewhere close to home. If you have to be on a phone call at work, why not stand up at your desk and walk on the spot?

Physical activity does not have to be confined to a gym. If you have a dog, commit to walking it every day. Replace an hour on the internet or a movie/TV series with a walk in the park. Clean your house, your bedroom or bathroom, instead of paying somebody else to do it. Take the opportunity to move! There are so many opportunities during the day to do so and the benefits that they bring add up like savings in a bank account, You will be building your health bank which will give guaranteed returns for your health and lower or negate the cost of paying for disease in the future.

The PAFFENBARGER STUDY, one of the most comprehensive investigations about exercise and its benefits to our health was conducted by Ralph

Paffenbarger of Harvard University in 1986. Data from 17 000 students was collected between 1916 and 1950 and determined that:

- People who ran or walked, exercised on a treadmill or played sports regularly, had 25% lower risk of heart disease compared to sedentary individuals.
- The mortality rate from cardiovascular disease decreased when the intensity of exercise decreased to 2000 calories lost per week (equivalent to running 32 km per week). People who maintained that intensity of exercise lived on average two and a half years longer than the sedentary ones. Among the people studied that burned over 2000 calories, 68% lived to be 80 years or older!
- Regular exercise equated to decreased rates of cholesterol, blood pressure and the development of diabetes mellitus (type 2). People who burned over 2000 calories a week had lower cancer mortality than those who burned only 500 calories per week.
- Moderate levels of exercise activate the immune system, which has many benefits, one of which is to help fight cancer cells before the development of tumours.

Many studies, including that of Paffenbarger, show that exercising reduces the incidence of cancer of the colon (large intestine). Exercise helps avoid constipation, and with food matter moving faster through the GI tract there is less time for carcinogens to transform normal cells into cancer cells.

Untreated hypertension can dramatically increase the risk of heart attack and cardiac arrest. According to the WHO (World Health Organisation), there are 600 million people in the world who suffer hypertension (high blood pressure) and this is the third leading risk factor associated with mortality worldwide. Exercising helps to lower blood pressure in several ways. The muscles worked by exercises generally have more capillaries (small blood channels between the arteries and veins). Capillaries facilitate the exchange of oxygen and nutrients between the blood and tissue cells and also help the blood to drain from the arteries in greater quantity and faster. This results in helping to keep blood pressure at healthy levels. The veins of physically active individuals also have larger diameters that help the return of blood from the body back to the heart.

Another important benefit of exercise is to reduce the risk of obesity and resistance to insulin – two factors that increase blood pressure.

Breast cancer is the second most common type of cancer worldwide. A study by the University of Southern California with 1,000 women showed that only 1 to 3 hours of exercise per week were sufficient to reduce the risk of breast cancer by 30% and in women who exercise four hours or more decreases the risk up to 50%.

Exercise reduces the risk of osteoporosis (a disease that affects bone density of our skeleton), which affects one in three women and one in ten men during their lives (statistics of WHO). The increased load combined with the effects of gravity that occur during exercise (especially the ones that are weight bearing) slows down bone demineralisation, keeping them strong and resistant to Osteoporosis.

GO AND WALK!

"Walking is the best medicine for man."

HIPPOCRATES

Walking is one of the best forms of exercise for our body and it aids many of it's functions: it benefits the spine, helps to control pain and other symptoms and reduces the risk of various diseases. It also makes us happy!

Walking is safe and costs nothing. Some of it's benefits include:

- helps control blood pressure, because it strengthens the heart and can pump more blood with less effort and thus lower the pressure placed on the arteries;
- reduces the risk of myocardial infarction – a study conducted by 77,000 nurses participating in the Nurse's Health Study for over twenty years showed that just three hours of walking a week helped in reducing the risk by 30–40% of cases;
- lowers LDL cholesterol, which when out of proportion with HDL cholesterol, promotes the accumulation of plaques (arteriosclerosis) in the arterial wall;
- protects against hip fractures because it reduces the likelihood of osteoporosis;
- helps control weight and reduce obesity, which prevents osteoarthrosis, diabetes mellitus (type 2), heart disease and stroke, among others;
- reduces the risk of breast cancer;
- strengthening the muscles of the feet, legs, hips and torso, which increases stability of the spine and the confidence to step;
- promotes the nutrition of discs, muscles, and other soft tissues;
- improves flexibility and posture – your spine stays straight the entire time while you walk, a great advantage when compared to other exercises;
- reduces pain and inflammation quicker than if the person remained

sedentary, therefore allowing them to return to work, physical activities, and normal life sooner.

Many people who suffer with back pain are afraid to walk because they believe that exercise will cause more discomfort and worsen their problem. If this is your case, start by walking as far as you can until it hurts. It doesn't have to be far, even 5 minutes is great to start off with. When it hurts, rest and wait and then walk back. With time you should be able to walk a little further and a little longer every day. Before you know it you will be walking longer than what you would have imagined a couple of weeks ago. If walking provokes a low-grade pain, especially if you haven't walked for a while, try and push through as the pain usually subsides with time. Don't let fear dominate your intention to restore function to the spine. The pain may continue with low intensity, but the spine will have the opportunity to move and function as it should. It will be easier with each walk, and the pain will diminish.

Walking is one of the safest forms of physical therapy. In some cases of acute crises, it may be one of the only activities that you may be able to do. Walking helps to reduce inflammation, which can be a fantastic adjunct to any other interventions that may be utilised. You can also ice after a walk to assist with the pain and reduce inflammation (see 'ice').

WALK THIS WAY ... back to basics!

We should walk at least 10 000 steps a day. Many of us struggle to do 1000 steps! Incorrect walking technique can accelerate bony degeneration (osteoarthritis), set up incorrect bio-mechanical chains between the foot, knee and the hip (allowing problems to occur in these joints and even the low back) and even worsen already challenged postural problems. Here are some useful tips:

The head should be aligned with the shoulders, allowing the eyes to look towards the horizon and not down. Many people who walk looking at the ground cause themselves problems in the neck and a worsening of their resting posture. To help this the shoulders should be relaxed, and not falling forwards. If this is a challenge for you, try rotating your hands slightly outward (external rotation) as you walk. This will open the chest a little, stretch the anterior muscles of the deltoid (which become shorter when the hands are constantly turned inwards) and allow the head to sit more comfortably over the shoulders.

The core should be activated to support the torso, especially in cases of acute low back pain. The gluteal muscles of the hind leg should also be activated. This allows the hind leg to 'push off' as it moves the foot to step forward, as opposed to allowing the front leg lead this action. This is extremely important to guarantee normal bio-mechanics. As each step can be a positive influence or a negative influence to the whole bio-mechanical function of our lower limbs, low back and even upper back, taking the time to consider your technique is an easy investment that delivers massive returns in the long run.

TIP – Touch the buttock (gluteal area) of the hind leg when the foot is on the ground to ensure that it is activated. Do this periodically during your walk. Touch the abdominal region to confirm that these muscles are also activated.

The arms should stay close to the body and swing back as the hind leg pushes forward. This creates a counter torque that encourages correct pelvic function and hip rotation, also allowing for the most efficient use of energy whilst walking.

Avoid stepping with a 'passive' foot strike on the ground, where the foot would be contacting as a solid unit. This increases the load through the heel and does not allow for the absorption of this load efficiently, also leading too heel spurs in the future. Use an 'active' foot that contacts first with the heel, then with the whole foot in contact with the ground and lastly with the toes flexed as the hind leg pushes forward for the next step. In order to be able to follow every detail described above we need to concentrate, especially if poor walking habits have developed.

Running shoes are best suited for the support they provide. They should be comfortable and have enough support (as a buffer) under the heel to absorb impact. Alternatively, if you are on a beach or a familiar grassy area, walking in bare feet is an absolute joy, allowing your feet to function as they were intentioned to whilst also giving you the benefits of grounding (receiving the energy of the earth's magnetic field).

When you buy running shoes the purchase should be made at the end of the day when your feet actually have a larger size than the morning, due to an increase in size that occurs from moving throughout the day. Take the socks you usually use and walk in the store before making a decision.

Creating a routine is very important when starting to walk. Choose a certain time of the day (in the morning is usually easier for most people, possibly before children wake etc.) to walk, that way it will be easy to remember and will become a part of your life before you know it. Those who are new to walking and don't lock in time for a walk often relate to being distracted by other priorities and chores during the day.

Choose surfaces such as grass, dirt or sand instead of concrete, which minimises the impact on your spine. That said, if the surface is uneven, take care or choose another area that is even. Many back problems are exacerbated by walking on an uneven beach or hill. If your back is still getting used to exercise after a long hiatus, be wary of excessively hilly areas. You can hit those next month when you are stronger and more prepared!

If walking seems to cause pain in any way, find the cause, do not blame the activity. It is most probably that it is an old problem that is only just now manifesting itself.

RUN THIS WAY

Humans are born to walk and run right? Well there's probably no need to learn how to walk correctly when we start as kids, however there is a need to learn how to run correctly, especially if you plan to do it as your chosen exercise or even competitively later on in life. As running comes as an easy and natural transition after the walking phase of childhood, most people understandably think that there is no need to learn how to run correctly. Unfortunately, the negative effects of an incorrect gate during running can rapidly wear out soft tissues such as ligaments and tendons, overload joints, and shorten their lifespan. Joints such as knees, hips and those of the lower back are the ones that suffer most, and not surprisingly are the most common areas targeted for surgery and replacements later on in life. If you enjoy running, the idea is to be able to run for a lifetime without being prevented by doing so by avoidable injury caused in the process. Many of these injuries can be avoided if we focus on our running technique earlier in life. The importance of being able to run and distribute your load evenly not only between both sides of the body, but also uniformly across areas of the intervertebral discs and articulations, is comparable to the importance of driving a car and having all wheels of the car equally aligned. As a large percentage of the population already have postural abnormalities and structural misalignment in the skeleton, it is even more important that these people are aware of the bio-mechanical challenges before they take up running as their new exercise or resume it again after a long hiatus. When pre-existing bio-mechanical problems occur in the skeleton of a person getting into running, quite commonly these problems will be exacerbated by the increased loads caused whilst running. Often and understandably the person will think that the pain and other symptoms were caused by running, instead of recognising that the problems were already present and that the new activity of running simply served as a way of advising the brain that there is an underlying problem.

The benefits of running for our physical and emotional health are enormous. From cardiac and circuitry health, to boosting the levels of serotonin, regulation of hormones, maintenance of normal muscle tone, flexibility and mobility.

It would be a shame to be impeded from receiving these benefits due to pre-existing problems that have been dormant previous to starting and have them only 'appear' when somebody starts to run. Understandably many people blame running as the cause if this occurs, as opposed to recognising that there are already problems that were simply exacerbated by the new loads and stresses on the body caused by running.

HOW TO RUN CORRECTLY

Posture is an extremely important thing to consider when we run. The head should be held high with the chest expanded, leaving the shoulders open. The centre of gravity line (previously described in this book) is maintained, albeit with a slight forward inclination.

Start by walking – accustom yourself to looking to the horizon and not down at the ground where your foot will land when you run. This will help maintain correct posture when you are running. Looking down at the ground in front of you will curve your shoulders and bring your head forward, increasing the load at the base of the neck, causing subsequent muscle tension here. If your head is too far back when you run it will promote heel strike and subsequent increase in load through the low back. Focus on your heel strike and toe off, as described extensively in the section on walking in this book. Now start walking faster until you eventually start running. Running increases the force so soften your knees a little. At this point landing with a mid foot contact will help absorb the shock and minimise loads through your low back, hips,knees and ankles. It is common to see people over striding, especially when they start running. This is easily recognisable, as the heel lands way out in front of the body, acting like a break and increasing the load even more. When your correct running posture has been found, the same foot will ideally be landing under the body whilst it's already starting to go backwards.

What you can do to improve your running style.

1. Running on the spot helps perfect the point mentioned above, helping you be conscious of where your foot is landing before and backwards.
2. Jog on the spot slowly. Be conscious of landing on the midfoot and using this area to push off when raising the knee again. After a few minutes of doing this, do it a little faster and raise the knees to the height of the hips.
3. Now move your hands to the back and touch your feet as they come up towards your buttock.
4. Maintaining your style, start to move forward, still leaving your hands around hip level and touching your feet lightly as they come up. Be conscious of your posture always with the chest expanded and your

tummy tucked in. This will make it easier for you to raise your knees whilst running. It is common to observe that beginners running postures worsen as they become tired. The drills mentioned above will help avoid this occurring, especially when they are done at the start of every run for a couple of minutes. If you feel yourself fatiguing, either slow down or stop, go back to the basics and then start again. If you are simply too tired to maintain correct technique, it is highly advisable to walk and leave the running until the next time, when you have more energy to maintain your proper technique.

OTHER TIPS

Moving your arms helps your momentum when you run. As one arm goes forward the opposite leg goes backwards. This is also incredible stimulation for processes in your brain that benefit from coordination, particularly the cerebellum.

Keeping your arms at 90° will ensure that they do not fall down and increase the chance of you losing your correct running posture. Focusing on how you breathe whilst you run is also extremely important. You can gain enormous health benefits by focusing on breathing through your nose. This helps keep your body in a parasympathetic state as opposed to a more stressful sympathetic state that can be invoked by breathing through your mouth. Our noses are meant for breathing. Breathing through your nose (and not your mouth) helps moisten the air we inhale. It also activates an essential molecule called Nitric Oxide, which acts on the inner layer of the blood vessels, the Endothelium. By infusing the underlying smooth muscle, it causes them to relax, which has an important role in controlling blood pressure and subsequent cardiovascular health. If you don't already breathe through your nose this is one very important reason to start doing so. TIP – taking the amino acids L-Arginine or L-Citrulline also helps to increase Nitric Oxide.

A suitable gauge to know what running pace is safe for you is one that allows you to breathe comfortably and hold a conversation while you run. If you feel that you need to gasp for air or cannot converse with a person you're running with, slow down, as you're more likely be maintaining yourself in a fight or flight stress state.

Be conscious of feeling your belly and getting air into your lower abdomen. This will help you avoid shallow chest breathing, which impedes us from a variety of benefits that come from full deep lung breathing.

Don't forget to use running shoes that are adequate to your running style. You wouldn't put cheap tyres on your car and expect them to enhance performance whilst you're driving. The same can be said for running shoes. Buy yours from a running store where the staff are informed on how to measure your foot and match it up with a suitable shoe.

If you would like to include sprinting into your workout regime for the incredible benefits it brings to our health be conscious of inclining your body further forward and using your arms more aggressively. Take shorter faster strides landing with the forefoot and propelling with the toes. Land with a soft impact to minimise jarring of the joints. Sprinting offers the amazing benefits of high intensity interval training that is perfect for those days that you only have a short amount of time to train. It activates type 2 muscle fibres, which stimulates the brain to secrete growth hormone.

IN THE GYM

The relationship between a gym and our spine can sometimes be a paradox, because we usually join a gym to improve fitness and to rehabilitate injuries however the irony is that, for many people, it often ends up negatively affecting the spine, especially when an exercise is performed incorrectly or excessive weights are used.

The vast majority of people old enough to start a program at the gym already have some type of pre-existing bio-mechanical dysfunction of their spines when they join. Like any machine, when there is a degree of dysfunction, the load ends up being concentrated on the weakest element. In the case of a spine with bio-mechanical dysfunction (caused by the factors that we discuss in this book), the increased load that a new gym program can place on the spine can not only exacerbate the pain but also contribute to bony or intervertebral disc degeneration.

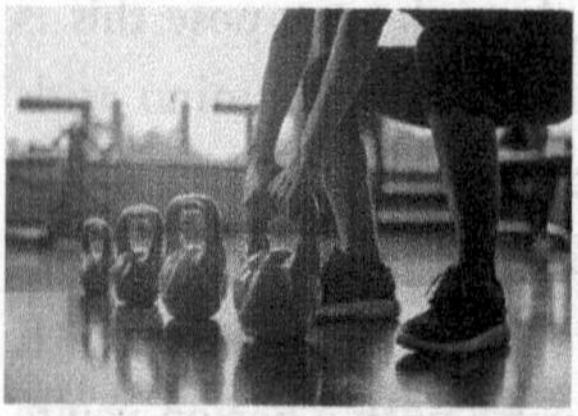

Frequently, the first time that many people become aware of a subluxation is soon after starting their workout program in the gym, and the body signals that a certain exercise or load may be detrimental via pain or joint restriction. It may also present itself in other ways (symptom), such as numbness in the arms or legs, stiff neck, headache or something else 'debilitating'. In fact, all this serves to draw your attention to the problem and the brain simply wants you to avoid doing what is potentially harming your body, whether you recognise that at the time or not.

TIPS

People starting a program at the gym should be prepared and get appropriate advice from professionals so that they know that they are fit to do so.

Always exercise after being instructed by a good trainer who not only knows how you should execute each exercise, but also recognises when you are pushing the limits and possibly damaging your spine.

Many injuries occur by not knowing exactly how to execute certain exercises when the load is increased. A common mistake that causes injury happens when somebody changes their posture or position to lift a heavier weight.

Independently of whether you stretch before or during your workout session, dedicate time specifically for stretching for at least 20 minutes, three times a week. Many people choose to vary their exercise routines by doing yoga classes, that are fun and interactive, whilst at the same time focus on core strength and flexibility. This can protect the spine from potential injury from heavy weights. The more flexibility you have, the less you will overload the muscles. When limbs lack flexibility, the load usually increases in the joint and tendon in the area closest to the joint.

SAVE YOURSELF FROM INJURY

Exerting your body, in spite of providing many benefits, invariably results in some negative ones. This should never be a deterrent to exercising or practising a sport that makes you happy. When injuries do occur, you must listen to your body, rest the area affected (this often means practising some other exercise that doesn't overload that particular tissue) and learn. Work with your spinal health specialist to restore spinal function to the tissues and help lower inflammation as fast as possible. Problems can be acute (of recent and easily identifiable causes) or chronic (caused by overloading certain tissues continuously over time, or from an incident that occurred previously that was never corrected. Chronic problems can happen without you being aware of them with the function of the spine or joints being affected little by little and the pain is often ignored or not felt due to the low severity of the aggravating factor. Chronic lesions may be discovered when the underlying problem is advanced and tissue degeneration in the form of intervertebral disc disease, cartilaginous degeneration or bony osteoarthritis has already occurred. These problems can sadly affect a person's health due to the fact that they may impede them from continuing with the exercise that they have always practiced (but was also responsible for the degeneration). As they can manifest many years after the problem actually started they can also impede all physical activity for a while, especially if surgery is indicated. It is for this reason that it is imperative that any ache or pain, no matter how slight it may appear, is taken seriously. Warning signs from the body often disappear for years before the devastating 'straw that breaks the camel's back' which can end a competitive career or simply limit the person from ever functioning at their peak.

Do not allow yourself to reach this stage. Using common sense and equipped with basic knowledge on how to exercise correctly, you may exercise the rest of your life and, most importantly, without pain or damage to your spine.

FACTORS THAT EXACERBATE AN INJURY

The duration and intensity of each exercise session in any given week greatly influences whether you are prone to an injury or not. You need to listen to your body. Don't strain or overload it thinking that simply because you've never had an injury before then what you are doing is OK. It may not be and may be gradually compromising tissue function until it gets to a point where it becomes symptomatic. Over training often results in fatigued muscles that are not efficient in protecting other surrounding tissues and joints. Fatigued muscles also increase the risk of damage to bones, cartilage, tendons and ligaments.

Many injuries are the result of previous injuries. Exercise requires a lot from your body, your spine and joints, and the weakest part often gives in first. After an injury, many people do not respect the time needed to allow the body to heal, recover and return to normal function, and as such do not respect the need to rehabilitate themselves through physical therapy, chiropractic or other modalities before they go back to exercise.

TIPS – on how to avoid injury

Do not train if you are tired. The risk of injury increases, because tired muscles fail to provide the support and protection required.

Minimise the number of consecutive training days. The interval between training allows the muscles and tissues to recover before the next session.

Take whatever time is necessary for recovery from injury. Use ice, do stretching exercises, seek the appropriate professional to help you return to your functional state.

Never take pain killers/analgesics in order to train without pain. Your body intelligently causes pain to warn you that something is not good. If you turn this signal off, you will not be aware of tissue damage when it occurs, worsening the situation and possibly leaving you injured for longer.

Go easy and take care when you start a new sport or physical activity. You're more susceptible to injuries, compared to someone who has done the same activity for years and who has had more time to strengthen their muscles, tendons and ligaments accordingly. Many people rush in to 'conquer' a new sport or simply become 'addicted' to the new activity that they are practising and their body simply isn't prepared for it. Build up to it and observe how your body is reacting. It may be fine up until 25 minutes of a certain activity but going past this time may throw it over the edge, leaving you inflamed and your muscles fatigued. This is a person to person phenomenon that is influenced by many factors, such as diet, hydration, consumption of alcohol, sleep quality and more.

Give apparently 'less serious' injuries due attention to ensure that they are not worse than what you imagine. Many serious injuries are caused by people unknowingly pushing through a little 'niggle' because it didn't incapacitate them only to find out further down the track that the original aggravation was worse than what they had imagined. Knee injuries can typically start slowly, sometimes with a tolerable 'click' however the bio-mechanics of the knee, if altered, can lead to an accelerated arthritic process. Always apply ice, rest and use compression as soon as possible as well as doing a diagnostic image such as an MRI (Magnetic Resonance Imaging) if there's any doubt about the state of the joint and it's surrounding tissues.

Increase your complex carbohydrate intake during training or heavy activities. Muscles need carbohydrates for energy. Muscles receiving low amounts of complex carbohydrates or an excess of simple carbohydrates, fatigue quickly and struggle to protect you from injury or withstand the loads on their joints.

Adequate hydration helps avoid muscle fatigue and fibre damage. 80% of a muscle's composition is water, so it makes perfect sense that in order to function correctly, it requires a sufficiency of this vital nutrient. The heart is a muscle and therefore it is no surprise to know that hydration helps avoid cardiac arrest, especially during exercise. According to the American College of Sport Medicine, athletes should be sufficiently hydrated before physical activity and this should be maintained at regular intervals during exercise to replace the water lost during exercise.

If you feel pain during your workout or activity, stop immediately, rest for a short period of time and then return to it. If it still hurts, listen to your body and stop. Revert to walking if it doesn't hurt and follow the protocols for dealing with inflammation, i.e., ice, rest etc. This approach makes much more sense than pushing on and risking permanent damage to your body and possibly an early retirement from your favourite sport or activity. If you need to, keep reminding yourself of the purpose behind the pain and why your body is causing it. To keep ignoring the pain will only worsen the problem and the prognosis!

Every sport or physical activity presents a threat to the spine simply because they involve physical activity which can compromise it's function. Each one requires something different from specific areas in our body. Learn about the risks and what you can do whilst practising the sport as well as what you must do afterwards to compensate for it.

Unilateral or asymmetrical sports such as tennis and golf overload one side of the body more than the other than the other. They also place uneven forces on some joints of the body than others and therefore contribute to more accelerated degeneration of these joints. Other sports such as soccer, jiu jitsu, rugby, and basketball cause traumas and impacts, often with other players, and the injuries are accumulated throughout life. They also involve fast movements and last minute changes of direction that overload certain articulations suddenly, often without allowing supporting muscles the time to prepare for the change in forces. The need for regular compensatory and preventative maintenance care with your chosen spinal practitioner is paramount.

Even a low impact sport such as swimming can cause joint dysfunction and muscle contraction if the swimmer's stroke is not correct, especially if freestyle is the predominant stroke. The main pitiful here is when the swimmer favours one particular side and turns their head to that side over and over in order to breathe. By not breathing towards the opposite side, chronic muscle shortening can occur on the side where the neck rotation repetitively occurs during breathing. If you are a swimmer, make sure you turn to breathe both to the left and right, even if you have been swimming your whole life and have become accustomed to breathing to the same side. If this is your case, yes, it will be more difficult to accustom yourself to breathing to both sides. However the benefit to your spine in the long run is undeniable. By doing this, you will save yourself suffering from pain and avoidable arthritic degeneration in the future.

Even though we have all run from early childhood, correct running technique doesn't come easily for may of us. This is understandable as most of us have never been taught. As such, it is something that needs to be focused on, especially if we want to run our whole lives without causing irreversible degenerative changes to areas of our skeleton. Runners also face their challenges in maintaining spinal function and avoiding the common problems that running long distances poses for the spine. Many people congenitally have a leg that is shorter than the other leg (Leg Length Discrepancy). Runners should check their leg lengths via a scan called a Leg Length scan, also known as a Scanogram, especially if they are suffering pain on one side of their body only. Many people dedicate themselves to running years and decades without questioning why certain aches and pains in their body only appear on one side of their body. By looking at possible leg length discrepancy and congenital problems of the spine that cause uneven loads on the lower limbs, suffering from the effects of Osteoarthritis and Degenerative Disc Disease can be avoided. A simple x-ray of the spine is a must for any runner, whether they be competitive or simply do it to get the body moving and the blood circulating. Runners should also study their gate and learn.

TIP

If you are an athlete or practice a sport standing/running etc., you need to know if your weight is being distributed evenly between both sides of your body. Get two scales, put them together, edge to edge and stand on the lateral edge of each scale. Get somebody to position your feet so that they are placed in the same position on each scale, look forward and ask the person helping you to read the measurements. See if you have a difference between left and right sides. If you do, a Scanogram is a great way to confirm if it is due to a leg length discrepancy.

The number and variety of sports and exercises is diverse and each one poses a different risk to the spine and other joints of the body. Be aware of the inherent risks of the ones that you practice and do your best to compensate for, or manage, the consequences of your chosen sport.

Sometimes we must accept that some simply aren't apt for our spine or our condition.

EXERCISE MAKES YOU HAPPY!

Multiple studies show that symptoms of depression decrease when the level of physical activity increases (see chapter – Emotional Causes).

Exercise improves self-esteem, confidence and emotional stability. Talk to friends who work out and ask how they feel!

Exercise raises levels of endorphins, which are neurotransmitters (chemicals that nerve cells use to communicate) with chemical structures and actions similar to those of opium. Endorphins reduce pain, resulting in a sense of tranquillity.

As little as 30 minutes of exercise is a sufficient amount of time to stimulate your brain to produce serotonin, a hormone that stabilises our mood and well-being as well as increasing our levels of happiness. It is no surprise to know that people who exercise are more resistance to stress!

There's more good news if you suffer from back pain as the extra serotonin produced during exercise also has an inhibitory effect on pain.

Exercise doesn't need to be intense to be able to benefit from the positive effects of serotonin. Walking as little as 30 minutes daily can be extremely beneficial for not only your back pain, but also many other physiological processes that contribute to good health.

SOME OF THE PHYSICAL CAUSES THAT YOU MAY NOT HAVE THOUGHT OF

KNITTING/SEWING/MACRAMÉ

As you would have already learned in this book, looking down for extended periods of time is a disaster for the neck. Those who knit, sew, do macramé or crochet often stay in this position for hours and hours! By being distracted by the activity that they are doing they are often not feeling the pain and other symptoms that it causes.

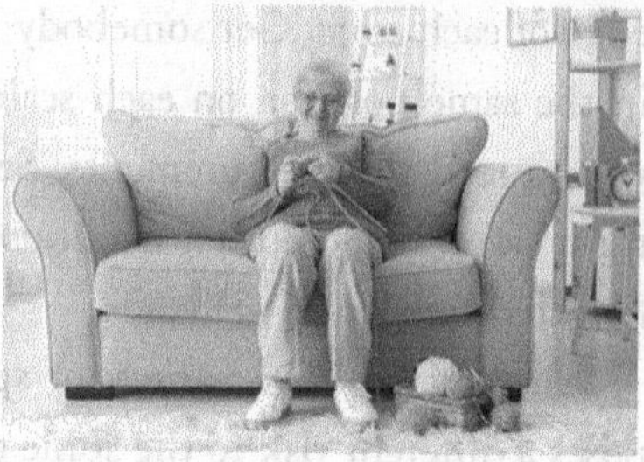

It's amazing how the remission of symptoms is rapid after temporary suspension of the activity. When the problem is chronic, some treatment with your physiotherapist, chiropractor osteopath is often required.

TIPS – Suspend the activity for a period of time until symptoms disappear. When you start again, slightly change your position and support the head against the chair or lounge that you were sitting in. Use a pillow or cushion to raise the elbows, leaving the hands higher. This will help you avoid looking down.

MUSICAL INSTRUMENTS

In the same way that athletes develop many problems in their spines and other joints, so too do musicians. And it's not just professional musicians that suffer. Both beginners and professionals record high incidence of problems.

Resultant problems depend on the type of instrument and how it's being played, and the ability to maintain correct posture. Those who sit to play their instruments tend to suffer more than those who stand as it is easier to move and maintain good posture when one is standing. This position also allows the body's weight to be distributed from one foot to another and allows the upper arms to be freer to move.

There are several causes of spinal dysfunction, common to all musicians if the spine hasn't been protected. The most common ones are:

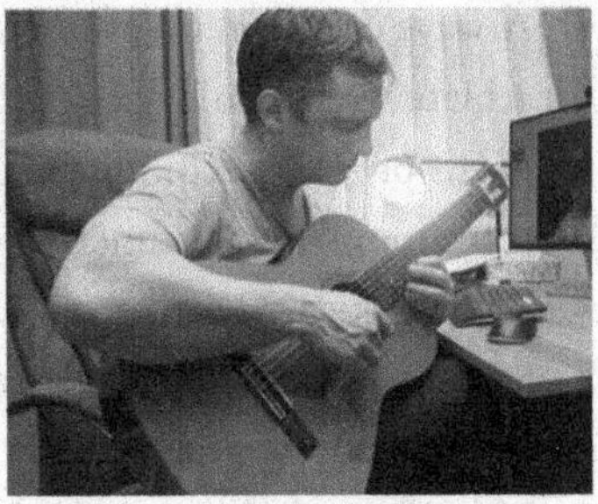

- The effects of gravity – playing most instruments requires resisting the effects of gravity. Whether it be whilst sitting down to play the piano or drums, or standing to play guitar, a musician's body is constantly fighting the force of gravity and the body's tendency to compromise it's posture. Imagine the spine of a violinist, holding and playing the violin with their head bowed to one side and the violin sandwiched between the shoulder and neck!
- Repetitive movements – cause injuries to joints and tendons. Especially when the technique is not correct, the load on the body in long hours of practice and performance is often very harmful. Characteristically, the first signs of the body that the activity is harmful come in the form of pain or intermittent numbness.

With time, if the musician does not modify the way he plays or rests enough to allow his body to heal, the symptoms usually worsen. Many people focus only on the effect of the problem rather than the problem itself, resorting to medication for relief.

Do not be fooled by the fact that painkillers can provide immediate relief. This may be good to get through a rehearsal or concert but the underlying problem will still be present, after the effects of the medication wear off.

Painkillers allow the musician to continue playing, but the underlying cause will usually be exacerbated. Many musicians do not interrupt their routine to rest and as a result end up having surgery, or worse still, retiring early because they allowed the problem to worsen.

Unfortunately, musicians with a full schedule of concerts often do not have time for an injury to heal or recover. Therefore, it is imperative to respect the body's needs and prepare the spine and joints before playing the instrument.

TIPS for minimising the impact on your spine and joints

- Exercise regularly: Your muscles shorten and joints lock up with the repetitive movements while playing your instrument. Choose activities that do not promote strong movements in the regions used when playing your instrument. Swimming, yoga (which can be done anywhere, including during the tour), Pilates and stretching are excellent both to lengthen shortened muscles and to promote extension of the spine (which is very important for people who play sitting down).

- Always do warm up exercises and stretches before each rehearsal, just as an athlete would do before each game. Start by stretching and playing slowly.
- Focus on your technique, a good technique is essential to play without compromising the function of joints and spine.
- Allow your body to move whilst playing. A musician's static posture and the fact that some instruments must be held against gravity, fatigue certain muscle groups.
- Musicians who are required to sit while playing should avoid the tendency of the shoulders to fall forward as this will aggravate the nerve roots that leave the neck and go to the shoulders, arms and hands.
- Try to avoid bending your head forward or to the side as this can overload the joints of the neck and also cause associated symptoms such as headache, numbness and pain in hands and fingers, dizziness and even insomnia.
- If you are suffering from inflammation caused by repetitive movements, resulting in tendinitis, bursitis or muscle contractures, apply ice as soon as possible. This practise minimises inflammation and possible severity of the injury and has allowed many musicians to finish a show or tour without quitting.

CARING FOR YOUR BACK WHEN YOU ARE ON THE BEACH

You may have never thought about how important it is to take care of your spine at the beach.

Lying and sitting on the sand for long periods of time can compromise your posture. It is important to get up and take a walk every now and then, the same way you would in the office. The beach is an excellent place for walking, to move around and compensate for the long hours you spent sitting at your job during the week.

Sitting on the sand often leaves the legs bent and our spine curved forward. This can be harmful to the joints of the lumbar spine. Prolonged periods of time in this position can fatigue the muscles of the low back causing stiffness and pain when we get up, and can also lock the joints of the spine and back. While a good beach chair can help, they are not the answer as they lack the support of a good office chair.

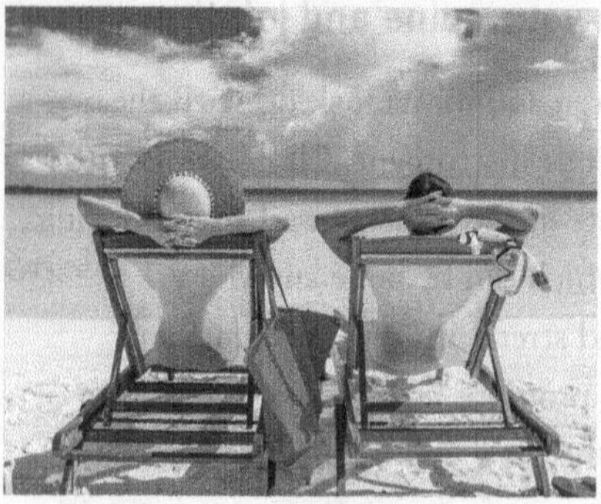

To negate the effects of being in one position for an extended time whilst sunbaking on the sand, rotate between lying on your stomach, on your back or on your side, and sitting cross-legged. Limit the time in each position to 15 minutes.

Be careful when you're lying on your stomach, do not lay with your head to one side for too long, this may lock up your neck. Switch between the two sides or simply make a hole under the towel that you can rest your face in while you look straight down. While lying face down in this way, you can breathe without difficulty and your head will be aligned with the rest of the spine.

You should be as careful on the sand as off the sand. Many injuries happen when you are surprised by a wave and thrown onto the sand. Do not exceed your limits by going in to the sea when there are large waves if you have spinal problems. If necessary or possible, go a little further into the ocean, where the waves are not breaking, and the sea is calmer.

Even the simple pleasure of playing with kids can be more dangerous than you think. Crouching while building sandcastles and digging holes can be great fun, so much fun that we do not notice the pain as a warning to our body at that time. When we are distracted we can spend a lot of time in the same position while maintaining a posture that is detrimental to the spine.

Games for adults, such as racquetball, volleyball, foot volley and soccer bring great benefits, but must be treated with caution and should not be undertaken without adequate preparation, they demand a lot, especially when practiced on an uneven surface such as sand.

WATCH YOUR ALCOHOL INTAKE

Alcohol is a muscle relaxant. This means that when consumed, it stimulates the relaxation of the muscles that have possibly been contracted in a manner to protect the spine and minimise the chance of further damage. When there are bio-mechanical problems of the spine provoking this contraction, it is called 'Muscle Guarding'. When we drink, relaxation of muscles allows gravity to have an even stronger impact on our spine, especially the lumbar (low back) and thoracic (mid back) spine.

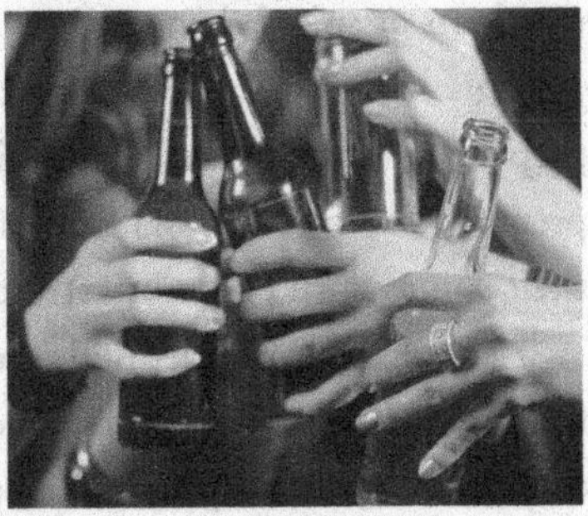

Muscle tension (as a result of the problems of the spine) serves to support the spine and joints, acting as natural protection. The brain causes this reflex to limit the movement because it could damage the spine and worsen the problem further.

Due to the sedative effects of alcohol, the person drinking often cannot feel anything. However, the additional load of the things we do in social situations, such as standing in high heels and dancing, without the protection of postural muscles, can really damage the spine, especially if there are already underlying problems.

For each alcoholic beverage consumed, have a glass of water and favour low-alcohol beverages such as beer instead of stronger ones such as spirits, especially if you are suffering from a back problem.

Water is a major constituent of our bodies (60%) and our muscles do not function correctly without it. If you experience cramps, you may be dehydrated and this potentially magnifies any problem in your spine. (Refer to the section on Water in the chapter Chemical Causes.)

Wearing high heels for hours standing or dancing and drinking at the same time, is a certain recipe for pain the next day. Worse still, it could lock the joints of your spine, leaving side effects for much longer.

SEX AND THE SPINE

We associate the act of having sex with pleasure, connection and well-being, however for those people suffering chronic back pain, it can be anything but.

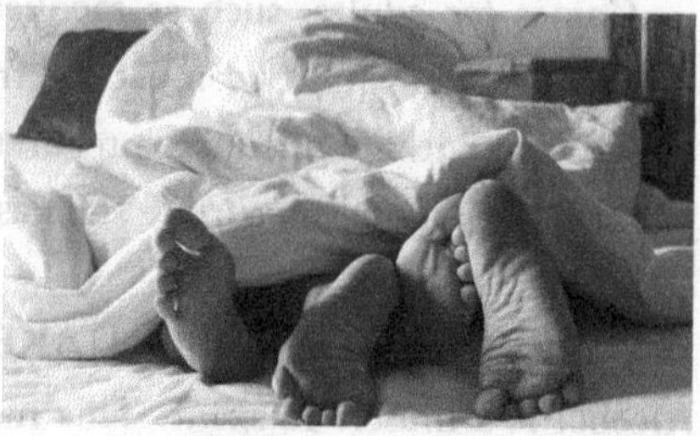

Compare your body to a car that goes really well up to about 80 km/h. However, in passing this speed, it starts to show some engine problems. Due to the noise of the car, the engine vibration and other factors that can distract us, we can be unaware of any damage that may be occuring.

People with bio-mechanical dysfunction of the spine, when having sex, go through a similar process. The pleasure and euphoria of the experience, combined with the repetitive, rapid, sudden and possibly strong movements, distract us from pain or other symptoms created by the body to warn of problems or spinal damage.

This is one more reason to prepare your body for sex, just as you would prepare for any exercise or physical activity. There is no difference. The best prepared athletes optimally perform and minimise occurrence of injuries in their spines with prepatory stretching and exercises.

Accordingly, people in better physical shape, with more strength and flexibility, are also better prepared for sexual performance. Like any other sport or exercise, exercise prepares a spine for sex. Listen to your body and, if any pain is present during intercourse, stop immediately and change positions. Remember that the pain indicates that something is not right, so it would be irresponsible to continue. If after changing positions the pain still does not go away, it's important to take a 'breather' and stop a little to loosen up and stretch.

Many people who do not observe these signs are left with the spine literally 'locked up' (called antalgia) until they receive some type of analgesic injection in the hospital. This is easy to avoid – simply listen to your body!

If for some reason, even following these recommendations, you feel pain after you have intercourse, ice the painful area for 20 minutes (see 'ice').

Try to make sex fun, because it is one of the best ways to receive pleasure and connect. It is also a great pain reliever if it doesn't overload pre-exisiting problems in your spine. Do not let your problems hinder your sex life, find different positions and support so you don't feel frustrated, depressed or isolated.

FEELING WELL ON FRIDAY, WORSE ON MONDAY

One of the most frustrating things that happens in my practice is seeing a patient return on Monday in much worse pain than what they were on the Friday.

After several years of wracking my brain to understand why this happens, I began to notice some common factors among patients who present themselves like that after the weekend. In general, they either overexert themselves to make up for lost time (working etc. during the week) on the weekend or do the opposite and spend too much time sitting.

First we have to remember that the pain does not appear by chance.

If you already spend five days a week sitting at work, you have to compensate over the weekend. So don't stay inside the house. Get out and go to the gym or meet up with friends for a walk or a game of tennis. Prolonged periods of sedentary time on the weekends is detrimental for your body in more ways than one.

The weekend is an excellent opportunity to organize, clean and restore order to the home environment, like the garden, attic, basement and pantry. It's amazing how many back injuries or exacerbation of pre-existing chronic problems occur during these activities because they overwhelm the spine in a way that it is not accustomed to.

Do not forget that if you're a weekend athlete and are used to a sedentary lifestyle, risking pain and stiffness on Monday, taking the risk of locking up of your spine during this process. This will include people who do activities such

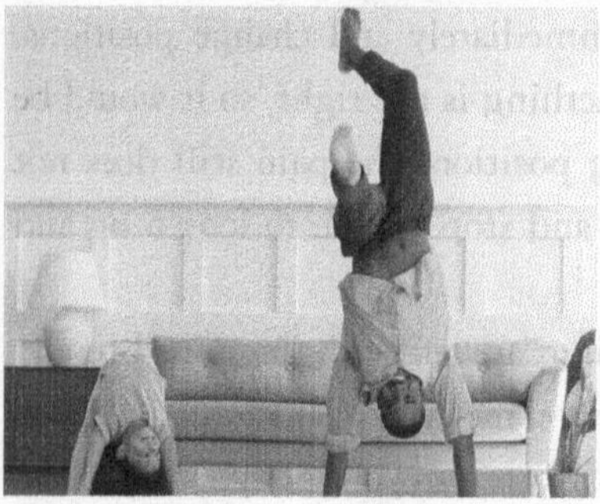

as horseback riding, riding motorcycles, sailing, or simply spending hours drawing or painting, playing piano or guitar. These activities, when not done regularly, may make your body react in the form of pain, muscle contractions or symptoms such as headache, numbness in hands, arms, feet or legs.

DO NOT PANIC

Your body is simply communicating with you and you should take this opportunity to find the root cause of your pain. This could be either a muscle spasm, inflamed muscle or joint or a new bio-mechanical problem caused by the chore undertaken.

If your problem is chronic and pain has returned, or a new pain appears on Monday, think about what you have done differently over the weekend. Almost always you will identify the cause, because your body will react to you simply because it was not prepared for that activity. It is wise then to adequately prepare by stretching with specific exercises or even set aside time during the week to practice and accustom your body to whatever you going to do on the weekend.

HEIGHT MATTERS

As a chiropractor, I notice the consequences that a tall person's life and trying to adapt to a shorter person's world, has on their spine. We definitely live in a 'one size fits all' world. Our world was not designed to take differing heights into consideration. Chairs in schools, beds, cars and buses are mostly not suitable for tall people, who need to constantly change their posture to accommodate themselves to the environment in which they are.

Offices, dentists and surgeon's equipment, trucks and boats, and many more. It's difficult to find situations that accommodate taller people. Tall people often have to flex their heads forward to communicate with shorter people and consequently lose the normal curve because of the intense and prolonged bending of the neck. This forward head carriage is one of the most predominant spinal problems that taller people suffer. They tend to have neck problems, headaches or dizziness as a result.

Many taller kids alter their posture as they simply do not want to stand out. In doing so, they compromise their spinal function at a time of life when the spine is growing and developing.

It is very difficult for a tall adult to recover good posture after bending down for years or not being mindful of their posture. Similar to misaligned teeth which need the influence of odontological braces for a long period of time to align the teeth to normal, the spine also needs a period of time to return to correct posture. Chiropractic, physiotherapy and osteopathy act on the spine in a similar way that braces act on the teeth. This correction is even more effective when combined with consistent stretching, yoga, Pilates and general exercises.

TIPS to help tall people to minimise the load on their neck that causes bad posture

Try to keep your eyes in line with the person you're chatting with or object in which you are concentrated on.

If needed, use a chair instead of standing.

You can also separate your feet to lower your body, while keeping the spine straight.

Buy a car that accommodates tall people as well as shorter people, to avoid spending five or ten years uncomfortable in a car that isn't suitable for you.

Furniture must also be well chosen, from the couch to the dining room table. Think of your needs first and not those of your guests. And don't forget a bed that is your size!

Many companies do not think about their staff's needs when they buy furniture for the office. You might have to talk to your boss or think of something that allows your spine to stay straight and aligned.

Other ways to compensate are to crouch down when dealing with children and pets as well as stretching regularly to compensate for the times when you have your posture compromised. Do stretches that promote extension to further extend the spine, which is the opposite movement of the stooped posture (flexion) that locks the upper spine.

THE WALLET IN THE BACK POCKET – A POTENTIAL PAIN IN YOUR BACKSIDE

Many of the simple things we do repeatedly for years cause many of the spinal problems that we suffer from. Carrying your wallet in the back pocket of your trousers and sitting on top of it is one of these examples. Yes, it may seem more appealing carrying it in the back, comparing to the alternative of carrying it in the front pocket, but the detrimental effect that it brings to our spine is very strong.

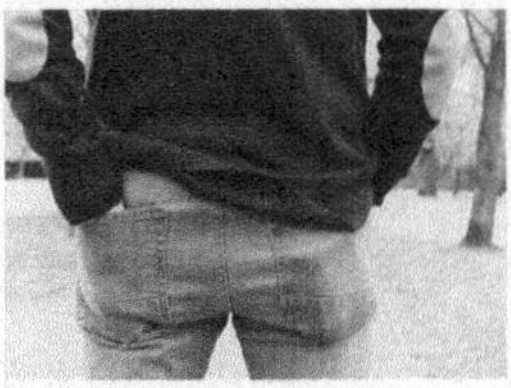

Good posture means good health and proper

functioning of the spine. Good posture means keeping the spine straight and aligned when one observes the person from behind, no different to observing a building from afar – it's straight!

This is also the case when we are sitting down. The weight falling on the pelvis and gluteal muscles should be distributed equally between the two sides. It is only when the weight is distributed in this manner that the lumbar spine can be aligned and able to distribute the load symmetrically between the two sides.

Now imagine a typical wallet, full of credit cards and business cards, in your back pocket, raising the pelvis on one side only when sitting down.

The wallet can put pressure on these muscles, particularly the piriformis muscle which encases the sciatic nerve in 30% of the population. Prolonged pressure (which occurs whilst sitting for long periods of time) can cause inflammation of the sciatic nerve, radiating pain down into the leg and the foot.

The change in symmetry causes an increased load on the sacroiliac joint, which connects the spine and the pelvis. Pain in the buttocks or low back and leg pain or numbness radiating to the foot are some of the common symptoms in men who usually carry the wallet in the back pocket. The ones that suffer most are those who drive long hours or who work sitting down.

This phenomenon was first described in the *New England Journal of Medicine* in 1966, when credit cards started to become popular, based on a case study of an attorney who suffered from pain in his left leg, on the same side as his wallet in the back trouser pocket. The sciatic pain worsened when his wallet was getting thicker because of all of the new credit cards. The condition was appropriately termed 'credit-carditis'.

TIP

The easiest way to avoid this problem is to prevent it from happening: remove your wallet from your back pocket and put it in your jacket pocket or front pocket, whilst sitting down.

CHEMICAL CAUSES OF BACK PAIN

Every living tissue needs to receive the nutrients that it was genetically programmed to receive. If it doesn't, it simply can't function the way nature intended it to. When this occurs, the cells cannot resist the aggravation and resultant inflammation that other factors, such as physical or emotional factors, invariably cause. Problems occur when we get too much of what we don't need and not enough of what we do need.

Most people who suffer from back pain fail to recognize just how important their diet is in the degree of pain and suffering that they may be experiencing. Incorrect food and diet choices cause inflammation in our body and inflammation restricts the way muscles function. As muscles span joints to give us movement, we want to make sure that we look after those muscles to ensure 100% function and of course, a pain-free existence. In the same way that you wouldn't expect dirty fuel to maintain or improve the function of your car, you can also imagine how dirty food, drink, and other factors can quickly compromise our health and inevitably our spinal health.

When most people think of back pain and its origins, they understandably think of factors such as the physical ones mentioned in the last chapter. We fall on our back. It hurts afterward. We fall asleep in the lounge with our head flopped to the side. We wake up with a sore neck. While many of the physical causes of back pain and spinal dysfunction are discreet and difficult to identify, the chemical causes of back pain are even harder for us to associate with our state of discomfort.

In the following pages, you will learn about extremely common causes of back pain that are rarely identified. However, removing them from the equation can have a profound effect on pain levels and for many people, can result in total resolution of their problem.

Chemical factors are those that induce a change in the way that the tissues of our body function. They alter homeostasis. As I have compared our body and spine to the intricate workings of a car numerous times up until now, I will continue with this comparison.

Imagine your car and how you'd be greatly inconvenienced without it. For argument's sake, let's imagine that your car runs on gasoline, however, you mistakenly fill it up with diesel. How would you expect it to run? If your car did continue to function for a while after introducing diesel, it would eventually stop dead and possibly show signs of irreparable engine damage. You would have exceeded the terms of the warranty and would be up for major repairs. Although this type of reaction doesn't generally happen quite as fast as this, when we introduce substances that we shouldn't into the human body, it most definitely occurs. While many foods can be ingested continually without any 'apparent' damage, inadequate foods and drinks cause a low-grade inflammatory action for years. As symptoms such as bloating and gas can be subtle and persistent for years or even decades, it can be extremely difficult to correlate the foods or drinks that cause these symptoms with physiological dysfunction. Inflammation 'feeds' inflammation. If a certain area of your spine is being inflamed due to physical causes, such as overloading of your joints, poor posture, or a fall, an inflammatory diet will most definitely worsen the scenario.

Factors that interfere with our body's biochemistry can range from more obvious ones such as pesticides, artificial food colouring and flavouring, and cigarettes to the less obvious ones that we may have been consuming for years or decades such as grains, gluten, and dairy. Factors that most of us wouldn't even stop to imagine are inflaming our already dysfunctional backs. Altering the body's biochemistry through synthetic or non-synthetic substances can have devastating effects on our health. It can impede the absorption of vital nutrients such as vitamins, minerals, fats, and amino acids. It can alter our hormonal levels resulting in increased levels of hormones such as cortisol or insulin that can promote inflammatory processes. Our microbiome (intestinal flora) that are essential for hundreds of our bodily processes are aggravated every time that we expose them to conditions that are not genetically congruent with their environment. While back pain and muscle aches are already bad enough, conditions such as heart disease, cancer, and type two diabetes are devastating. These lifestyle diseases can be dramatically improved as well as the painful musculoskeletal problems that often accompany them.

The human body requires a genetically pre-determined quantity of vitamins, minerals, amino acids, fatty acids, proteins, and carbohydrates from the food we eat to perform all of its vital functions. Dead cells must be replaced for newer, healthier cells to guarantee homeostasis (100% normal cell function) and avoid the downward tendency towards illness. Without adequate nutrition, this healthy replication of cells is simply not possible, and then the cells replacing old ones are of the same or even worse in quality than the ones they are replacing. There are actually many obvious signs that our body is busy replacing old cells with new ones regularly. For example, if we cut our finger, we see it heal within weeks. We wash our hair and see strands of hair in our hands on the shower floor, however, we do not go bald. Bone cells (osteoclasts) are being replaced every two weeks, contributing to a 10% change in our skeleton annually. Small intestine epithelial cells take 2–4 days, stomach cells take nine days and in the lung, alveoli cells are replaced every eight days. The quality of the food you consume and the success you have in avoiding or eliminating toxins from your body determines your overall health. This in turn influences the 'new you'. Cellular turnover, or cell replication, should result in cells that are as capable of maintaining normal function as the cells that they replaced. Understanding how your biochemistry affects your health and how you can directly affect your body's chemical environment is vital if you aim to get or stay healthy and recover from back pain.

Remember that good health isn't the result of good luck. The pain or disease picture that we paint for ourselves is predominantly determined by the artist, *you*, except in a very small percentage of genetic conditions. *The Lancet* medical journal conducted a study on 195 countries, 249 causes of death, 315 diseases, and 79 risk factors. They found that 71.3% of deaths were caused by conditions such as heart disease, stroke, cancer, and diabetes, all of which are avoidable!

There is no surprise in regards to the contributing factors they identified, with smoking, high blood glucose levels, sedentary lifestyle, obesity, and drinking too much alcohol topping the list. These factors are all 100% under our control. In other words, we have a choice in regards to whether we incorporate them into our lives or not.

It is also interesting to note that while many people assume that increased lifespan would indicate a parallel improvement in the state of people's health, Lancet recognized that tens of millions of people are spending their final years in poor health, citing that women can expect to pass the final 10 years of their lives in a poor state of health. Men will spend the last nine years of their lives in a bad state of health and disability.

So what does the state of your health have to do with your back pain and muscle aches? Plenty. When you look beyond the daunting names of the diagnoses and the tissues such as intervertebral disks, paravertebral muscles, spinal nerves, bones, and joints that have been affected, you see the underlying causes of damage to those tissues.

The accumulative effects of poor posture, modified bio-mechanical function after impacts or traumas, prolonged sitting and sedentary lifestyle, and many more factors that have been discussed in the chapter 'Physical Causes of back pain' which all contribute. Obesity was also focused on in this chapter. However, look at the factors that are responsible for obesity such as the typical western diet of excessive sugar, simple carbohydrates, and alcohol. Foods and drinks that are inflammatory. They spike our blood sugar levels obliging our bodies to convert it to fat. Then there are the substances that are toxic and overload our detoxification organs such as the liver, kidneys, and lymphatic system. When these organs can no longer deal with the load, the ability to eliminate effectively is compromised and toxins flow back into our bloodstream. Muscle aches and pains, fibromyalgia, poor sleep quality, headaches, and psychological alterations result, which are all bad news for those who are already suffering from back pain or those who wish to avoid suffering it. Inflammation from the poor diet and lifestyle routines feeds the inflammation that is caused by biomechanical, physical problems.

Back pain is such a broad, nondescript label for a symptom that is influenced by multiple factors. Look up 'Back Pain' on Dr. Google and you will soon discover that it's causes are grossly misunderstood. Western society has focused way too much time on suppressing the pain reflexes that a properly functioning body provokes instead of actually looking for and dealing with its causes. Most underlying causes, aside from the physical factors, are given very little attention. These include chemical factors such as inadequate diet (including the excessive consumption of sugar, trans fats/vegetable oils) dehydration, inflammatory foods (such as those containing gluten and dairy for most people), alcohol, smoking, pharmaceutical drugs and more. Chronic inflammation and organ dysfunction are commonly overlooked by someone who is suffering from back pain and wanting a solution.

TIP

Our taste buds relish the taste of sugar, oily french fries, and fatty hamburgers. For many of us that started life with a less than perfect diet, eating these foods is as gratifying now as it was back in childhood. Even though they may contain zero nutrients, knowing this doesn't make it any easier to drop them from our diets. Even though there is no lack of evidence linking them to almost all degenerative chronic illnesses, it still doesn't help when we see them on a menu or on somebody else's plate. If you can relate to this and want to move your health in a less toxic direction, don't try and eliminate all of the bad stuff at once. You'll be much more successful if you introduce healthy foods and habits first, maintaining your less healthy ones and gradually eliminating them with time. Your body has adapted over many years, allowing substances that are deleterious to our health to be ingested without apparent symptoms. This is why it is important to remove them from your diet slowly and in a coordinated fashion. You may be accustomed to pieces of chocolate at night but could you change it for one that has a higher percentage of cocoa or is sugar-free? If you feel addicted to fizzy drinks try including a glass of water in between them. Is the hamburger maybe non-negotiable? Then could you walk down to the restaurant and walk back after eating it? It's so much easier introducing healthy habits instead of trying to remove the unhealthy ones straight away. When most people think about getting healthy, they immediately think about the things that they are going to have to quit and this, unfortunately, discourages many from even trying at all. Remember that health means 100% cell function, and this is only possible with a sufficiency of nutrients and elimination of toxins. If you find it hard to eliminate toxins at the start that does not mean that you shouldn't try and introduce the nutrients. Many of the 'naughty' foods that have contributed to your loss of health contain substances designed to make you want more. Try and remove candy from a child's hand and witness just how addictive sugar is. Most kids (and some adults) will throw a tantrum if you try. Monosodium glutamate (MSG) is an ingredient that countless foods contain and is highly addictive. Corn chips, crisps, and many processed foods contain it as it improves the taste and removes hunger. Sounds like the perfect product if you are in the food industry and want to promote sales. It is highly addictive and if you are accustomed to consuming it regularly, realize that it will be difficult to eliminate it all at once, in the same way as someone who smokes will find it difficult to quit suddenly. So go slow, eliminate slowly and consciously and start by introducing healthy habits into your life instead of being too radical and removing everything that you've been accustomed to straight away.

If what you are reading on these pages is enough to convince you to make the change, do it knowing that a body free of pain, with a surplus of energy and vitality, awaits you. Certain 'realities' that you previously accepted as normal in years and decades gone by (such as insomnia, headaches, bloating, constipation, sexual dysfunction, fatigue, and autoimmune diseases) may be proving to be misconceptions and not your reality at all. The most gratifying experience for me is listening to patients who have made the change, from a sedentary lifestyle to exercising, from soft drinks to water or vegetable juice, or after quitting sugar and hearing how these simple changes have prompted drastic improvement. Weight loss, vitality, increased libido, improved health, deeper sleep, and clearer concentration are some of the many benefits to occur after making these simple changes in your lifestyle.

You can rest assured that the day you smoke your last cigarette or eat your last fried meal, your health will move in a positive direction immediately. Do it for long enough (sometimes only a matter of a few days) and you will actually feel the difference. A healthy body will always take us to a better place, and this includes being less sensitive to back pain and other musculoskeletal conditions.

CASE STUDY

Felicity had been a patient of mine for over a decade. She had always been overweight but not obese. I hadn't seen her for three months since her last appointment and instantly noticed that she had lost weight. When I asked how she had done it she said that she had simply stopped drinking fizzy drinks and eating bread, pizza, and pasta. I was truly impressed as she looked amazing with a healthy glow and shiny eyes. I asked her if any of her other symptoms have improved, as she had been suffering low-grade pain in her lower back for as long as I knew her. She said that she hadn't felt any pain for the last two months and that her sleep had never been better. She was waking up with energy instead of waking up feeling fatigued, something that she said she had felt for many years. Her constipation had disappeared and with higher energy levels her drive to do exercise allowed her to walk daily, which was her favourite exercise.

The human body is composed of biological tissue. You know the words 'living cells' and 'tissues'. In the past 40,000 years, our genetic makeup hasn't changed. Our cells still have the same genetic requirements that they had thousands of years ago. The question is, are we living congruently with our genetic needs? Are we providing them with what they genetically require? Sadly, the answer is no in almost all of society. Our environment has changed so much that our genes, without the pre-requisite proportion and quantity of nutrients, are expressing themselves differently from what they would have in those times. They are adapting to an environment that is genetically foreign to them and therefore they end up expressing themselves differently from what they would have thousands of years ago in Palaeolithic times. Cancer, heart disease, diabetes, and even obesity were almost certainly unheard-of in prehistoric times, as these diseases are lifestyle-related, and the lifestyles of Palaeolithic humans provided them with their genetic needs. Humans ate only fresh and natural foods, without toxic preservatives, colouring agents, pesticides, flavourings, and other chemicals to help them last longer and taste better. The soil was rich in minerals allowing plants to contain the number of vitamins and nutrients that they were meant to contain. Modern-day agricultural methods have stripped our soil of its nutrients and added toxins via pesticides, fungicides, and synthetic fertilizers. All of this gets taken up by the root system or through the leaves to the plant. Previously, humans only hunted for fresh meat. We farm our meat, adding hormones to make cattle grow faster and antibiotics to fend off infections that only animals kept in enclosures would have to contend with. These days most of our food contains toxins from a variety of sources, whether it be preservatives to make it last longer, artificial colours to make it look more attractive and flavours to trick our taste buds into making us think that it is appealing. The problem is that while it is appealing to our receptors on our tongues, the living cells of our bodies do not recognize it. This causes a reaction, usually a low-grade inflammatory reaction. Some of our heating methods are also incongruent with providing healthy food to our bodies. We radiate food in the microwave or ruin it by cooking it in hydrogenated fat and still expect to stay healthy. The ultimate consequence for a cell that doesn't receive enough of what it needs and too much of what it doesn't is decreased function and accelerated cell death.

When muscle aches, inflamed joints, stiffness, and cramps, bloating, constipation, and other symptoms occur they are actually healthy warning signs from our body that are trying to advise us not to continue damaging our body in that way. Pain is always a signal. The problem is that not many of us use it as a way to find out the true cause of the problem. A diet causing these types of symptoms is a diet incongruent with the inherent needs of the body. This situation is worsened by other factors such as dehydration, certain medications, excessive sugar, smoking, and alcohol. Read on and you may discover that the cause of your lower back pain isn't just that old deformed mattress that you are sleeping on, but a myriad of influences that only you can identify and correct.

BACK PAIN BUT NOT A BACK PROBLEM

It's easy to understand how a bad diet, too much alcohol, or trans-fats can cause pathology in your organs (viscera) such as your liver, stomach, heart, or intestines. However, the fact that these and other organs of your body can cause pain in your back, neck, and even your limbs is commonly forgotten. VISCEROSOMATIC PAIN occurs since nerves that send and receive messages between the spinal cord and the organs connect with nerves that supply the muscles, blood vessels, and the skin of the back. Being closely related, distress signals originating in the organs can also cause painful responses in the tissues of the spine around the nerve roots that supply those organs. This is why people who suffer from kidney infection can also suffer horrible pain in the lower back. Or how one of the first symptoms of a heart attack could actually be a sharp ache down the left arm. Women are subject to many forms of this pain during their reproductive life, with premenstrual pain often being felt in the lower back and other gynaecological pathologies also referring to this area. Being aware of the relationship between the viscera and the spine can greatly help when speedy attention needs to be given to the organs and not the spine. Take a heart attack for example. Many people have mistaken the left arm pain with a problem in the actual arm or pain from the neck, ignoring the heart completely and therefore risking great damage to the heart or even death by not giving it deserved attention. It's believed that in general, by the time organ pathology causes reflex pain in other tissue (whether it be skin, muscle, or blood vessels) the process has already been established for quite some time. Taking pain medication and unintentionally ignoring a more serious, deep-rooted vessel problem could present a grave danger to a person's health. The difficulty localizing visceral pain is due to a substantially lower proportion of pain receptors in the organs when compared to somatic structures, such as those found in the arms, legs, and head. When organ dysfunction reaches a stage where it is more serious it is diffuse in nature and difficult to localize. Contrary to the nerves that innervate our legs (just think of sciatic pain, ouch!), arms, back, or skin, all of which have a far greater numbers of pain receptors, our organs have very few.

I have seen countless cases throughout my career where a person presented with a muscle ache or contracture in the spine that was actually manifesting the body's way of advising the person that they had potential organ pathology that needed attention. For instance, endometriosis cases that cause low back pain, kidney infection or tumours that cause thoraco-lumbar pain, and digestive organ dysfunction that is reflected on the spine. You may have even felt one of the most common viscera-somatic pains, that being an uncomfortable pain in your mid-back when you suffer indigestion. There are many other examples as each organ can show a distinct pattern of spinal pain. The key is to be able to recognize when somebody is showing signs of pathology and not simply a bio-mechanical cause of the back pain. This is often easier said than done as the pain sensation experienced in the muscles of the spine can feel exactly the same for both. A study involving 5,000 patients done over a five-year period showed that the majority of those whose disease is caused by pain experience it on the same side as the affected organ and that the number of musculoskeletal structures affected are related to the duration of the disease[1].

CASE STUDY

Martin was a 48-year-old journalist who I had successfully treated for neck pain and headaches for over a year. As his job required him to be in front of the computer for hours at a time and this compromised the bio-mechanical function

1 'A double-blind clinical study of osteopathic findings in hospital patients: progress report'. A.F. Kelso, *J Am Osteopath Assoc.*, 1971.

of his upper back and neck, he would visit me monthly for maintenance. On one particular visit the muscles of his upper back were extremely tense and sensitive. I obviously knew his spine well due to the amount of time I had been caring for it but this particular time it was as 'stiff as a rod'. He had arrived with X-rays and an MRI because he felt that it was 'different' from any other pain in the back that he had felt before. I also believe that we are our own best doctors. If a patient says that the pain is distinct and as practitioners we ignore that thinking that it is the same thing that we have been regularly treating, we could be doing a great disservice to them. We did some deep massage work and adjustments twice in one week. It was difficult to adjust his spine and relieve the muscle tension through massage, however, he reported relief on the day of the treatment. This relief was only short-lived, however, as he woke with the pain much more intense in the morning. When I asked him if he had made any correlation between an increase in pain intensity in anything that he may be doing, he mentioned a spicy curry that he and his wife had eaten. He had also noticed that lying down would worsen the pain. This was the 'aha!' moment that helps a practitioner join the dots, and in this case, leading me to suspect the problem with one of his digestive organs. I helped him find a gastroenterologist who ordered an endoscopy. Sure enough, the examination revealed a problem with the oesophageal sphincter (valve located between the oesophagus and stomach) and this allowed stomach acids to go up to the oesophagus, burning it and reflecting as pain to the midback as the muscles of the spine shared common nerves with the nerves from the sphincter. Martin's back pain disappeared in less than a week after taking the medication that his specialist had recommended.

Remember the word homeostasis from the first chapter? Our cells function 100% correctly (which, yes, is actually possible) when they receive the sufficient amount of nutrients that they genetically require whilst being spared of toxic influences. We are unintentionally shifting our cells and invariably our body's homeostasis through multiple factors, many of which are being focused on in this book. On a chemical level, inadequate foods do not provide us with what they innately require while at the same time and simultaneously in many cases, are aggravating them with toxins. Ultimately inflammation that results from this unintentional assault leaves our bodies spending more energy fighting that low-grade inflammation. This leaves it with less energy in building immunity, repairing damaged muscle fibres, replicating old cells with newer healthy cells, removing toxic waste, and many other consequences. The cellular fitness of our cells unfortunately falls and then back pain and spine-related complaints inevitably go with it.

The following excerpt from the World Health Organization (WHO) could be seen as news in the scientific community, however, our genetic requirements haven't changed in thousands of years.

> *"Affluent populations habitually consume a diet that was unknown to the human species a mere 10 generations ago. Compared with the diet that fuelled human evolution, the so-called 'affluent' diet of today has twice the amount of fat, a much higher ratio of saturated to unsaturated fatty acids, a third of the former daily fibre intake, much more sugar and sodium, fewer complex (fruit and vegetable) carbohydrates and reduced intake of micronutrients. Worldwide, the adoption of this diet has been accompanied by a major increase in coronary heart disease, stroke, various cancers, diabetes, and other chronic diseases."*[2]

Our cells are genetically programmed to receive optimal nutrition and nature provided us with what we need for optimal health and fulfilled lives thousands of years before our civilizations formed. Please look at, understand, and provide your body with what it needs. There is a huge mismatch nowadays, which we need to be aware of and compensate for. DNA evidence shows that genetically, humans have hardly changed at all, being virtually the same as what we were 20,000 years ago.[3]

CORTISOL AND HOW IT CONTRIBUTES TO BACK PAIN

Understanding why we suffer from back pain, headaches, and the other unpleasant symptoms associated with the spine can be greatly aided in knowing a little more about cortisol. Cortisol is a hormone secreted by the adrenal glands (also known as the super renal gland) which sit on top of each kidney.

Despite cortisol being most commonly known as the stress hormone, optimal cortisol levels are essential for homeostasis. Some of these functions include the regulation of energy levels by selecting how the body uses carbohydrates, proteins, or fats, regulating sleep cycles, and controlling blood pressure. When the body is subject to stressful situations (see STRESS in Emotional Causes of back pain) the adrenal glands secrete cortisol, which consequently increases BP and heart rate, helping us deal with the situation. In prehistoric times, that may have been to physiologically prepare us to defend ourselves from predators (fight) or run from them to be able to survive (flight). Hence the phrase 'fight

2 *The World Health Report 1997: conquering suffering, enriching humanity*. WHO, 1997.

3 'Palaeolithic Nutrition: what can we learn from the past?', N.J. Mann, *Asia Pacific Journal of Clinical Nutrition,* 2004.

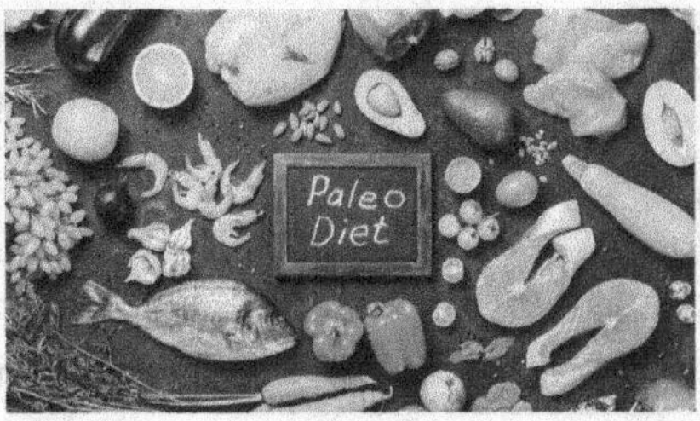

or flight' response. In these moments, our physiological response was fully focused on survival and cortisol was only momentarily secreted. This represents a perfectly healthy reaction to a potentially dangerous situation. However, in modern times, with stressful factors (stressors) frequently affecting us, cortisol is being stimulated at chronic levels. While the relationship between stress and cortisol will be discussed in more detail in the chapter on the Emotional Causes of back pain, there is an equally important relationship between the biochemical stress that certain substances exert on our body that inevitably increase cortisol levels too. When functioning as was intended, in other words, in response to acutely stressful situations, cortisol is a potent anti-inflammatory hormone. In the past, this may have been useful in cases of tissue damage whilst fighting with Sabre-toothed Tigers or dinosaurs. However, this role quickly changes when the body is under continual, chronic stress. When this happens, cortisol's influence becomes an inflammatory one due to a change in tissue sensitivity. To learn more detail about this vital process, refer to an excellent research paper 'How stress influences disease', Sheldon Cohan et al, *Science Daily* 2012.

Specifically, immune cells become insensitive to the cortisol regulatory effect, allowing inflammation to develop. Now, what about if this chronic, continual stress was being generated by your diet? Yes, your diet. The western diet has deviated substantially from the foods that our ancestors were accustomed to eating in prehistoric times. If we recognize that our genes have not changed in 20,000 years then we can assume that genes accustomed to certain foods in those times are definitely not accustomed to foods that predominate the western diet.

The Paleo diet contains an abundance of plant fibre that our biome (gut bacteria) depends on to fill the numerous physiological processes that they contribute to. It also contains complex carbohydrates found in unprocessed plant foods, animal protein from unfarmed meat, whether it be red meat, chicken, fish, or other game. Historically, this animal protein diet did not contain hormones or antibiotics (used to promote faster growth or resist infections that keeping animals in confined conditions causes). There was negligible toxicity and an abundance of nutrients! It is therefore easy to understand that if our body is not receiving the nutrients that it genetically requires to function optimally, this could be perceived as a 'stressor' and consequently provoke a stress response.

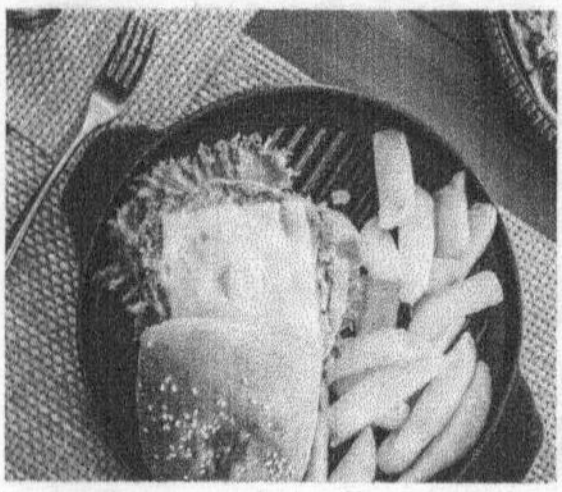

Think of all of the 'foods' that the western diet offers. From refined flour products such as bread, pasta, and pizza to fizzy drinks full of sugar and preservatives. Also consider breakfast cereals full of sugar, microwave dinners, French fries fried in hydrogenated fat, dairy products that are derived from the milk of cows that have had their hormones manipulated to keep them lactating. 'Foods' that have been cooked excessively or cooked inadequately (for example deep-fried). 'Foods' that have been coloured, artificially flavoured, and enhanced in an attempt to make them resemble real food, or simply make their taste irresistible to most mere mortals. A diet lacking in vegetables and fruit (and often when these are consumed, they have been poisoned by pesticides and fertilizers). Foods high in the wrong fats and lacking good fats (our cell walls and brain are predominantly lipid and need an adequate amount of the correct fats to function correctly). Alcohol, prescription drugs, polluted water, polluted air, and the list goes on and on. Can you see how this deviation from what our cells were accustomed to in prehistoric times could be stressful for our cells? Cells that were accustomed to a vastly different source of nutrients. We have to change the substrate (fuel) that every cellular function relies on to do its job!

When you eat meals that are high in simple carbohydrates your body produces more insulin to decrease blood sugar levels. This results in a crash. Cortisol is then released to increase the blood sugar level to provide you with the energy you need to perform your everyday activities. What is also interesting to know is that your body produces catecholamines, which actually make you feel stressed out as well as making you crave more carbohydrates. It's a vicious cycle! While this happens, your feel-good hormone, serotonin is drastically lowered. Serotonin has an inhibitory effect on pain, so if, let's say, you have a bio-mechanical dysfunction in your spine of a physical nature that's potentially causing pain, higher levels of serotonin can actually keep it in check. In other words, serotonin helps lower the way your body perceives that bio-mechanical stress. When these levels lower, combined with an elevation of cortisol, which is pro-inflammatory, the situation can be devastating for anyone who suffers from back pain.

CASE STUDY

Dave loves drinking a well-known fizzy drink. I have been treating him for years and always noticed how the muscles supporting his spine, the paravertebral muscles, were extremely tense. The relief that he received from his treatments wouldn't last very long. He received deep soft tissue massage and hot packs among other things, as his spine felt like a rod and would never release through manual manipulation. Although I have talked to Dave for years about improving his diet, he admitted that he was addicted to sugar, citing desserts and junk food as his weakness. I would remind him of his favourite soft drink and he would admit that he would drink it all day as he didn't like the taste of water! (That may sound strange but I have worked with numerous patients over the years who simply didn't drink water).

When Dave turned 40 his life insurance required him to do a general medical examination, testing all of his basic markers to determine his level of risk. After doing his blood exams and his physical, he was informed that he would not be insured in his present state of health! His blood sugar levels (glucose) and insulin levels were through the roof! His blood pressure, cholesterol, and triglyceride were also off the charts. I was not surprised to learn that his cortisol levels and markers of inflammation such as C-reactive protein, were also extremely elevated.

Dave was finally obliged to take the situation more seriously. He decided to consult a functional nutritionist and of course, the fizzy drinks were top of the list of foods to be avoided. Only a month after cleaning up his diet, removing toxins, and introducing real food nutrients, the musculature on Dave's back had completely relaxed. His pain levels had subsided substantially and the bio-mechanical work that I did on him was more effective and lasted longer.

Many foods and liquids stimulate our body to produce excessive levels of cortisol and these place us in a stressful state. It simply doesn't make sense to continue aggravating your body if it is reacting negatively to something that you are ingesting. Remember that many of these foods or drinks either taste incredible or make us feel incredible. Sadly, they are not incredible for our health. Their deleterious effects compound over time, keeping blood sugar levels high, insulin high, and creating insulin resistance. They continually aggravate our biome (the gut bacteria responsible for literally thousands of bodily processes). Toxins accumulate in our liver and our adipose tissue (fat) and our lymphatic system becomes congested.

If you suffer back pain or related symptoms such as headaches, fibromyalgia, or muscle aches, you must remove any foods or drinks that chronically elevate cortisol levels. It is incredible just how fast an inflamed and pain-sensitive body reacts when it receives the nutrients that are genetically required and is saved from the toxins that it genetically doesn't recognize. No matter how severe it is or how long you have been suffering, trust your body. Go back to basics and let your body do its healing.

ALCOHOL AND BACK PAIN

"What harm could a couple of drinks do?" I hear you ask. In reality, none or minimal harm if it was simply a couple of drinks. Alcohol, however, just like many other toxins we ingest, is generally consumed more than once, often

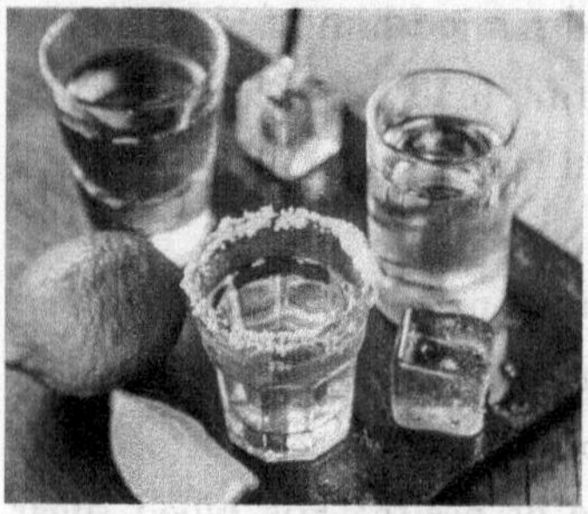

daily. Although some studies show a positive correlation between alcohol consumption and pain relief, this should not be used as a motivating factor to have a few drinks and forget your problem. If you do forget, it will most certainly be temporary, as the cause behind the chronic spinal problems will persist in the morning. Additionally, drinking alcohol to reduce pain can quickly turn into dependence, accelerating the consumer to alcoholism and opening up Pandora's box full of painful consequences, both physical and emotional.

There are many great reasons to avoid drinking alcohol if you suffer from back pain or related symptoms.

Alcohol is a muscle relaxant. This may sound encouraging if you have taken muscle relaxants before and found relief. However, those muscles are tight and protective for a reason. It's called a muscle guarding reflex, stimulated by your brain to minimise possible damage to the spine that could occur through movement or posture. Those tight muscles act like a splint and when we drink enough to relax those muscles, they can no longer protect the spine, at least not while your body is affected by alcohol. Those of you who suffer lower back or neck pain and have had a few too many will be able to relate to this occurrence from waking up the next day in pain. The lumbar spine (low back) suffers more when standing, which is common in most social events and gatherings, worse still for those who go out dancing and drinking. Neck problems are frequently aggravated since the tight muscles were helping to maintain a posture that was least overloading the spine. Those extra drinks relax the muscles that support our posture, the head moves forward and the articulations of the neck work overtime to protect the strain in the spinal cord caused by the forward head carriage.

Alcohol also affects sleep patterns, especially our REM (Rapid Eye Movement) sleep. Bad sleep quality is related to an increased likelihood of back pain and an exacerbation of pre-existing back pain. Even though alcohol may make it slightly easier to get to sleep, it affects the regenerative phases of our sleep, lowering the amount of time the brain can dedicate to fighting inflammation and promoting tissue regeneration. Read more about sleep in 'Emotional causes of back pain'.

Alcohol can also interact dangerously with certain medications, exacerbating side-effects which may include back pain, muscle aches, cramps, or circulatory problems.

COFFEE – HOW IT CONTRIBUTES TO BACK PAIN

'Everything in moderation' is a phrase that most of us have heard multiple times in our lives. This certainly rings true for coffee consumption. If you are a coffee drinker, do you drink it to enjoy it or are you somebody who relies on it to get you into and maybe through the day? If you rely on it for a boost and mental clarity there's a good chance the coffee consumption has become a habit for you. That's fine if not consumed excessively and you are adequately hydrated before drinking it. The boost our body feels when it receives coffee is from the release of cortisol from the adrenal glands, which sit above the kidneys. Cortisol is a vital hormone that helps control blood sugar levels, regulate our metabolism, and is anti-inflammatory when stimulated occasionally. Coffee stimulates the adrenal glands to release cortisol and if this occurs continually throughout the day or compounds with other factors that elevate cortisol (such as emotional and physical stress, sugar, or alcohol) it can quickly influence cortisol's function to be inflammatory. Inflammation feeds inflammation, meaning that factors that have an inflammatory response in our body can compound, worsen, and even perpetuate pre-existing inflammation in the body. Various studies have linked caffeine to chronic back pain showing that patients with chronic lower back pain consume on average, over twice as much caffeine as patients without chronic low back pain.[4]

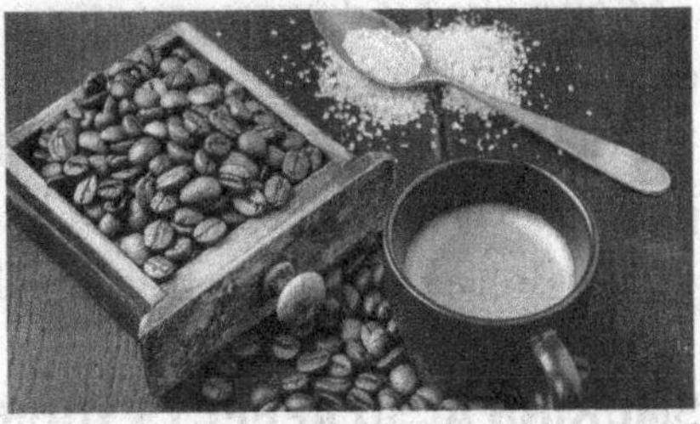

Besides enhancing pre-existing back pain and other conditions, the cortisol spike caused by caffeine can also increase muscle tension. As most chronic bio-mechanical problems have an increased degree of muscle tone, increasing this tension further restricts normal joint mobility and function, contributing further to the problem.

For many people, drinking coffee affects the quality of their sleep. As sleep is a time for repair and regeneration, impaired sleep leaves an already painful problem potentially without improvement when the person wakes up (Refer to the section on sleep in the chapter Emotional Causes of Back Pain).

4 'Caffeine and chronic back pain.' J. McPartland and J. Mitchell, *Archives of Physical Medicine and Rehabilitation*. Volume 78, issue one, January 1997.

TIP

If you are confused as to whether your love of coffee is contributing to your back pain, try stopping for a while. Minimising any factor that may be contributing to your stress levels (whether you are conscious of them doing so or not) will invariably help your body deal with any inflammatory process occurring in your spine or joints.

As well as being highly addictive, coffee can irritate the intestinal wall. When consumed excessively, coffee can stimulate the peristaltic movement of the intestines in an attempt to eliminate the caffeine from the body, loosening the bowels and promoting bowel movements or even diarrhoea in some cases. This, combined with the fact that it is acidic, can result in inflammation of the intestinal walls and stomach. If this continues, gastritis, reflux, and other inflammatory conditions can arise, which in many cases set up a viscera somatic reaction, reflecting pain to the spine, generally the lower back.

Coffee also has diuretic properties, which means that excessive consumption can leave you dehydrated.

As dehydrated muscles can't fulfil their role of protecting your joints or providing normal mobility, it is a good idea to be aware of this pitfall if you are a coffee drinker who also suffers from back pain.

SMOKING ALSO AFFECTS YOUR BACK

"It's easier to overcome a bad habit today, than tomorrow."
CONFUCIUS

Individuals with office jobs easily identify their work posture in front of a computer as the cause of their neck pain. Similarly, a taxi driver who sits all day driving could understand and relate their back pain to the seat or prolonged sitting. However, if either of these two people smoked, smoking would quite possibly be one other factor that would have to be considered in the aetiology of their back pain. If there aren't already enough reasons to stop smoking, here are a few more.

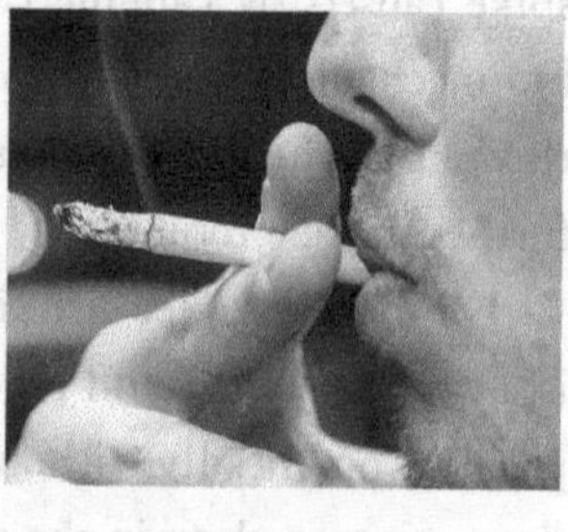

Back pain and other spinal problems are additional consequences associated with smoking cigarettes, as it increases the chance of a smoker suffering back pain by 2.7 times compared to non-smokers.[5] [6]

5 'The association between smoking and low back pain: a meta-analysis', Rahman Shiri et al. *The American Journal of Medicine*. Volume 123, number one, January 2010.

6 'Association between smoking and back pain in a cross-section of adult Americans.'

Even though most smokers would be aware of the fact that smoking deleteriously affects many systems of their body, most do not consider it as a possible cause of back pain. A group of British researchers have studied 13,000 people and their lifestyles. They concluded that smoking increased smokers' chances of suffering debilitating pain by 30%.[7] This study isn't the only one making this correlation. A review of 40 studies published in the journal *Spine* concluded that smoking is undeniably associated with back pain.

HOW?

The harmful effects of smoking can affect the function of the spine in many ways.

- Smoking reduces pulmonary capacity. With time and less than optimal lung expansion when inhaling, the relative limitations mean that the rib cage simply cannot expand to full capacity. This can occur through more obvious mechanisms such as emphysema or simply the gradual loss of physical conditioning. The lungs of smokers lose their elasticity with time, which is a property that is vital for respiration. Intercostal muscles are shortened due to lack of full use. As these muscles join adjacent ribs and the ribs attached to the dorsal spine, overall loss of mobility and flexibility of the thoracic cage results, making a smoker increasingly vulnerable to pain and bio-mechanical dysfunction in this area. They are consequently less resistant under poor posture, during traumas or impacts, etc., and therefore more susceptible to back problems. This fact combined with a smoker's cough, which many chronic smokers can experience, drastically overloads the costovertebral joints, increasing the chance of inflammation.
- Smoking compromises the ability of the blood vessels to nourish important structures associated with normal spinal function. Carbon monoxide is a toxic substance given off by cigarettes and compromises haemoglobin's (the component in the blood responsible for transporting oxygen) ability to nourish the body. Oxygen is absolutely vital for the function and regeneration of the cells of the muscles, bones, ligaments, and tendons, and limiting its delivery will invariably reduce the function of the tissues. As such, this leaves the spine unable to fully recuperate from the loads that a normal life puts on it.

B. Green et al, *CUREUS* 2016 Sept 8(9).

7 'Smoking and musculoskeletal disorders. Findings from a British national survey', K.T. Palmer, et al, *Annals of Rheumatic Disease*, Jan 2003.

- Cigarettes contain nicotine, which is a vasoconstrictor, narrowing blood vessels and restricting blood flow to arteries and veins in the vertebral column and surrounding muscles, further complicating the healing processes that occur in this area daily.
- Smoking damages the intervertebral discs. As previously mentioned in the first chapter, the intervertebral discs act as shock absorbers and separate the vertebrae. The separation is imperative for the correct function of the nervous system, as the nerve roots pass through the intervertebral foramen created by the separation. Smoking can contribute to this degeneration (think protrusion and hernia, grossly known as a 'bulging disc'). This breakdown can occur due to the reduced nutrient exchange in the disc, worsened by the decrease in oxygen and the consequent effects of nicotine explained above. With a reduction in blood flow to the surrounding muscles, the support role is compromised in the spine is less equipped to absorb the loads and traumas that a healthy spine is perfectly prepared to deal with.
- Smoking is inflammatory. As is the case with the other inflammatory factors mentioned in this chapter, smoking induces an elevation in cortisol levels, which when chronically elevated can make the body more prone to inflammation. Bad news for anybody who is already fighting an inflammatory response in their body.
- Smoking contributes to osteoporosis. Whether it be via the generation of free radicals, the stimulation of cortisol and resulting hormonal imbalance, or the fact that nicotine kills osteoblasts, smoking strongly promotes demineralization of the bone. When a smoker suffers a fracture as a result of osteoporosis, repeat fractures are more likely since poor blood supply impedes healing.

TIP – It's not hard to guess that the strongest recommendation here is a cessation of the habit. That said, smoking is one of the most difficult habits to let go of. If you plan to stop smoking remember that your body is addicted to nicotine, so quitting gradually is the key.

Be very clear of your reason for quitting and all of the benefits that it will bring you (such as more energy, agility, self-esteem, etc.). Nicotine replacement therapy has proved to be extremely effective for many people. At this time a full body detox, change of diet, and a new exercise routine would aid in sticking to your goals.

SUGAR – PUBLIC ENEMY NUMBER 1

As the consumption of sugar has increased over the last decades so too has the incidence of obesity, Type II diabetes, and chronic illness in general.[8] While this may not be a surprise to most people, many wouldn't associate sugar with back pain or chronic joint pain, and inflammation.

As pain information has the same subjective quality, independent of its causes, it is extremely difficult for most people to associate the sugar that they consume with their pain. Sugar can exacerbate everything from muscle pain to joint stiffness, headaches to fibromyalgia, and of course, digestive dysfunction and many other inflammatory conditions such as rheumatoid arthritis and psoriasis. If that task isn't hard enough, it is just as difficult to identify the source of the sugar in our diets as it is well disguised in many foods that are 'supposedly' healthy and labelled accordingly. Most of us are that accustomed to sugar in our diet, that when we eat truly healthy foods that don't contain sugar, we think they are tasteless or worse still, unpleasant-tasting. It's actually quite sad to recognize that a substance with absolutely no nutrient value dominates the taste of our food and our health in such a profound way. Even scarier is the fact that the average person consumes 82 grams (19.5 teaspoons) of sugar a day!

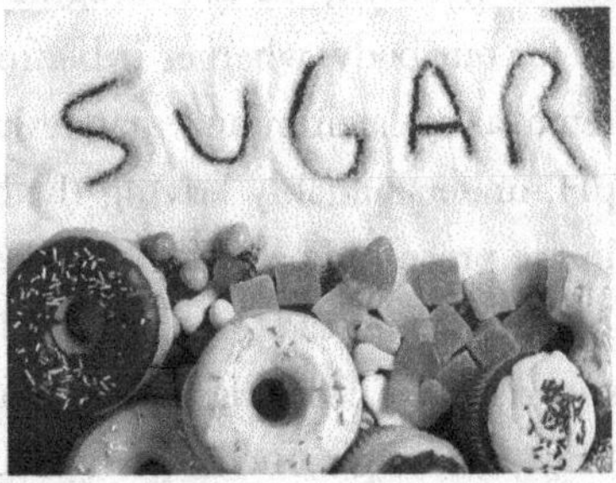

Our body uses sugar for energy in the form of glucose. When blood glucose levels rise and stay elevated for prolonged periods of time (the continual sugar consumption via fruit juices, alcohol, sweets, products with high fructose corn syrup, etc.) glycogen is stored in the liver. When the level of glycogen in the liver is excessive, it passes back into the bloodstream where it is stored in other tissues of the body, in particular, adipose tissue (fat) hence contributing to obesity. Obesity is a major source of back pain and will be discussed later in this chapter. Back in Palaeolithic times, sugar was only consumed in the form of fruits and berries and even then, these would have been a rare treat. Nowadays many people consume sugar for breakfast, lunch, and dinner, leaving our blood glucose at dangerously high levels. With an increase in blood glucose a proportionate increase in the levels of cortisol occurs as well as a chain reaction. This affects multiple other bodily processes as well. These consequences are all unfortunately negative for our health.

8 'Stress, food, and inflammation: psychoneuroimmunology and nutrition at the cutting edge', Janice K Kiecolt-Glaser, *Journal of Psychosomatic Medicine,* 2010.

One of the devastating consequences is bone demineralization, or even worse, osteoporosis. This occurs as sugar and other artificial sweeteners are highly acidic. Vinegar is one of the most acidic compounds that we consume with a pH of 2. Sugar in sweets, fizzy drinks/sodas, cakes, etc. come in at a very close pH of 3! In an attempt to neutralize the acidity, minerals such as calcium are leached from the bones while magnesium is leached from the muscles. Remembering that the heart is also muscle and magnesium is vital for its function, we can recognize just how devastating demineralization can be for our body, whether it be from bones, the heart, or any other organ. The removal of calcium and magnesium occurs in an attempt to neutralize blood pH, understandably leaving the bones weakened and consequently can result in the process of osteopenia and osteoporosis.

It makes me sad to see our children consuming 'foods' that are predominantly sugar such as breakfast cereals, flavoured milk, cakes, candies, and other foods laden with high fructose corn syrup. Kids rely on adults to make their dietary decisions for them, and many well-meaning parents have absolutely no idea of the devastation they are causing their children's health. My consultations always include an in-depth conversation on a person's history and I have encountered hundreds of people whose parents prohibited them from consuming sugar when they were children, correlating their state of health and vitality throughout their lives to the absence of sugar. Conversely, the greater majority of people, myself included, who consumed high quantities of sugar during childhood also had or have had health issues that accompany high sugar consumption.

SO HOW MUCH SUGAR IS ACCEPTABLE?

This is the question that I know so many health professionals have difficulties in answering (the other one is how much alcohol is acceptable before it has a deleterious effect on our health). When you consider that sugar negatively impacts our gut health (biome) and intestinal flora directly influences almost every vital function of our body, from our sleep to our body weight, our pH to our cardiac health, the degree of bone demineralization, our levels of inflammation and our pain sensitivity, one would have to recommend zero is an acceptable level of sugar consumption. As even small amounts will have negative effects on these processes, this recommendation would be even more relevant if somebody has any underlying health disfunctions, whether they are conscious of it or not. Admittedly, removing sugar from our diets is not easy, as it is disguised under many names (fructose, glucose, maltose, dextrose, and more) and is contained in corn syrup, molasses, honey, maple syrup, and brown sugar among a few. There is no healthy form of sugar or any other substance that enhances sweetness. Artificial sweeteners such as saccharin, acesulfame, aspartame, xylitol, sucralose, and stevia can be worse still, as the way the brain responds to these is very complex, with many causing side-effects that are worse than sugar.

TIP

The only safe way to consume sugar is via fruit and berries. Think like a palaeolithic caveman and eat them in moderation. Don't drink fruit juice thinking that it is healthier than fizzy drinks. If you consider that there may be three or four oranges in an orange juice, think how long it would've taken to eat those oranges. Now consider how long it took to drink. Even though the sugar is of a natural source, fruits were never intended to be consumed at such a high concentration.

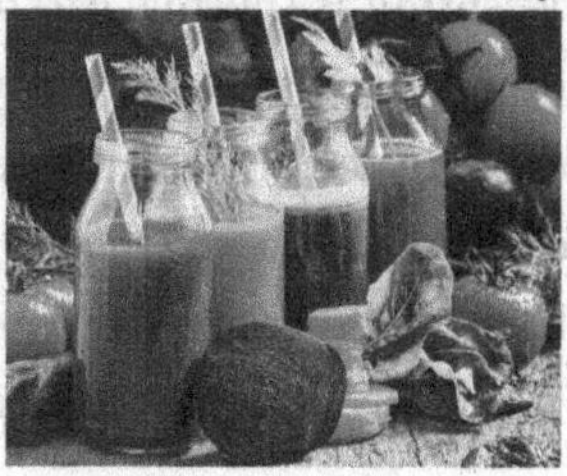

DRINK YOUR VEGETABLES AND EAT YOUR FRUIT

Look for sugar in apparently inconspicuous foods and beverages such as alcohol, pasta, bread, pizza, cheese products, and fruit juices. If you eat fruit and want to minimise your sugar intake, choose low glycemic fruits, (e.g., pears and apples) over higher glycemic fruits (for example bananas and grapes). It's also a good idea to stay away from prepacked and processed foods, as they are usually high in sugar, making them tastier and influencing our desire to eat them again in the future. Sugar also stimulates the release of opioids in dopamine from our brain making its consumption, especially in higher quantities, addictive.

The stimulation of the substances is the same reason that makes many illicit drugs highly addictive. These neurotransmitters make us feel good and give a person a desirable 'high' sensation after eating or drinking them. With continued consumption, the brain actually releases less and less of these feel-good neurotransmitters, increasing the amount of sugar needed to give the intensity of the previous 'highs' felt by the consumer. Remember that it is not only adults that have these neurotransmitters. Kids are even more sensitive to this reaction and this may explain the temper tantrums that these children may have when they do not get any. Lastly, in relation to people who have underlying spinal dysfunction or painful processes occurring, these neurotransmitters play a vital role in pain modulation. This allows them a certain degree of increased tolerance in dealing with their condition. Allowing sugar to unnecessarily stimulate the secretion of these neurotransmitters to leave these people with much less tolerance.

OSTEOPOROSIS – WHAT IS IT AND HOW TO AVOID IT

Osteoporosis is a disease that we as a society are becoming too accustomed to accepting as a normal part of the ageing process. In reality, this couldn't be further from the truth. Like many other degenerative illnesses, for most people who are diagnosed with it, osteoporosis results from poor lifestyle choices. What's exciting for those who are afraid of getting it or those who already know they have it, is that it is preventable or can be improved via correct lifestyle choices. When we look at the causes of osteoporosis documented in publications from medical journals to laymen's websites, we see that almost all of its causative factors are under our control. From smoking, sedentary lifestyle, inadequate diet including excessive sugar and alcohol, and certain medications. Many of these medications are taken for preventable lifestyle diseases, such as glucocorticoids (for lowering inflammation), aromatize inhibitors (used for breast cancer) proton pump inhibitors (for indigestion), and Comodin (for blood thinning). Other diseases such as coeliac disease, inflammatory bowel disease, kidney disease (which also affects vitamin D absorption) thyroid problems as well as hormonal problems that affect normal oestrogen levels (such as menopause) are also causative factors. Sadly, many people diagnosed with osteopenia or osteoporosis will be prescribed drugs such as Actonel, Boniva, and Fosomax, without understanding that they can improve their diagnosis via lifestyle changes.

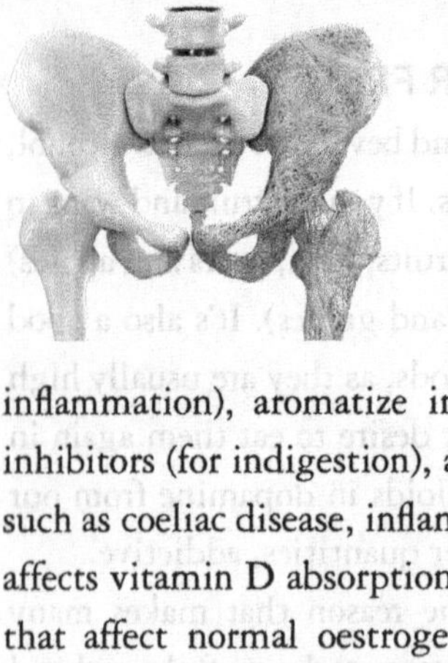

Osteoporosis occurs when your body absorbs more bone than it produces. In a healthy body, there is a psychological removal of unhealthy bone followed by the replacement of new bone. This keeps the bones of our skeleton strong. The drugs taken to treat osteoporosis do not actually help the body build new bone. They function by activating the cells (called osteoclasts) that break bone down. This sounds good on paper, however, without the cells, the bone becomes denser but not necessarily stronger. Without the ability to regenerate, the bones of women who have been taking these bisphosphonate-tight drugs for five years or more significantly increases their risk of fracture.

According to the World Health Organization (WHO), around 30% of women and 10% of men over 50 have an osteoporotic process occurring. The American Chiropractic Association quotes that one in five women will suffer a vertebral fracture in their lives, however, the majority don't even know, as they show no apparent symptoms or they simply don't look for help if they are in pain.

So, is osteoporosis a painful process? The loss of bone density is actually an asymptomatic process. It's incredible how many patients that I have consulted over the years that attributed their back pain to their osteopenia or osteoporosis. They think they are condemned to a life of suffering because they suffer from a condition that, in their mind, is incurable. Thankfully this is not the case.

CASE STUDY

Betty was 65 years old when she first presented to my clinic with back pain. She had suffered for years and had minimal success with any of the treatments she had done. She also showed a loss in bone density. One of her doctors asked for a bone density exam looking for answers. With years of minimal success in treating the problem and a new diagnosis of osteopenia, she was informed that the reason for her suffering was the fact that she had demobilization of her bones occurring. She was also told that the only way to treat it and have any chance of being pain-free was to use phosphate drugs. She understandably took the drugs. A year later her pain had increased to a point where her low back pain was now causing sciatic pain down her left leg.

On examination, I noted that her left sacroiliac joint was sensitive to palpation and restricted in extension. I asked if this area over the joint was where she had been suffering. She answered yes and affirmed that it had always been over that exact area. When I asked about the origin of her pain and when it had started, she said that it was after playing golf one day (golf is particularly demanding on the sacroiliac joints due to the rotation of the upper body and the pelvis that wasn't designed for this kind of rotation). As she had played her whole life, she understandably didn't relate golf to being the cause of her problem. As the pain worsened over time, she exercised less and less to a point where she became completely sedentary, thinking that that would be the best thing for her pain. This started a year ago, the exact time that she started taking medication for osteoporosis. We treated Betsy twice a week for a month. Her sacroiliac joint was easy to release. We focused on relaxing the muscles that were surrounding the sciatic nerve and the stabilizing muscles in her spine and core. Her leg pain subsided quickly. From day one of treatment, I recommended that she walk twice a day for 40 minutes. This not only became easier with time but actually helped the pain in the earlier days while she was still suffering. We talked about the importance of her lifestyle including advice on an anti-inflammatory diet, resisted exercise with weights, and supplementation with vitamins such as vitamin D3 and K2, to maximize the disposition of new bone cells. She spoke with her doctor and discontinued medication, telling him that she preferred to focus on her bone health via exercise and a change in diet. She was pain-free after a month of treatment and two years later shows normal bone density results.

Too many people relate back pain to be a consequence of osteopenia or osteoporosis. As sarcopenia (loss of muscle mass) is often associated with the same causative factors as osteoporosis, especially in the elderly[9] a vicious cycle often forms.

This includes a sedentary lifestyle, less than optimal diet, incorrect posture, osteoporosis, and sarcopenia. With time the cycle worsens unless the person suffering takes conscious steps to focus on the actual causative factors and not the resultant diagnosis. In these cases, the vicious cycle understandably results in pain, as spinal bio-mechanics are compromised due to lack of movement, abnormal posture and loss of muscle mass, all factors that can be easily and positively influenced if the person is sufficiently well-informed and motivated. The pain is ultimately a cause of bio-mechanical dysfunction and not osteopenia or osteoporosis.

Osteoporosis only results in symptoms when the loss of bone density leads to a bone's inability to withstand the loads that a normal life places on it or trauma such as falls and other impacts. When the collapse of the vertebra, whether it be total or partial, is compromised by the mechanical function of the articulation or interferes with the transmission of nervous impulses, severe pain can be experienced. These cases, however, are rare. Whenever a fracture is suspected, it is highly recommended to do an X-ray or other diagnostic imaging to confirm this and determine its severity. A bone density test will determine the degree of demineralization (bone loss) whether it be osteopenia or osteoporosis.

HOW TO SLOW DOWN OR REVERSE BONE LOSS NATURALLY

- Bones actually increase their bone density when a load on them demands more strength from the bone. This is why weight-bearing exercise is one of the most effective ways of improving bone density. This could be done as easily as walking or via the use of resisted exercise, such as weight training. Numerous studies have shown that strength training, whether it

9 'Management of chronic pain in osteoporosis: challenges and solutions', Teresa Paolucci et al., *Journal of Pain Research,* 2016.

be with weights or your own body weight, can slow the rate of bone loss and even built bone. With a list of benefits that's already extensive, this is one more to add to that list.

- **Exercise is an essential component of health and not a temporary intervention to treat the effects of an underlying problem by masking its symptoms.**
- Choose what exercise you dedicate yourself to carefully, taking into consideration your state of health, what stage of bone loss you're at, and what your musculoskeletal-system is capable of. While sprinting and lunges will be great for some people, walking and yoga will be more appropriate for others, such as those who are out of condition. Weight training is an excellent way of loading your skeleton and can be started with lighter weights before building up to more resistance. Other ideas include playing tennis or golf (without the golf buggy!) Dancing, high-intensity interval training, step machines, and treadmills. Even climbing stairs will quickly build your skeletal and muscular strength whilst making your muscles stronger. One of my favourite exercises is whole-body vibration, using a platform that vibrates between 30–60 times a second. NASA works with this simple technology to help astronaut's bone density levels go back to normal levels after returning from space. Their bones suffer demineralization since they have been in a zero-gravity environment whilst in space. The vibrating platform also improves balance, growth hormone levels, increases blood flow, and serves as excellent lymphatic drainage whilst improving bone density and muscle mass.

TIP

Please don't take a calcium supplement or increase your consumption of dairy products thinking that they will treat your osteoporosis. Your body removes calcium from the bones for a reason. Unless you identify what that reason is and focus on it, simply increasing your intake of calcium, whether it be through supplementation or diet, will unfortunately not lead to an increase in bone density. Following on with the theme of this book, focus on the cause and rectify it. Your body will do the rest. Some studies even indicate that calcium supplementation (non-dietary) can actually increase the risk of heart attack and other cardiovascular diseases.

- Don't underestimate the role that incorrect lifestyle choices have in the evolution of the osteoporotic process. There are reasons why some people suffer a loss of bone density and others of the same age don't. If you have an osteoporotic process occurring there is also a reason why your body decided to remove calcium from your bones. The cause needs to be identified and rectified. If we recognize that optimal health can only be achieved by providing the nutrients that the cells of our body are genetically programmed to receive, while at the same time minimising or avoiding the toxins that it was never programmed to receive, we have a fair shot at obtaining optimal health. If a body is healthy, it does not suffer from osteoporosis in the same way that a healthy body does not suffer from cardiovascular disease cancer, diabetes or obesity. If a healthy lifestyle is being followed, the cells of your body simply have sufficient required nutrients while at the same time experience minimal or zero effect from toxins. Deficiencies of nutrients such as Omega 3, calcium, vitamin D3, K2, and magnesium occur from diets that are high in sugar, processed foods, and trans-fats. Remember that raised cortisol levels lead to insulin resistance, raising blood sugar levels and contributing to the depletion of calcium. Stress raises cortisol levels; therefore, it also contributes to the demineralization of bone. Avoid the obvious sources of sugar such as soft drinks and sweets, but also, the not so obvious ones such as high glycemic index foods including fruit juices. Alcohol is also high in sugar and should be avoided.

- Vitamin D3 is necessary to absorb calcium and this occurs when we get healthy levels of sunlight directly on our body. For people with fair skin, the time in the sun doesn't need to be long (around 20 minutes) and can be in the morning while the more worrying UV rays are weaker. If time in the sun is not a possibility, supplementation vitamin D is vital. There are many degenerative illnesses linked to low levels of vitamin D, making it an essential supplement to include in your daily routine.
- Check your hormone levels! While menopause can contribute to bone loss in women, so too can andropause in men. In addition to checking the SHGB level (sex hormones) also check cortisol, insulin and parathyroid hormone levels as alterations in any of these can indicate a possible contributing factor to the depletion of calcium from the bones.
- As mentioned previously, when the body promotes the removal of calcium from the bones, it is often done in an attempt to neutralize acidity. Most people already know that a typical western diet high in sugar, processed foods, trans-fats, etc. is highly acidic. Our physiological processes operate in a narrow range of pH, tending towards neutrality. With an acidic environment caused by the food we eat, the body removes calcium from the bones (and magnesium from the muscles and heart) in an attempt to buffer this consequent acidity.

- The average western diet is also high in protein, which also generates acidity, mainly as sulphates and phosphates according to an article from the *Journal of Nutrition*[10] Similarly, alkali buffers, whether they be chemical salts or dietary fruits and vegetables high in potassium can reverse the acid-induced calcium loss caused by the factors mentioned in this chapter.

MILK – FRIEND OR FOE?

Milk has been the standard advice (as well as calcium supplements) that I have heard relayed to my osteoporotic clients over the years by their health practitioners and MDs. The *American Journal of Epidemiology* in the study titled, 'Case-control study of risk factors for hip fractures in the elderly'[11] found that the consumption of dairy products increases the risk of hip fracture.
Another study from Harvard concluded that those people who had the majority of their calcium from dairy foods broke more bones than those who rarely drank milk. The study was conducted on 77,761 women between the ages of 34–59 years of age. Milk is not a viable intervention for the treatment or prevention of osteopenia or osteoporosis, contrary to what western medicine promotes. It is highly acidic and actually does the opposite to what it is recommended for, that being the removal of calcium from the bones and lowering of bone density.
Milk is produced by lactating mammal mothers to breastfeed their babies. Mothers' milk is rich in nutrients such as vitamins, minerals, and antibodies to promote the healthy development of their offspring. When the growth of the animal reaches a certain point and it can receive its nourishment via eating (because its gastrointestinal tract is developed accordingly) it is naturally weaned off milk. Nature never intended any animal to continue consuming its mother's milk past that early phase of life. Nature most definitely didn't intend for the milk of one type of animal to be consumed by another (sound familiar?). The milk of each species is specific to that species. Cow's milk, for example, contains around three times the amount of protein as human milk, making it perfect for baby cows but unsuitable for humans who require a totally different composition of nutrients. It's little wonder then, after reading the studies relating high-protein consumption, acidity, and the resulting bone loss, that milk would be considered one of the worst things to introduce into an already osteoporotic person's body.

---

10 'Excess dietary protein can adversely affect bone', Uriel Barzel, Linda Massey, *Journal of Nutrition,* Volume 28, issue 6, June 1998.

11 'Case-control study of risk factors for hip fractures in the elderly', Pei-Ju Huang, Shu-Hsin Lee, *American Journal of Epidemiology,* Volume 39, number five, 1994.

MEDICATION – THE GOOD, THE BAD AND THE UGLY

"If we try to suppress pain it is possible that we will duplicate it."
JEAN MOLIÈRE

Medication is the most common intervention that people use to deal with their back pain. Sadly, the majority believe that it will 'cure' them of their suffering, similar to the way that antibiotics may resolve an infection after they have dealt with the bacterial infection. This of course is not the case as the pain and unpleasant symptoms are the consequence of an underlying physical, chemical or emotional cause. All medication has side effects, whether you feel it or not,

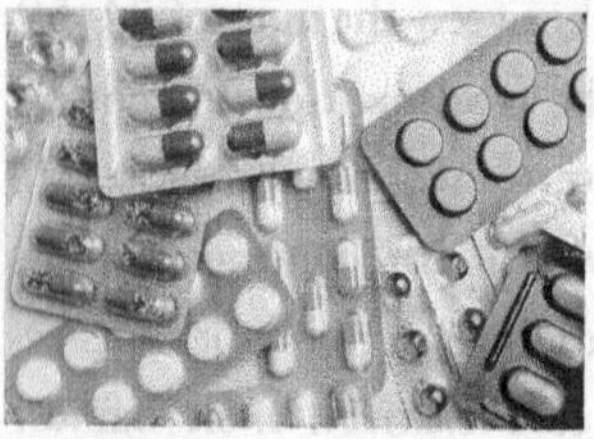

as our body will always react to substances that it is not genetically meant to be exposed to. This doesn't mean that medication is not necessary for appropriate moments or specific problems however the use of medication to treat back pain is poorly understood and has been grossly abused. Joint pain, back pain, muscle aches, and headaches are common side-effects from several different types of medication, however, they are rarely considered when people are looking for the cause of their problem. Most people never read up about the possible side effects of the drugs they are taking. Many medications have dozens of side effects documented in the instructions for use, ranging from a sudden heart attack and death to less serious ones such as skin irritation, constipation, dizziness, joint pain, and muscle aches.

TIP

If you suffer musculoskeletal problems, back pain, joint aches, headaches, and are taking medication, please investigate whether your symptoms are a side-effect of that particular medication.

Here are just a few everyday medications that may be causing your joint pain, muscle aches, or headaches[12 13]

---

12 'Drug-Induced Musculoskeletal Disorders', B. Bannwarth, *Drug-Safety* 30, 27–46, 2007.

13 'Musculoskeletal adverse drug reactions: a review of literature and data from ADR spontaneous reporting databases', A. Conforti, et al., *Drug Safety* 2(1) 47–63, 2007.

- Antidepressants such as Venlafaxine EP (Effexor XR) which increases the level of the neurotransmitter serotonin Norepinephrine. 10% of people taking this will experience joint pain.
- Osteoporosis medication such as Risedronate contributes to joint aches and pains in 30% of people taking it.
- The asthma inhaler Fluticasone (Flovent) increases the chance of suffering joint pain by 19%.
- Cholesterol-lowering medication (statins). Between 5 to 10% of all those taking Crestor, Lipitor, or Altoprev will suffer joint pain.
- Antibiotics such as levofloxacin (Levaquin) are commonly prescribed for sinus infections and ammonia. Research shows that 25% of people will suffer joint aches within three days of starting and those aches subside within seven days of finishing.
- The list goes on and on with less obvious drugs such as the contraceptive pill causing headaches.

PAINKILLERS

Opioids are the most common medication used to treat chronic pain. Their use has become so widespread that it has become a serious cause of addiction. Unfortunately, opioid use causes the body to increase the number of opioid receptors and, in an attempt to allow the pain signal to continue to function in the way that it was intended to, advise us via unpleasant signals that something isn't right. So, with time, as people take more and more painkillers, they become less effective in those taking them to become even more sensitive to pain. Our body makes its own opioids called endorphins that eventually decrease with the continued use of opioid medication. It's a vicious circle. Endorphins are also vital for healthy sleep and our happiness, and both of these suffer drastically after long-term (over 4 weeks) opioid use.

Commonly prescribed opioids include fentanyl, oxycodone, hydrocodone, methadone, oxymorphone, codeine, and morphine. Heroin is also an opioid. It is therefore not a surprise to recognize that a drug that stimulates a sensation of pleasure and pain relief, once addicted to it, users feel a compulsive urge to consume them, even when the original problem has been resolved. Addiction can obviously lead to overdose, which causes breathing to slow down and the heart to eventually stop. Back pain and symptoms related to spinal dysfunction are the most common reasons people start taking opioid drugs in the first place. In reality, painkillers of any type, if they are to be taken, should be taken to relieve the severe pain that inhibits someone from moving more and therefore restoring function to the effect of joint or joints. According to the National Institute of Drug Abuse, roughly 21 to 29% of patients prescribed opioids for chronic pain misuse them. Between 8 and 12% developed an opioid disorder. An estimated 4–6% who misuse prescription opioids transition to heroin.[14]

Pain is not the only symptom that results from joint dysfunction. Our brain also provokes muscle contraction to limit movement and therefore subsequent possible damage to a joint. Inflammation is promoted to speed the healing process. The brain obviously causes these reactions for a good reason, however, there are also medications to override the bodies in intelligence and interfere with the healing process.

ANTI-INFLAMMATORIES

Anti-inflammatories can cause miracle results when used in certain situations. However, as many are over-the-counter medications, most people auto–prescribed, which may be to their detriment. Non-steroidal anti-inflammatory drugs (NSAIDs) such as ibuprofen, naproxen, and diclofenac are the most common of these anti-inflammatories. They often cause stomach ache, and if taken over long periods of time, can increase the possibility of developing a stomach ulcer. I have worked with countless people over the years that simply didn't understand how detrimental continual use of NSAIDs could be to their health. Many of these ended up with stomach ulcers. Some people even end up with cardiac problems. When we override the inflammatory process, reducing it via anti-inflammatories, we must also look for the original cause of the symptoms. When it's a fall, trauma, or obvious event, joint dysfunction may have also occurred at the time. Medication may remove symptoms promptly, however, without unpleasant pain stimuli, muscle contraction, or inflammation, it is understandably very easy to forget to investigate the problem when the pain has disappeared. By suppressing symptoms, we may allow degenerative processes such as osteoarthritis and degenerative disc disease to occur. Acetaminophen (paracetamol) is another common painkiller. However, studies have shown that it is no more effective than placebo while damaging the liver and even causing liver failure when used excessively.[15] Acetaminophen is also an over-the-counter drug.

---

14 'Heroin DrugFacts', National Institute on Drug Abuse (NIH) nida.nih.gov/publications/drugfacts/heroin

15 'Low back pain: What role does medication play in the treatment of non-specific back?' www.ncbi.nlm.nih.gov/books/NBK284957

MUSCLE RELAXANTS

These do exactly what the name suggests – relax muscles. Have you ever sprained your ankle or knee, had it braced or bandaged to feel supported and suddenly removed that support? If you have experienced this feeling, you'd be able to relate to the sensation of lack of support and instability. Muscle relaxers do something similar by overriding the central nervous system's command to contract those muscles. When these muscles spasm, joints such as the intervertebral joints, shoulder, knee, or hip the resulting muscle relaxation can drastically increase the load on the joint, due to the fact that the muscles were sharing the load when they were contracted. This could exacerbate the problem, both in an acute, short-term sense and in a chronic, long-term matter.

TIP

Try walking to restore joint function, decrease inflammation, and relax muscles instead of taking anti-inflammatories or muscle relaxants and resting your body. Prolonged absence from physical activity (movement) will lead to muscle atrophy, and even more joint dysfunction and pain.

Muscle relaxants also have undesirable side effects from dizziness, drowsiness, and headache from short-term use to seizures, cardiac arrest, coma, and death for long-term users. When mixing with alcohol the dangers are even greater.

Some chronic pain sufferers are also recommended ANTIDEPRESSANTS when other pharmaceutical interventions have failed. Interestingly, most antidepressants have never been proven to be effective in treating back pain. Nociceptive pain signals directly affect serotonin levels. Pain is stressful and while serotonin is high enough (naturally produced) quantities of serotonin naturally produced by the body would suppress these stressful, cortisol producing pain signals.

Artificial stimulation via antidepressants soon exhausts our bodies' ability to produce serotonin. Common side-effects can range from low blood pressure, reduction in libido, insomnia, constipation, anxiety, and many more. Would it be easier to simply focus on rectifying the cause and allowing the body to do what it does best – self-regulate?

CASE STUDY

Helen had suffered constant headaches for three years without finding success from any of the treatments she had tried. She received regular massage and acupuncture, which gave her relief for a short period of time, but the headaches would always return.

Her doctor recommended painkillers; however, the symptoms would return when she stopped taking them. The doctor asked for a computerized tomography exam of the brain to investigate the possibility of something more serious. All clear.

When I asked her if she was taking any medications, she mentioned that she was taking blood pressure medication more as a precaution than anything else. Three years ago, she suffered from traumatic events with her brother's death and a marriage break up, leaving her feeling stressed out and overwhelmed. Her blood pressure at the time was slightly elevated her doctor recommended medication. I asked her to bring in the box and instructions, which we read together. Headaches were one of the first side-effects that we encountered. I asked her how she had been feeling emotionally and she said that all of her stress had passed two years ago. She said that she was feeling better than ever. She had also become healthier with regular exercise and a nutritious diet. She returned to her doctor and ask for her blood pressure to be measured again. It was actually lower than normal! She said that she would like to cease the medication and he agreed. Eureka! After only one week without taking the medication, she had a total cessation of her headaches.

THE ROLE OF MEDICATION IN YOUR LIFE

"The art of medicine distracts while nature deals with a disease."
VOLTAIRE

Most of us have taken medication in our lives. Probably multiple times over the years. I remember painful or life-threatening events in my own life were calmed by medication. I have had spinal surgery where intravenous medication after the surgery calms the pain and I've taken DMPS (a chelation medication to remove heavy metals) for the mercury toxicity that I received from the incorrect extraction of my amalgam fillings. I have taken codeine for wisdom tooth infection and antibiotics over the years for severe infections. I have felt excruciating pain a couple of times in my life that thankfully was settled by some type of analgesic. Anti-inflammatories were taken before my spinal surgery to minimise possible damage that my intervertebral disk herniation may have caused to the neighbouring nerve root. Every time that I've taken medication, I've researched the benefit as well as the side-effects, and then decided whether to take it or not. I've also taken them knowing what my problems were and that in general, the medication would distract me from the pain while my own body did the healing or I removed myself from the environment that was actually causing the problem. The decision to take medication of any type is a personal one. Pain and other symptoms are extremely subjective, with some people being slightly impacted and others being incapacitated. I have been very thankful for the benefit that medication has given me at certain times in my life. I have also been very thankful that those times were short-lived and that I have never needed to chronically depend on medication. When somebody's livelihood depends on them showing up for work or they have to take care of a family, it is totally understandable why they may decide to medicate themselves. However, too many people consume medication thinking that it is curing their problem. This is understandable considering they are overriding unpleasant reflexes that our brain intelligently causes to call attention to a problem. It is important to highlight that symptoms are intended to guide us away from aggravating the original problem further. For example, if your back hurts when you move, does it make sense to take a painkiller to be able to exercise or walk? We may push on and seriously damage the tissue since it didn't hurt to do so whilst under the influence of the medication. If we felt the pain, it may have impeded us from exacerbating the problem. Maybe our body is trying to tell us something? Our innate intelligence is more intelligent than our conscious mind. It decides when it is in our bodies' favour to be warned via unpleasant symptoms and when the problem gets to a point where it is no longer a threat and therefore diminishing painful and unpleasant symptoms is advantageous.

Our innate intelligence causes indigestion when we eat food such as hotdogs, fried food or hamburgers, or any other food that simply doesn't agree with our body. Our decision is whether to listen to the conscious science and change our behaviour in regards to our diet or ignore them and swallow an antacid. Decisions like this can have life-threatening implications on our health in the long term.

Our innate intelligence also causes our blood pressure to rise when our body is being subject to a situation that it needs to adapt to, such as a stressful situation. My decision is whether to look for the cause (whether it be a stressful event, inadequate diet, sedentary lifestyle, or any other stimulus) or take a beta-blocker to force it down. This would obviously be against the body's will. Understandably, in cases where a blood pressure increase may threaten somebody's life, many opt for medication. Unfortunately, most also opt not to look for the true cause of the high blood pressure.

In another example, when our insulin levels elevate, they do so for a reason. Do you look for the cause, whether it be dietary, hormonal, stress, etc. or do you follow a diabetic treatment protocol via medication?

Symptoms such as constipation, insomnia, erectile dysfunction, high cholesterol, depression, osteoporosis, and many, many other symptoms will all pose a similar question to the people suffering them. The decision that is necessary to be made every time is whether you'll look for the cause and solve it or ignore it and take the medication. Of course, you may also choose to take the medication while you are searching for a cause. Once again, that decision is yours, and looking for the cause is the only way to actually improve your health. Focusing on symptoms and dealing with them via allopathy gives no attention to our health and strengthening it by listening to what our body is actually trying to say.

If your head is aching, maybe it is doing so for a good reason. Maybe all you have to do is stop sleeping on your belly or refrain from watching TV in bed before you go to sleep. If your lower back is sore, is it because you're sitting for too long? Or sitting on a couch that doesn't support your back? Maybe your sciatic pain down the leg isn't as serious as a sharp pain may indicate. Maybe it's just the fact that your wallet is in your back pocket on the same side as the pain.

Asking the right question is crucial if you desire maximum longevity from your spine and joints. You could ask "How do I relieve this pain?" and be directed towards an appropriate medication. Alternatively, you could also ask "What am I doing that could aggravate my spine to cause this pain?" and be guided towards a solution. A solution that will not only result in the disappearance of symptoms but also the preservation of joint function and homeostasis.

Pain can save you years of suffering on multiple levels. It's not advisable to simply turn it off. Would you turn off your car's oil light if it was advising you that your motor was out of oil? I know that's a rhetorical question as you would of course add more oil and not simply turn the light off. However, that is not necessarily the case in the way that most of us treat our spinal health and general health for that matter.

The decision if and when you take medication is based on each problem. By considering the benefits and the risks and then making the decision you'll be putting your health first and not your disease or symptom. In a career spanning over 25 years, I have seen very few people ask the correct questions. Most things are being 'cured' by a certain medication and almost all are unaware of the side effects.

According to the investigation *Death by Medicine*, 783,936 people die annually due to medical error in the United States. Led by Dr. Greg Null, the investigation revises thousands of medical reports of death caused by a medical error. As a considerable percentage of medical errors are not documented, the report comments that the above figure is a conservative estimate and that the number could be up to 20 times greater.

Of the 783,936 deaths in the year of the study, 2003, 106,000 were due to medication. This number is also conservative since many adverse reactions caused by medication are probably not reported. Most people are aware that there are risks involved when taking medication, however, these figures are much greater than most people would expect. In the United States, one person dies every five minutes due to incorrect use of medication. Errors of conventional medicine are the leading cause of death and incorrect use of medication is the fourth leading cause.

OBESITY – BEING OVERWEIGHT OVERLOADS YOUR SPINE

"True happiness is impossible without true health and true health is impossible without a rigorous control of our gluttony."

MAHATMA GANDHI

Obesity is a word that we have become very accustomed to hearing in modern-day society. What does it actually mean? Obesity means that you have too much body fat and it is a condition where our natural energy reserve, which is stored in fatty tissue, has been raised to a point where it is a risk to human health or increases mortality. To confirm if somebody has too much body fat, a calculation is made based on a person's body mass index (BMI). This compares somebody's weight to their height, with a score of 25 to 29.9 classifying somebody as being OVERWEIGHT. A BMI of 30 or more puts some in the OBESE range. A BMI greater than 40 is considered to be MORBIDLY OBESE. According to the Centre for Disease Control and Prevention, obesity affects 42.8% of middle-aged adults. Around 39% of the world's population over 18 years of age were overweight in 2016. Around 30% of the adult population was obese. Frighteningly the prevalence of obesity nearly tripled between 1975 and 2016! Obesity is now associated with the leading cause of death worldwide, as it is a major risk factor in diseases such as cardiovascular diseases (heart disease and stroke), diabetes, and many cancers. Musculoskeletal disorders such as osteoarthritis, degenerative disc disease, and back pain are right up there on the list with heart disease and diabetes, as consequences of obesity.

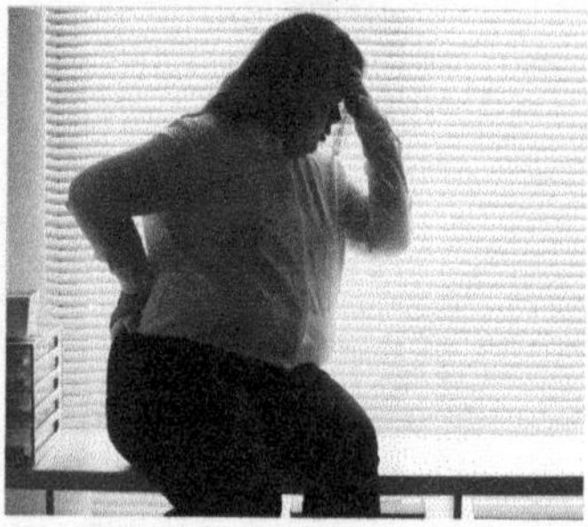

To place the bio-mechanical influence of obesity on the musculoskeletal system in a clear perspective, imagine increasing the load that your car carries by 30% or more. Can you imagine how much harder the engine (heart) would have to work, or the load on the wheels (bones) and shock absorbers (discs and cartridge) would increase? Now imagine if the fuel that you were filling the tank up with was less than optimal to satisfy the increase in the output the car would require for the excessive load it is carrying. Or independently of what your actual weight is, imagine carrying a shopping bag of only 5 kg in each hand for one day. This would represent an increased weight of only 12.5% or less for anybody weighing 80 kg or less. Anybody carrying this type of load would be able to relate to the fact that after a very short amount of time your body reacts. The forearms and hands tire first, the shoulders roll forward, taking the head with them and worsening your posture. Carrying the bags for long enough would make the muscles of the back work harder and eventually tighten, restricting joint function and leading to restriction of movement. All of these effects would occur in less than a day! Imagine if the load was continual, day in, day out.

It's easy to understand how the increase in the load placed on the joints of the body would wear them out faster. It is also very easy to understand how people in the overweight and obese range would also have their range of normal motion restricted. When articulations are impeded from functioning in the way that they were intended to, many deleterious consequences commence, such as edema, low-grade inflammation, Increased pain sensitivity, and many more.

It has to be remembered also that many other factors that contributed to an increase in BMI are inflammatory. Topics already discussed in this chapter such as sugar and alcohol consumption, cigarette smoking, dehydration, and the standard western diet all contribute to raising inflammation in the body. INFLAMMATION FEEDS INFLAMMATION, making somebody who is overweight or obese even more prone to suffering back pain, joint, and muscle aches as well as all of the other degenerative conditions they contribute to.

CASE STUDY

Throughout my career, I have lost count of how many overweight patients I've worked with that suffered from the symptoms of loss of bio-mechanical function of the low back. Symptoms such as lumbalgia, sciatic pain down one or both of the legs, pins and needles in the toes, pain irradiating to the groin and of the buttocks. In many of these cases, no obvious signs of dysfunction or degeneration were found on diagnostic images such as X-rays, computerized tomography (CT), or magnetic resonance imaging (MRI) that could explain the degree of pain suffered by the patient.

Wendy had suffered considerable lower back pain radiating down the left leg for five years. She was 160 cm tall and weighed 90 kg. Her BMI was 35.16 (90 ÷ 1.6 squared). After examining her spine and the tissues that were affected, we talked about the influence of her weight on her current state of suffering.

She recognized immediately that her pain and discomfort had increased since she started to put on weight. We talked about factors that contribute to obesity and sedentary lifestyle, inadequate diet, alcohol, and stress. She was determined to turn things around and remove the excessive load from her spine, and as a bonus get healthy. She went from 98 kg to 76 kg in 6 months, simply from refraining from drinking fizzy drinks, and eating sugary sweets, fried food, and dairy while at the same time walking 40 minutes twice a day. By losing more than 20% of her weight she had removed a significant load from her spine and other joints, such as the hips and knees. She observed that her pain gradually subsided week by week as she lightened the load. As a bonus, she also said that her general health had improved significantly, noting that she hadn't been sick with the flu, her allergies had disappeared and her sleep was better than ever. Her doctor also said that her blood tests were the best they had been in years.

Admittedly, it's not this easy for most people to lose weight. Is that because they aren't as disciplined as Wendy? Or do they have other influences such as hormonal imbalance (e.g., menopause) occurring? Maybe there is a psychological or emotional component involved. Recognizing what factors are most relevant in your case is no different from dealing with any of the other symptoms discussed in this book. Ask the correct questions and you'll be directed to the most relevant answers. If you are overweight or obese, the need to lose this weight is undeniable. There is no shortage of weight-loss advice out there. Important health benefits will invariably occur as a bonus alongside any efforts to lose weight. It is important not to desist if you don't get immediate results. Be mindful of the fact that your present state of health took years and maybe decades to arrive at. Why wouldn't it be feasible to accept that it will take time to revert to a healthier state? Even if you are not shifting the kilos from day one, this does not mean that you are not getting healthier. The day you shift your health towards homeostasis (100% cell function) you'll be becoming healthier, whether you feel it or not. Avoid using the parameters of how you look or how you feel as a gauge of the success of your health strategies. Health is how you are functioning and ideally, it should be at 100%. That said, during the process of moving your body towards a healthier state, you will invariably discover other factors contributing to the state of health you're in. Commonly, someone starting out on a detox will feel terrible. Does this mean that detoxifying our body of toxins is not healthy? Of course not. The road to homeostasis takes time and patience, and having a deeper knowledge of what is going on at a cellular level will help you stay on track.

The following is a list of some strategies that aren't as commonly talked about as 'burning more calories than you ingest' or 'increasing the amount of exercise you do'. Avoiding sugar, alcohol, trans-fats and fried food are fundamental pieces of advice. So too is increasing your hydration and the amount of fibre and whole foods you ingest. And, of course, exercise is a given, not just for weight loss but for our health in general.

TIPS

- Chew your food slowly and mindfully. This gives your brain sufficient time to measure blood glucose levels and stimulate a feeling of satiety (which helps avoid overheating).
- Practice intermittent fasting. Consider the fact that our genes haven't changed in the last 10,000 years or more. They have been genetically programmed to certain conditions in our environment. One of these conditions was not knowing when our next meal would be. Palaeolithic humans would leave to hunt or gather and not know when they would be consuming their next meal. Intermittent fasting limits the consumption of food to a window of usually eight hours, but sometimes less. Several studies[16] have shown that intermittent fasting helps overweight people lose weight. Other options include alternate day fasting and a 5:2 diet in which fasting occurs for two days out of seven.
- Eat for your bacteria – Viome (viome.com) is a company that tests the genetic needs of your own biome (intestinal flora). It's hands-down the best way to know if you're eating concurrently with the genetic requirements of your biome. It lists what foods you should avoid, what foods are your particular superfoods, and provides a ranking for all other foods. It also tests several metabolic processes which can be used as a parameter to measure improvement when future exams are done.
- Look at the liver – as it's often overlooked in its importance in the process of losing weight. In reality, it should be one of the first ports of call since it relates to various vital bodily processes. Firstly, it is our principal filter of toxins. Modern life, independent of how healthy you live it, puts an extremely toxic load on our bodies. Whether it be in the food we eat, the liquids we drink, the air we breathe, or what comes into contact with our skin. Toxic elements not recognized by our genes and incongruent with our health, enter our body. Similar to the filter for the pool that fills up with leaves, our livers are loaded with toxins, which often go back into the system and lodge in tissue such as fat, sexual organs, skin, and even

---

16 'The effects of intermittent or continuous energy restriction on weight loss and metabolic disease risk markers: a randomised trial in young overweight women', Michelle N. Harvie et al., *International Journal of Obesity.*

the brain. Medication, alcohol, trans-fats, food colouring, flavours, and aromas, preservatives, chemicals in our cleaning and personal hygiene products, air pollution, toxins in our water, and many, many more sources explain why our liver can't keep up. The liver also aids in digestion by producing bile to help break down fat and absorb fat-soluble vitamin C and minerals. It regulates glucose, insulin, oestrogen, testosterone, BP and immunity, blood cholesterol production, and elimination. It's way more important than what most people recognize and most of us unintentionally abuse it during our lives.

- Milk thistle is a herbal remedy derived from the milk thistle plant, also known as *Silybum marianum*. It can be taken every day as a liver tonic. Goldenseal and dandelion are two other herbs that can be taken with milk thistle for their detoxification and nurturing properties on the liver.
- Focus on your sleep – as it is probably the most important nutrient for your body. Poor quality sleep slows the body's metabolism down, meaning that it is more likely to store unused energy as fat – not good for those wanting or needing to lose weight.
- Exercise mindfully – after deciding that they want to lose weight and recognizing that exercising is an important tool, many people throw themselves into excessive amounts of exercise. They are only thinking that if a little bit is good, then a lot must be better. It's common to hear many of these people complain about not losing weight despite jogging copious distances. After a certain period of time when exercise is recognized as being excessive by the brain, it becomes a stressor that the body needs to adapt to. At this time, the production of extremely beneficial hormones such as testosterone and growth hormone is substituted by an increase in cortisol, insulin, and even cholesterol! The body interprets the situation as a fight or flight response and prepares itself accordingly. This can promote the storage of fat instead of actually burning it off. As discussed in other chapters, the body is regulated by a complicated system of hormones. If they are thrown out of synchronicity, serious consequences can result. Exercise performed at a moderate intensity for prolonged periods of time can do this. The solution is to look to high-intensity interval training (HIIT) which involves exercising intensely for short periods of time, to stimulate growth hormone. Growth hormone contributes to burning fat through its actions on two key enzymes that control lipolysis (the breakdown of stored triglycerides into three fatty acids). These enzymes are Lipoprotein Lipase (LPL) and Hormone Sensitive Lipase (HSL). On other days, lower the intensity completely for long walks

which don't wreak havoc on your hormone system and keep your weight loss aspirations alive.

- Probiotics – are live bacteria that can be taken in supplement form to help build our own biome, while at the same time helping to suppress parasites (bad bacteria). Our gut bacteria (micro-biome) are essential to our health in the same way that bacteria in the soil is essential for the soil's health and its ability to allow certain plants to flourish. Numerous studies have shown that gut bacteria play an influential role in weight regulation. For people needing to lose weight, supporting their micro-biome via supplementation is a big plus. Buy spore based supplements instead of refrigerated probiotics. The spores will hatch where they need to be active while the refrigerated bacteria will likely die before they have left the stomach. Their action of course needs to be in the intestine which is further down in the gastrointestinal tract.
- Drink your vegetables and eat your fruit. Fruit juice is high in fructose and elevates blood sugar levels as much as fizzy drinks. Cold-pressed vegetable juices provide a bomb of nutrients including vitamins, minerals, and enzymes. Many overweight people are overfed but undernourished and vegetable juices are an incredible way to revert this.

EMOTIONAL CAUSES OF BACK PAIN

Have you ever had to perform or be on your best game only to fall short due to poor sleep the previous night? Does anything ever work out the way it should when we are stressed out or angry? These are two of the many emotional factors that can affect every cell of our body negatively. That includes our muscle and connective tissue cells and the cells of the nervous system and bones. When we add negative emotional input to a spine that is already less than optimal, we set ourselves up for even more pain, inflammation, and restriction.

In this section you will be guided through fundamental concepts regarding the emotional factors involved in back pain and other bio-mechanical problems of the skeleton. By understanding what factors in your life may be affecting your current spinal health, you'll be able to remove the emotional factors that are negative and/or focus on the emotional factors that are positive. By doing

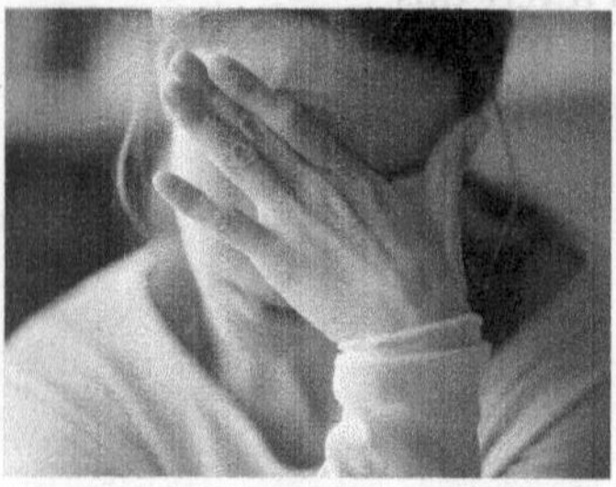

this you will take yourself to an improved level of function, decreasing back pain, restriction of movement and degeneration. Understanding the emotional causes of back pain is a valuable investment in the longevity of your spine and the highest possible performance you can obtain from it.

HOW TO KNOW WHEN YOUR PAIN IS 'IN YOUR HEAD'

"Diseases are the result not only of our actions, but also of our thoughts."
MAHATMA GANDHI

Have you ever been told that its in your head, in response to a certain health problem, pain or symptom or even the way you perceive a situation? Whilst the person telling you that its in your head, will never really know how your pain or discomfort feels, they are accurate when they make that link between our mind and what we feel physically.

Problems such as back pain, headache, symptoms from disease and even lack of sleep, can and do impact upon our emotional body, (our mind). Similarly, problems that originate in our mind, such as depression, fear, grief and countless other emotions can manifest themselves throughout the physical body in many ways such as headaches, digestive disorders, heart palpitations, hormonal imbalance and many more.

While you and I have inherently been aware of this connection for most of our lives, science is now catching up with what people have always suspected, that what we feel and how we think can and does effect the way our body functions physiologically. If you suffer from musculoskeletal disorders such as back pain, muscle pain and stiffness or even illness or disease that you and your health professional simply cannot get to the bottom of, don't ignore the possibility that your mind and in particular your emotions, may be influencing the situation more than what you imagine.

HOW DO YOU KNOW WHEN YOUR PAIN IS IN YOUR HEAD?

Figuring out the cause of our symptoms is always a challenge. It is like asking a dentist what the cause of somebody's tooth cavity is. Someone could ask if it was the soda pop, others may ask if it was the chocolate and both would be correct. The cause of the cavity is multi-factorial. We are always the most appropriate people to objectively look at our lives and determine what may be causing our suffering.

This is even more accurate when our physical pain has coincided with emotional events. The effect of a hard fall or impact are easy to measure. We see a bruise or lump when we fall, we may limp for a while after it and a fracture may even be visible on the x-ray. However, the consequence of emotional trauma is much more difficult to determine as only you can relate to the effect that traumatic events had on you. Breaking up with a partner may be traumatic for one person but a relief for somebody else. The death of a loved one who has been suffering whilst alive may be a relief for some people, whilst the unexpected passing of someone special in a car accident would be understandably more potentially devastating for somebody else.

There is no diagnostic medical equipment that can measure the degree of emotional trauma or the physiological effects it has over your body. There are many variables that determine how somebody deals with a traumatic event from gender, ethnicity, other psychological influences, the consequences of that trauma on somebody's life and the effect of previous emotional trauma on that person. As we are so genetically diverse, so too is the way that each of our minds deals with emotional trauma. As such, the physical effects of emotional trauma are also varied and so particular for each individual.

If you can relate the onset or worsening of your symptoms to an emotionally charged event, even though you may already be aware of others physical factors that could be at play, consider that event as an important contributing factor to your condition. If this is so, it is advisable to focus on this emotionally traumatic event, via therapy, mindfulness practices, yoga or a visit to a psychologist in the same way that you would consult a physical therapist or do physical activity to solve a physical problem.

Now let's imagine the case of somebody who has a physical condition such as osteoarthritis in the neck or a non-bio-mechanical problem such as psoriasis. The symptoms that these conditions provoke may lay dormant for a considerable period of time. Many people who have been diagnosed with these problems and many more can go months or years without feeling their effects. Until that one fine day when they experience an emotional event, which can once again bring the existence of those conditions to their attention. Other people report these same conditions becoming more apparent when they are angry or lose their temper. The pain experience can be profoundly influenced by emotional states. This can confuse many people who also notice that their pain may disappear whilst on holidays or during moments of emotional calm.

The way we choose to think and the thoughts that we feed our minds stimulate very real and measurable changes in our body, These changes can influence a variety of functions in our body, from heart rate and blood pressure to our levels of insulin and thyroid functions and of course to the way our body deals with the biochemical and physiological problems it already has.

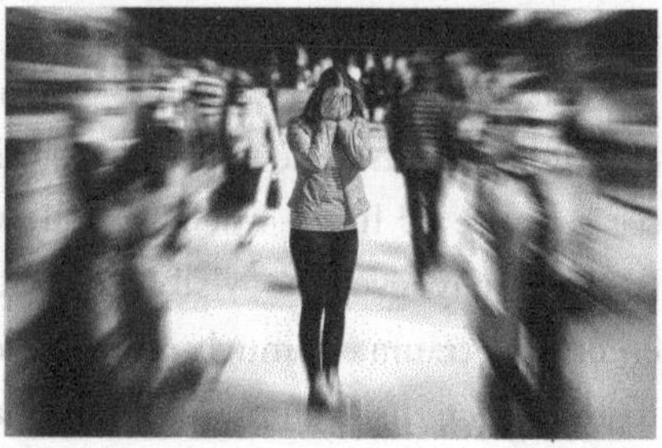

THE TRUTH ABOUT STRESS

Most of us would understandably associate stress with being negative. Our body's stress response was never intended to be harmful. Imagine our Neanderthal ancestors relaxing by a lake and suddenly confronted by a Sabre-toothed Tiger. Do you think that they would have had a fair chance of survival with their body and all their functions such as blood pressure, heart rate and insulin metabolism in relax mode? You guessed it; they wouldn't have lasted long! This would be considered acute stress and it involves rapid changes within your body that greatly increases its chances of survival in a threatening situation. Factors

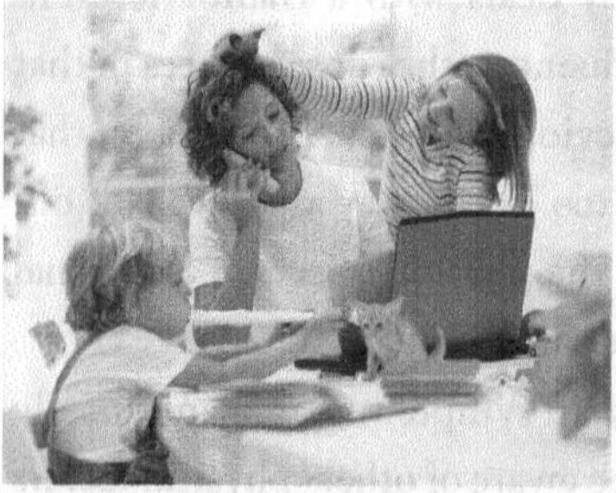

such as an increase in heart rate, blood pressure, muscle tension and respiration rate, enable us (and our ancestors when faced with the imminent attack of a prehistoric animal) to remove ourselves from potential danger as fast as possible.

At these times, other physiological conditions such as cognition (memory) and immunity are down regulated, because remembering a shopping list and fighting disease are not high on the list of the body's priorities. Insulin and cholesterol levels are also increased to evoke rapid utilization of glucose as a fuel and an increase in cholesterol to aid in clotting/blood coagulation (in case the Sabre-toothed Tiger removes a limb, the chances of survival will be greatly increase if blood loss is minimised via clotting).

However can you imagine what effect a continual elevation of these functions would have on our health? It would be extremely detrimental, and in reality the body does not deal with this situation very well, as continual increase in these markers, such as heart rate and blood pressure and hormones such as cortisol, cholesterol and insulin will greatly increase the likelihood of cardiac disease, hypertension, type 2 diabetes, obesity, depression and PAIN. These alterations occur when acute stress turns to chronic stress. When short-term bodily reactions to a near-miss in the traffic or a one off argument with a loved one, turn into day-in, day out traffic or somebody in a toxic relationship, turns into chronic stress.

Chronic stress can cause pain due to increased muscle tension and postural alterations which at the same time lower our body's resistance to pre-existing conditions that may otherwise be unnoticed if the person was not stressed!

CASE STUDY

Emily was a 42 year old CEO who had been suffering continual episodes of neck pain for more than 8 years. She worked late, slept late and struggled to follow a healthy diet. She had been to numerous health professionals over the years and had done everything from massage, acupuncture, taken medication to lower her high cortisol levels, chiropractic, physiotherapy and even psychotherapy. Nothing had given her long lasting relief. Even though her cervical spine (neck) had a small degree of degenerative osteoarthritis, I had seen thousands of other patients with more advanced arthritis that were asymptomatic.

When I asked her about the times of the day or week that her neck was more manageable, she said that she often woke up without pain on the weekends. We started to connect the dots and recognized that when she was stressed her pain increased. This 'Aha' moment that lead her to recognize the importance of bringing her holidays forward so that she could pass 2–3 weeks in a truly stress-free environment. She travelled to Greece and spent her holidays going to the beach, sleeping early, waking after 8–10 hours of restorative sleep and eating well. When she returned, she reported passing her holidays completely pain free.

Many people in this situation jump back into their routines and observe a speedy return of their symptoms. We talked about this and Emily agreed to work less, eat better and value her sleep. We also programmed regular mindfulness practices, such as yoga, breathwork and meditation to regulate the stress levels that a high-pressure job, such as hers, would obviously promote. She has now gone 5 years without a single episode of neck pain!

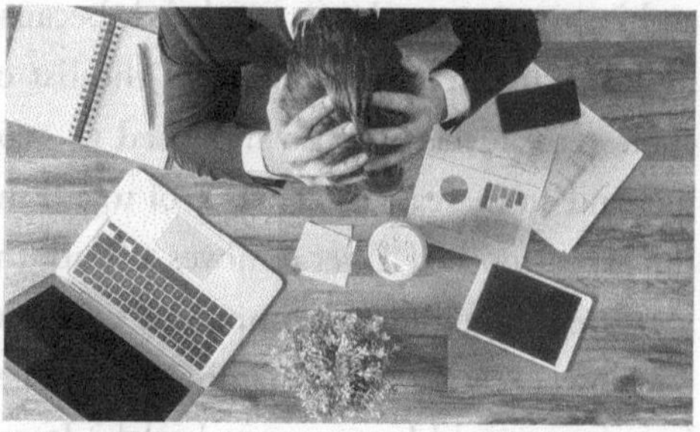

There is a comprehensive body of evidence focused on the connection between chronic stress and pain.

Being affected by stressful situations is obviously unavoidable, however we must endeavour to modify the factors in our environment that are stressful and also the way that we react to them.

CORTISOL AND STRESS

Cortisol is often referred to as our stress hormone as it is released by the adrenal glands when we perceive a threat to our wellbeing (known as a stressor). Cortisol triggers the 'flight or fight' response that an acute stressful situation evokes, this is perfectly normal and healthy as it allows us to remove ourselves from perceived threats. As mentioned, in these situations, changes to blood pressure and heart rate occur, stimulated by cortisol.

Cortisol also increases the body's metabolism of glucose, inhibits pain and reduces inflammation. Once again, this is when stress is acute and short lasting (think of how you feel straight after somebody frightens you). When stressors have a continuous, long lasting (chronic) effect on you, they also result in a continuous, long lasting stimulation of cortisol from your adrenal glands.

This is when stress (on a physiological level) becomes dangerous and can cause many negative changes to your health such as weight gain or loss, hypertension, continual fatigue, skin problems such as acne or fragile skin, and alteration of normal hormonal balance. Hormones work like the instruments of an orchestra. They rely on each other for normal function and if one falls out of sync then the others are almost always directly affected. This obviously affects every system in the body, as almost every cell of our body has cortisol receptors, and as such a myriad of health problems can result. Chronic elevation of cortisol also increases inflammation (the opposite effect of what acute stress evokes) and increased pain.[17]

Cortisol is also a key player in our circadian rhythm (our sleep cycle) and chronic elevation of cortisol causes insomnia. Every pathological process of the body that may be occurring, including those that cause pain and other symptoms, will therefore also be worsened with lack of sleep. Chronic stress sets up a vicious cycle that is much more prejudicial than simply losing your temper. With cortisol at the helm, stress is similar to an ocean liner that cannot change its direction easily once set on its course. The thoughts we allow our mind to occupy itself with determine whether we maintain that course or change it for calmer waters.

CASE STUDY

Isabel was a self-confessed stress-a-holic. She never stopped to analyse the effects that her anxious demeanour and tendency towards negative thoughts had on her life until she was physically stopped in her tracks by chronic headaches.

She visited me for a spinal examination to investigate a possible relationship to her headaches. None of my treatment resulted in any long lasting benefits for her. After a couple of weeks of worsening headaches, she burst into tears after one of her treatments. I asked her what was wrong, and she said that she had discovered that her ex-boyfriend was having a baby with the woman that he left Isabel for. It had been 3 years since the breakup and Isabel blamed him for 'ruining her life'.

When I dived a little deeper into the conversation and asked whether she had suffered headaches before the break-up she said that she hadn't. She said that she had worked with a therapist for most of this time and assumed that because her headaches hadn't improved, that they were unrelated to the emotional trauma she had experienced. This was an understandable assumption. I suggested she consult her GP and ask for a blood test. Her results showed that her cortisol levels were off the charts. Her doctor diagnosed her with adrenal fatigue, the adrenal glands were exhausted from the demands that her stress put on them for the production of cortisol. She also had high cholesterol and elevated insulin levels, which had elevated as expected with the elevation of cortisol.

Isabel got her life back on track. She took medication for a short period of time whilst starting meditation and regular walking. I also suggested seeing

17 'Cortisol level dysregulation and its prevalence – Is it nature's alarm clock?' C. Jones, C Gwenin – *Physiological Reports* 2021– Wiley Online Library.

a naturopath to aid in lowering her cortisol levels in a way that didn't depend on pharmaceuticals. She hadn't exercised for years so I suggested walking as it could be done at the pace that suited her.

Physically demanding exercise actually raises cortisol levels and holds them there, so we decided against jogging even though she used to be a marathon runner, as this would be one additional stressor. She continued with therapy and made a conscious effort to favour positive thoughts and emotions over dwelling over the trauma she had experienced.

Fortunately for Isabel, the intensity of her headaches decreased with the normalizing of her cortisol levels. After 4 months and considerable dedication to her health, Isabel was free of the agony that the headaches had been causing her.

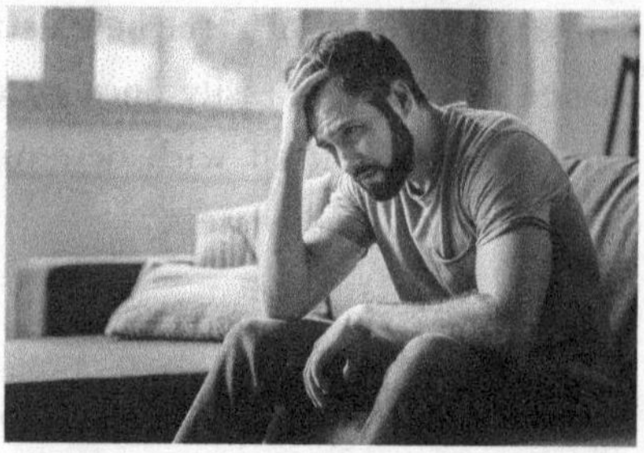

TIP – Look outside the box

If you have a recurring symptom or a disease that won't improve and have been doing the same thing to treat it for a long time (3–6 months) then look for other causes. Consult other specialists, do your own research and challenge what you've been advised to do if necessary. Never accept your symptoms as normal even though they are common in the general population, and always consider the possibility that two or more contributing factors are at play.

PAIN AND DEPRESSION – WHAT'S THE LINK?

Have you ever felt intense physical pain that lasted longer than a couple of weeks? If you have, you know that it gets you down, big time! It becomes difficult to remain positive, everything irritates you, restful sleep is a challenge and the joy of life is simply difficult to experience. Believe me, I know the feeling as I have passed months of excruciating pain that ended in spinal surgery. The link between pain and depression could be physiologically explained due to a shared neurological pathway.[18]

Our brain reacts to powerful physical stimuli via serotonin and hormones which also influence our mood. As previously discussed, hormonal imbalance can lower our sensitivity to pain which alone is enough to affect our level of happiness. Conversely, following the same rational, a person who suffers depression can (and does) complain of physical pain.

18 'Pain and Depression: a systematic review', WW IsHak, RY Wen, L Naghdechi, et al., *Harvard Review of Psychiatry*: 11/12 2018 Volume 26 issue 6, journals.lww.com

When somebody is depressed their drive/motivation for doing the everyday that most of us take for granted diminishes. They lose the drive to exercise, to maintain a healthy diet, to be disciplined with their sleep routine, libido and to spend time in nature (under the healing energy or the suns rays). If they are taking medication, a myriad of side effects including muscle aches and pains, fatigue and head aches can also complicate their will to do the actual activities and routines that their body needs to stay healthy and stay out of pain.

Early stages of depression can be difficult to diagnose, as a high percentage of people report only physical symptoms such as chronic joint pain, limb pain and back pain. This can make depression and hence, the origin of physical pain difficult to diagnose in many cases.[19]

In a review that analyzed a World Health Organization study of physical symptoms of that suffering depression showed that of 1146 patients in 14 countries that consulted a professional for depression, 69% reported only physical symptoms such as pain on their visit.

Now that the link between depression and one of its consequences, pain is clear, lets focus on its reverse relationship where pain can result in depression. According to *Medical Journal of Australia*[20], chronic pain is reported by 18.6% of Australian adults, remember that pain is considered to be chronic when it persists for 1 month or longer, often tissue halting or if it has been present for at least 3 of the previous 6 months[21].

Lets pause here to imagine how one day of being in pain feels. Imagine the activities that you cannot do, the ones that you enjoy and can only particularly execute, moments that give you joy and satisfaction. Like playing with your children, exercising, enjoying sexual relations, things that make you happy and make those people around you happy. Now imagine being in pain for a week, then a month. Think of the difficulty sleeping and the way that lack of sleep impacts upon your vitality. Walking, running, sitting and even thinking are just a few of the many aspects of daily life. It is no challenge to understand how pain can discourage, frighten, distress, demoralize and even depress the person who is suffering from it.

---

19 'Side effects of antidepressants: an overview', Elias A. Khawam, Georgia Laurencic, Donald Malone, *Journal of Current Drug Therapy*.

20 'Depression and chronic pain', Alex Holmes, Nicholas Christelis and Carolyn Arnold, *Med J Aust*, 2013.

21 'Chronic pain in Australia: a prevalence study', F M Blyth, L M March, A J Brnabic, L R Jorm, M Williamson, M J Cousins, *Pain* Jan 2001.

CASE STUDY

Mike was aware of back pain and the sciatica he had been suffering from for the last 8 years. He knew that it severely affected the quality of his life and the subsequent joy of living. He also recognized how it limited him from doing things in his life that were important to him such as physically participating in his young children's lives and maintaining the calibre of his relationship with his wife. It even affected his mood, leaving him with less patience with those that were close to him.

What Mike didn't know was that the effects of depression, were influencing his thoughts and behaviour. After chatting at our first consultation it was evident that Mike was fearful of trying to do everyday activities that he previously didn't even think about doing. His dialogue was generally negative, describing his anger and anxiety with being in this situation. He admitted to passing hours during the day cooped up in his room as 'there was nothing worth going outside for'. When I suggested that depression may be one more factor at play and that a strategy to combat it would be advisable, he initially scoffed at the idea. After a little more persuasion, he agreed to visiting his GP to 'check his health'. In a letter to his doctor, I detailed his case and suggested a full blood count plus hormones such as cortisol and insulin. After receiving the results and showing Mike how high his cortisol levels were he admitted that he may be suffering depression. His GP prescribed and anti-depressant and he visited a psychologist who had previously worked with many of my patients.

Working in a multi-disciplinary scenario, Mike progressively improved. He became more active, more conscious of the quality of his thoughts and his pain began to subside. The whole process took 6 months with considerable work done by myself and the other health professional involved.

TIP: If you feel that your physical pain or state of health are bringing you down emotionally, please consider the possibility that you are also suffering from depression and seek the most appropriate health professional accordingly.

According to the American Psychiatric Association – Depression is defined as a common and serious medical illness that negatively affects how you feel and the way you think.

Symptoms are varied and can include:

- Feeling sad or having a depressed mood
- Loss of interest in the activities that once brought joy to the person
- Changes in appetite and changes in normal body weight
- Difficulty sleeping

- Being excessively tired/fatigued
- Slow speech and movements
- Negative emotions such as feeling worthless or guilty
- Difficulty with concentration
- Suicidality.

Symptoms must be present for 2 weeks or more.

Dealing with any degree of depression that may be influencing you will help you enormously when it comes to:

- Dedicating yourself to do exercises and rehabilitation necessary to restore normal bio-mechanical function
- Improve the quality of your sleep. Sleep is arguably the most important factor in all illness and is absolutely vital for restoration of health, both physical and emotional
- Will override nociceptive (pain) pathways in your brain that are activated when depression starts
- Balance your hormones in favour of serotonin (your feel good hormone) which greatly inhibits pain pathways in the brain that are activated when depression starts
- Balance your hormones in favour of serotonin (your feel good hormone), which greatly inhibits pain pathways in the brain.

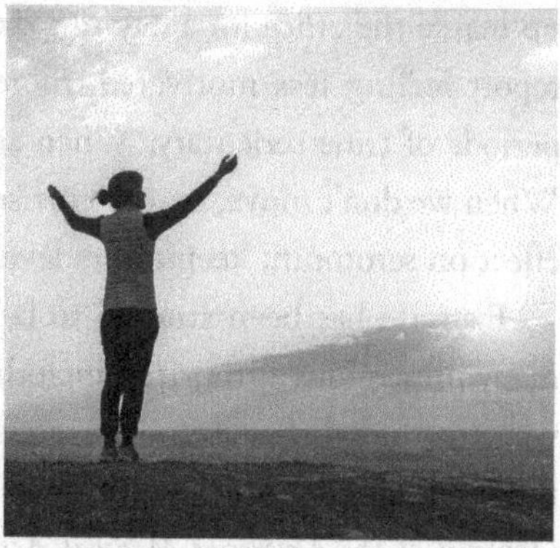

HOW TO REDUCE PHYSICAL SUFFERING AND LOWER THE EFFECTS OF DEPRESSION AT THE SAME TIME

The health of our mind and the quality of our thoughts is vital for the human body to be in a state of homeostasis. A positive mindset is beneficial in preventing a myriad of health problems. Conversely, a compromised mental and emotional state can severely impact on our health. In many ways. One of the more serious but often overlooked psychological problems is depression. Its impact and devastation on society cannot be overlooked. If you are suffering from depression or suspect that you may be showing signs of it do not hesitate to find the most appropriate support and health professionals to assist you in dealing with it. The factors that cause it are vast. The intensity that each person is affected by these factors and the way that they perceive them is extremely diverse between sufferers. For this reason effective treatment options are unique to each person.

Like all symptoms previously discussed in this book, pain and depression are symptoms that result from a lack of function (dysfunction) or more easily put, a lack of health. These interventions, while increasing the health of anybody practicing them have an especially potent effect on those who suffer pain and depression.

EXERCISE AND PHYSICAL ACTIVITY

This one is a no-brainer … *move!* Exercise increases the production of serotonin, our feel good hormone.

Stop for a minute to compare how you feel on a day where you are cooped up inside the office for a day to a day where you are moving. Most people will report feeling less motivated, more tired and unhappy when they pass long periods of time sedentary. When serotonin is increased, our mood improves! When we don't move, or, our cortisol levels actually rise, causing an inhibitory effect on serotonin, keeping its levels low.

Exercise has been studied to be an effective 'treatment' for depression by many prestigious authorities including the *American Journal of Sports Medicine*[22], who concluded that Aerobic exercise can produce substantial improvement in mood in patients with major depression disorders in a short time and *JAMA (Journal of the American Medical Association)* reported that an exercise training program may be considered an alternative to anti-depressants for treatment of depression in older persons. This is incredible as mainstream, traditional organizations such as both the American and Australian Medical Associations (AMA), are now recognizing that properly executed exercise programs can be an alternative to anti-depressants!

TIP: Intense exercise for prolonged periods (approximately 20 minutes or more) will increase cortisol levels. In other words, exercise becomes stressful (a stressor) and will be perceived as stressor by your body. The body's physiology will respond accordingly cortisol levels go up, serotonin levels go down and exercise will no longer be an effective tool to fight depression.

GET SOME SUN!

It is easy to underestimate just how vital sunlight is for life, not just human, but also the lives of plants and animals. Plants need it to generate energy through photosynthesis and animals will bask under its rays every day. Why would we humans be any different? The sun has been demonised in the last

22 'Benefits from aerobic exercise in patients with major depression: a pilot study', F Dimeo, M Bauer, I Varahram, G Proest, U Halter, *Br J Sports Med*, Apr 2001.

couple of decades and this has resulted in massive consequences on our health. While too much of anything is never a good thing, including the sun, our bodies require the right amount for optimal health.

Water is also a necessary requirement for optimal health, however water has not been utilized in the same way the sun has, even though too much water will negatively affect cell function and possibly death.

You don't need to be afraid of the sun. Rather, embrace it as a important factor in the maintenance of your health and if you do suffer from depression or pain, know that its beneficial effects have been studied and documented. A team of researchers from the Baker Research Institute in Melbourne Australia, found that the blood samples of 101 healthy men were compared with various weather factors (such as the amount of sunlight they were exposed to, temperature, rainfall and atmospheric), and showed that independent of what season the sample was taken the amount of serotonin produced the brain was affected by the amount of sunlight they were exposed to.[23]

As previously discussed, serotonin levels fall when people suffer depression and pain, so being able to influence serotonin levels naturally, without the intervention of pharmaceutical drugs is a game changer for breaking the pain/ depression cycle. Our happiness hormone, Serotonin also regulates level of our sleep hoormone, Melatonin. Melatonin , regulates day/night circadian rhythm and is necessary to induce sleep.[24]

CHECK YOUR VITAMIN D3 LEVELS

While low levels of Vit D3 have been related to a myriad of health problems the relationship with chronic pain and depression is undeniable and has been extensively documented. Vit D3 is vital for cell function, is anti-inflammatory and influences the immune and neuromuscular systems.[25]

---

23 'Effect of Sunlight and Season on Serotonin Turnover in the Brain', G.W. Lambert, C. Reid, D.M. Kaye, G.L. Jennings, M D Esler, *Lancet*, volume 360, Issue 934, 2002.

24 'Molecular Tools to Study Melatonin Pathways and Actions', J.A. Boutin, V. Audinot, G. Ferry, P. Delagrange, *Trends in Pharmacological Sciences,* Volume 26, 2005.

25 'Dietary Reference Intakes for Calcium and Vitamin', D. Ross AC, Taylor CL, Yaktine AL, Del Valle HB, editors. Institute of Medicine (US) Committee to Review Dietary Reference Intakes for Vitamin D and Calcium. Washington (DC): National Academies Press (US); 2011. PMID: 21796828.

THE IMPORTANCE OF SLEEP TO YOUR SPINE

UNDERSTANDING SLEEP

Our body possesses an innate intelligence that coordinates the function of every cell, tissue, and organ. Processes that are vital to our health and survival are coordinated by this intelligence in a way that obliges us to collaborate. Such processes include hunger, which reminds us to eat, and fever/malaise when we are sick, which guide us to rest. Sleep is another vital bodily process that is promoted by making us feel tired. It is that important to our health that it needs to occur every day and consumes between 25 to 30% of our life. Our health would surely suffer if something this important was neglected. And it does.

Sadly, 2/3 of adults in developed countries sleep less than the recommended eight hours of nightly sleep. When we consider just how many functions are reliant on a person sleeping those eight hours recommended by the World Health Organization (WHO), we can start to correlate how many problems that we suffer from with poor sleep. Sleep deprivation can be fatal and numerous experiments on animals over the years show this. While we sleep, our brain re-organizes neural networks and processes events that occur in our lives. It stores what's important in our memories and develops our emotional state. Not surprisingly, sleep disruption contributes to all of the principal psychiatric conditions including anxiety, depression, and suicidality. It affects our ability to learn and make logical decisions. The risk of suffering from Alzheimer's is increased if somebody is consistently having their sleep quality compromised. Sleep allows the cells of our body to reorganize, allowing new ones to regenerate and old, inefficient cells to be removed (apoptosis). The removal of these cells (senescent cells) is vital if we are to slow the effects of ageing. Poor sleep severely compromises our immune system's ability to function correctly, more than doubling a person's risk of cancer. It also plays havoc with blood sugar levels, increasing someone's chance of becoming diabetic. It increases the chance of blockage of the coronary arteries, thereby increasing the chance of cardiovascular disease and stroke. Insufficient sleep is stressful to our body and not surprisingly increases cortisol levels, which activate a cascade of negative psychological reactions including hormonal imbalance, increased inflammation, and more. The list goes on and on and when looking at it in this manner, it is easily recognized that receiving good quality sleep in sufficient doses is the most important factor determining whether we enjoy good quality health or not. Simply put, the less sleep you have, the less life you live.

Not surprisingly, poor quality sleep also strongly contributes to an aggravation of back pain on all levels.

The complexities of sleep can be broken down into a few fundamental concepts. Of course, there are many facets behind a healthy sleep pattern however the following are some of the most important ones.

SLEEP PRESSURE

Every waking minute of the day a chemical called ADENOSINE builds up in your brain. Quantities of adenosine become more and more concentrated the longer you are awake. As levels of adenosine increase your desire to sleep becomes greater and greater, and so the term 'sleep pressure' is used to describe it. It would come as no surprise to learn that caffeine blocks the receptors for adenosine uptake, thereby blocking its effects. This is why coffee can negate the desire to sleep. While we sleep, adenosine levels lower completely, starting to build again the following day after we wake up.

CIRCADIAN RHYTHM

Is a 24-hour sleep/wake cycle that makes up part of our body's internal clock. The brain is the master clock and ensures that certain physiological processes are stimulated and optimized at certain times within this 24-hour cycle. Understanding how sunrise, meal timing, exercise, your moods, core body temperature, and many hormones fit into this cycle enables us to 'hack' it and optimize your health. The body's 24-hour cycle also influences when you wake and when you sleep. Many sleep scientists, such as Dr. Matthew Walker, author of the book 'Why we sleep', believe that almost every living species adapted a Circadian Rhythm to synchronize themselves and their activities with the sun. Activities such as temperature regulation, feeding, exercise, and even social interactions can also be used to influence our circadian rhythm and 'reset' our biological clock. It is crucial for our health that this clock works around a 24-hour cycle. This 'clock' sits in the middle of the brain and is called the Suprachiasmatic Nucleus (SCN), located in the hypothalamus. Throughout the day, genes in the SCN send signals to coordinate processes in the body. Some of these processes and the times that they occur are noted below:

6 am – our cortisol levels rise. This wakes us up, increasing heart rate and glucose uptake in the brain. These processes promote the delivery of more blood, oxygen, and nutrients to the tissues and cells of the body, including the brain. We are now ready for the day!

From 6–11 am – our sex hormones peak, which will slowly diminish during the day, until they are replenished again that night during the REM sleep cycle.

2.30–5.30 pm – muscle coordination peaks, making this time a perfect time of the day to exercise when our body reaches its peak cardiovascular efficiency. Blood pressure and body temperature also peak at this time.

9–10 pm – the secretion of melatonin increases, stimulating sleep. This crucial process can be negated by emotional stress, working in front of the computer, or blue light from household lighting, computers, or smartphones.

11 pm – digestive processes decline in order to negate the need to wake up during the night to evacuate the bowels.

Midnight – the hormone Leptin enters the hypothalamus and releases fat reserves as well as stimulating the mitochondria of the cells to produce heat, meaning that they can burn fat. This is important because as we sleep our core body temperature falls and this fat uptake ensures that the lower body temperature will not affect mitochondrial function.

TEMPERATURE

The drop in core body temperature starts around bedtime and reaches its lowest point around 2 hours after sleep onset. The fall in body temperature helps to initiate sleep and is also coordinated by the SCN. A lower body temperature permits the repair of neurological tissue, reduces inflammation, and boosts immune function by increasing T cells (Killer Cells). This is why sleeping in a cooler environment is imperative for good quality, restorative sleep. Some people use devices such as the ChilliPAD to keep body temperature at this required lower range of temperature. Having a warm bath or shower before bed also helps as the core body temperature drops significantly after getting out. Avoiding an excessive covering of blankets and comforters also ensures that your body does not get too warm during the night. Many people are accustomed to sleeping too warm and this affects their health much more than what they would imagine.

CHRONOBIOLOGY

Even though we are all influenced by the 24-hour circadian cycle described above, each person possesses distinct moments of wakefulness and sleepiness during this cycle. They have a unique CHRONOTYPE that determines if they are 'morning types' or 'evening types'. The terminology 'early bird' and 'night owl' may be more familiar to you. If you are one of these types you will already understand what your chronotype is. If you are an 'early bird' you'll probably have your favourite time to go to bed and know that if you go to bed any later, you'll pay for it the following day. Similarly, if you are a 'night owl' you'll be accustomed to sleeping later and waking up at a certain time, and if you wake up earlier than this time you probably feel the effects during the day. Night owls may also struggle to fall asleep if they go to bed earlier than the time that their body is attuned to and stay awake for hours until that time comes around. These are patterns that are innate and distinct and not under voluntary control. 40% of the population are 'early birds' and 30% are 'night owls'. The rest of the population has varying times between these morning and evening types. Independently of the time that they go to bed, independently of what chronotype they are, they still require a minimum amount of sleep (usually 6 to 8 hours) to fulfil all of the body's physiological requirements. People who are night owls, contrary to the way that they may have been judged by many people, are not lazy. They go to bed later and therefore wake up later. It is extremely important to recognize this fact if your children are night owls and respect the time that the natural sleep cycle induces sleepiness and accordingly, the later times that they will wake. As society in general, is scheduled around early start times, especially schools and work, these children could be hugely disadvantaged, risking behavioural problems, learning difficulties, less than optimal levels of happiness, and even depression.

SLEEP STAGES

Believe it or not, during sleep, while our bodies are inactive our brain is far from it. The brain goes through phases that are repeated during the night, characterized by some stages where it is extremely active and others where it's completely inactive. Brain wave patterns measured by an EEG (electroencephalogram) recognize two types of sleep, each with distinct brainwave patterns. Rapid eye movement (REM) and non-rapid eye movement (NREM) reflect the activity of the brain while we sleep.

REM sleep is composed of Alpha and Beta brainwaves and involves movement of the eyes and a relaxed muscle tone. It is also where lucid dreams occur. REM sleep is repeated 4 to 5 times during the night, increasing in length as the night progresses. It occupies up to 25% of total sleep time. During REM sleep, brainwave activity almost exactly resembles wakefulness, with some regions of the brain being 30% more active. It's for this reason that REM sleep is also known as 'Paradoxical' sleep, where the brain is far from resting and the body is totally inactive. REM sleep is a time for processing information. Whether it be events from that day, memories, and emotions that are deemed to be important and worthy of storing or unimportant and therefore discarded.

In NREM sleep, those events that are deemed important are stored. For example, if you had received a speeding fine during the day, REM sleep may process that while remembering the actual act of receiving the fine from the police offer is not important, however remembering where and why it happened is. During NREM sleep this important fact would be stored for future reference.

NREM SLEEP IS COMPRISED OF THREE DISTINCT STAGES

N1 is the lightest sleep phase, characterized by the first sensation of drowsiness you feel when you are transitioning between wakefulness and sleep. Brainwaves slowly transition from Gamma and Beta frequencies to Alpha and Theta, which are slower.

Alpha brainwaves are indicative of more relaxed brain activity and are what people who meditate frequently strive to immerse themselves into. This is a state of presence and is extremely beneficial for people who are stressed and have higher cortisol levels due to their stress. In this chronic state, the brain allows cortisol levels to lower, taking the person from a sympathetic state towards a para-sympathetic, rest, and regeneration state.

Theta brainwaves are those that encourage creativity. Have you ever been falling asleep only to have ideas appear in your mind? Successful people say that you should always have a pen and paper handy to write those ideas down. This is a Theta brainwave state and is important in contributing to mental and emotional health. When stressed out or in chronic pain, our brain may not stay in this state for very long. N1 sleep doesn't last very long and represents about 5% of total sleep time. Those muscle twitches and sudden movements that you would've felt before occurring in this stage of sleep, just before you dip into the following deeper stages of sleep.

N2 is the second stage of NREM sleep and is predominantly Theta brainwaves. In this stage, short bursts of brainwaves occur to block out external stimuli such as outside noise, which helps ensure that vital sleep processes, such as memory processing, occurring without being distracted. Up to 50% of our sleep time is spent in this state.

The deepest state of sleep is N3 sleep, characterized by Delta or slow-wave sleep which occupies up to 20% of our sleep time. Consolidating events of the day, forming memories as well as processing information is what this stage is most important for.

It takes around 90 minutes to pass through all of the stages described above. To maintain our health and all of our body's processes occurring at the optimal levels, there should be 4 to 5 cycles within 24 hours. Some researchers claim that broken sleep at night may be complemented by a 'siesta' or short nap during the day which allows the brain to pass through these states. The longevity of many cultures is attributed partly to the habit of having an afternoon nap.

BACK PAIN AND SLEEP – WHAT IS THE CORRELATION?

Can you think of anything that isn't affected when you are suffering back pain? Anyone who has suffered will recognize that almost everything important in our life is affected when we suffer back pain. Sleep is one of the most affected things and as it is crucial for health, back pain for those who are suffering ends up being more than simply a problem for the back. It is for this reason that anybody suffering back pain must do whatever is necessary to encourage regenerative sleep, as this is also imperative for their back to heal. Good quality sleep also allows the body to stay on top of inflammation. Poor sleep increases inflammation which creates a vicious cycle and severely complicates healing. It's a double-edged sword, as the back pain sufferer must also improve the situation as soon as possible before it compromises their sleep any more than necessary. This will also increase the chance of suffering other health problems previously described.

So if you are one of those people in this catch 22 situations follow the following points to break this vicious cycle.

1. Sleep position – this is one circumstance where ignoring the rules for the correct sleeping position is OK. If sleeping on your belly (supported by cushions, etc.) is the only position that you receive relief from your pain, then sleep on your belly! It is common to be woken due to the pain when changing position while sleeping. If you have your 'go-to' position which has previously shown to give you relief, go back to that position after being woken so that you can jump back into your sleep.
2. Move! If you simply cannot feel a sufficient amount of relief from the pain to fall asleep, get out of bed and move. Walk around your house, support yourself against the wall and alternate lifting your knees or refer to the warm-up stretches earlier in the book. When your back pain subsides go back to bed, hopefully with less pain than before, and let your body fall asleep.
3. Breathe! Similarly, if the pain is impeding you from sleeping, go back to the breath. Following my breathing exercises which will help bring you back from a sympathetic nervous system state, which accentuates pain, to a parasympathetic state that naturally helps to calm the pain.

MEDICATION

Even if you are somebody who tries their best to avoid medication there are times that you simply have to bite the bullet and take it. When back pain is strong enough to compromise normal sleep it's time to consider taking a pain killer, anti-inflammatory, muscle relaxant, or a combination of these three. It can make a massive difference. By being out of pain and able to get into a restorative sleep state, you give your body the chance to rest, regenerate, and lower levels of inflammation. This can be a game-changer for those who are stuck in the visual cycle and have been suffering from poor sleep as a result of the pain.

AVOID ALCOHOL

Alcohol severely affects REM sleep quality. It is also inflammatory, as it opens up blood vessels and allows blood to rush to areas of the spine that may already be inflamed. Interestingly, many people that drink alcohol do it thinking that it may relieve the pain. This actually may happen temporarily however when any positive effects of alcohol have worn off the pain may come back stronger than what it was previously. Avoid alcohol at all costs during this time.

MATTRESS

A mattress that fails to provide support for the spine can cause serious back problems as well as contributing to poor sleep quality. If you already have back problems and difficulty with your sleep, an inadequate mattress can become the straw that breaks the camel's back (literally!), throwing the sufferer into a challenging situation. If you think that your mattress may be unsuitable for you, buy a new one. Refer to the following sections on mattresses and pillows to guide you towards one that is most apt for you. If this can't be done immediately, prepare blankets and comforters on the floor to provide sufficient, firm support for the spine. This tip is extremely effective so please don't underestimate the degree to which an incorrect mattress can affect both your sleep and back pain. Jump on the floor and give it a go.

HACKS TO IMPROVE SLEEP QUALITY

1. Avoid eating within three hours of going to bed. Make lunch your biggest meal and ensure that your evening meal is smaller. Eating a heavy meal too late increases blood glucose levels and consequently insulin. Growth hormone, which is released at night during sleep and is vital for the regeneration of cells and growth, is suppressed if insulin levels are high. This happens when we eat too close to bedtime. Eating late also increases core body temperature, which needs to be cooler to fall asleep and reach a

deep sleep state. Also, if your body is using energy to digest food it has less energy available for the regeneration of the cells that need special attention from the day's activities.

2. Favour foods that enhance sleep. Foods such as sardines, salmon and mackerel, avocados and nuts, coconut oil, and ghee are high in vitamin D3 and omega 3 fatty acids which help regulate serotonin.
3. Stay away from blue light. Blue light is emitted by computers, LED lights, Smartphones, and televisions. Blue light negatively affects the production of melatonin and makes the brain think that it is daytime. Use blue light blocking glasses if you are using the above-mentioned technologies. Turn off all electrical devices at least two hours before going to bed.
4. Make your room as dark as possible. Use blackout curtains to impede outside light coming in. Many electrical devices have lights that stay on permanently. It is for this reason that it is important to turn all electrical appliances off. If you need to get up during the night and go to the fridge, do your best not to look directly at the light as this will trick your body into thinking that it is time to wake up. Don't turn lights on if you go to the bathroom or walk around your home.
5. Put your phone onto Airplane Mode. Sleeping with your phone near your head has been shown to negatively affect brain function as we sleep.
6. Calm your mind – meditation before bedtime, breathwork, or reading under a dim light can help calm your mind after a busy eventful day. Our brain doesn't necessarily leave work matters at work when you get home and relies on you to calm it down, keep it present and set it up to focus on what's necessary at night time. Your conscious thoughts related to your day's activities may stimulate it too much and make getting to sleep more difficult.
7. Try high-tech technology such as BrainTap, which can stimulate your brain waves into deep restorative Delta waves. Alpha and Theta brainwaves can also be stimulated if you'd like to gain the benefits that they offer to your health.
8. Respect your Chronotype. If you are an early bird who is consistently sleeping later than you should, not only your sleep will suffer. Your health will too.
9. Use the right pillow. Most people aren't happy with a pillow that they are using however they usually don't know where to find one that supports their neck well enough to be comfortable and at the same time ergonomic. Many people are using pillows that are way too old and worn out. Just like shoes, pillows wear out and have a used date. Refer to the section on

pillows to find out how to choose the correct pillow for your body type and favoured sleeping position.

10. Supplements. As pharmaceutical medication for sleep can cause many side-effects (among these include dependency) it makes sense to use something natural first. Dozens of supplements and nutrients improve sleep quality, latency (the time it takes to fall asleep), and the amount of deep and REM sleep. Different nutrients and supplements work in different ways for each person.

While some people have huge success with melatonin, others may be kept awake by it. There are a few that are essential for good sleep such as Magnesium, Vitamin D3, and Zinc. Herbs such as Valerian, Chamomile, Hops as well as compounds such as 5 HTP can be extremely beneficial. 5 HTP for example is a precursor of serotonin. Many compounds, such as Tryptophan, which converts to 5 HTP in the body, are found in the foods we eat. Tryptophan is found in protein. B vitamins are also produced from Tryptophan, so taking certain B vitamins such as Niacin ensures that more Tryptophan is available to synthesize Serotonin. Melatonin levels also rely on a sufficient amount of Zinc in the diet to reach their optimum levels. It is important to look at your diet and what you are already taking in regards to supplements and determine what you may be lacking in or what may be beneficial for you. Many people are also getting great results from using CBD oil. Supplementation can make an incredible difference to somebody's sleep and is well worth considering for not only healthy sleep, but also our general health and longevity.

THE AUTHOR'S EXPERIENCE WITH EXTREME BACK PAIN

Life is full of ironies and my personal experience with disabling back pain is one of them. The weekend that I had reserved to review my book and prepare to hand it to the editor began with a big fall. As ridiculous as it sounds, I, the author of this book, was playing football barefoot on wet tiles. Not at all safe for your back, especially if you fall! I knew that it was not a good idea and had expressed my reservations, however a very energetic and enthusiastic 13-year-old boy convinced me otherwise.

Accidents happen so fast and before I knew it, I was lying on the ground, with excruciating pain in my lower back and unable to move. If you have ever been in a situation similar to this you will relate to that feeling of knowing that something serious has happened.

To cut a long story short, I spent the next three days lying down in intolerable pain with difficulty moving. It is not only a fall that can cause this, and I had seen so many patients with chronic problems or injuries at work or sport, but only when one goes through it can they really understand the severity of the pain.

I took advantage of the situation to review this book because I was unable to do anything else – while grateful to be able to perform this task even when immobilized. I did not take anti-inflammatories or painkillers. This wasn't because I didn't believe they could have helped me. On the contrary, they would have helped a lot, but I needed to take advantage of this situation and understand my patients, know what to do, what not to do, how to move, sleep, shower, etc.

Nobody can truly understand how disabling pain can be until they actually suffer from it. Pain intensity can be that intense and intolerable that it makes us fear that something very serious to our health is occurring, something that could be life-threatening.

I understand why many people who go through this experience for long enough would be willing to try any medication or would submit to any surgery that could offer them a release from this terrible situation.

Stop! Do not panic and remember that your brain intelligently caused this pain to protect you and prevent you from doing something that could possibly worsen the situation. At this time, your brain does not know if serious tissue damage has occurred or if the pain is from local inflammation resulting from the impact or trauma. As such, it does not want to risk allowing you to aggravate the situation until it knows that it is safe to do so. Reflex muscle spasm and debilitating pain are mechanisms that your brain uses to ensure this.

If you suffered a fall or other trauma, investigate the possibility of a fracture or other serious tissue damage via an X-ray or MRI (magnetic resonance image). If this is not the first crisis and you are already aware of a pre-existing problem, do not despair as stress and anxiety are likely to exacerbate the existing problem. If this is the first crisis, but you were already receiving warning signs (pain or stiffness) for some time, follow these steps, as you can safely assume that there is no need for an emergency X-ray or other diagnostic image.

1. Give your body a chance to heal itself without aggravating it. Rest and use ice (see following chapter). Do not underestimate the power of ice until you try it yourself. It's amazing how something so simple could help you so much in a situation like this, acting as an analgesic and anti-inflammatory at the same time.
2. In this state, even seemingly simple tasks such as drying the body after bathing, putting shoes on, or dressing yourself, can cause excruciating pain. This is because these actions overload the spine more than you would imagine. You have to think about every movement and action before trying to do it. This greatly decreases the stabbing pain that you will feel as you can brace yourself, focus on your breathing, and support your body in a way that will minimise the load on the affected area.
3. Ask for help. Asking someone close to you to help you do the chores, put your socks on or even help you bathe yourself will help you enormously, which will lower the risk of you aggravating your problem and delaying your recovery.
4. If you have a lower back problem, don't bend over or twist your spine. If you can't squat down flexing from the knees without causing pain, it is better just to wait until you can. This action overloads the lumbar intervertebral discs considerably as well as straining the intrinsic lower back muscles.
5. Sitting will generally aggravate lower back pain whilst in crisis. Unfortunately, you will need to sit to perform some activities like eating or traveling in a car so follow these rules. Keep your buttocks in contact with the backrest and your spine upright. When you eat, bring the chair as close as possible to the table. If it hurts too much, ask someone for help or, using the strength in your arms, pull the table towards where you are sitting (if it is light). Do not sit for more than 20 minutes at any given

time. Do not sit on sofas as they do not offer the necessary support.

6. Sneezing will increase your pain when you have a fracture or acute disc inflammation, so stay away from pets or other factors that may irritate any allergies that you may have.
7. In this practically immobilized crisis state it is normal for your metabolism to slow down as you will not be moving as much as what you are usually accustomed to. You will be more prone to suffer from constipation. Defecation can be an extremely painful activity because the abdominal force you use can highly irritate your spine, especially your lower back. Avoid foods that clog you up, such as white flour products (bread, pizza, cakes, etc.). Favour foods and drinks that will encourage a normal stool such as drinking sufficient amounts of water and juice that you may already know to be beneficial for you if you have previously suffered constipation. Beetroot and paw paw juice works for many people.
8. If you can, avoid traveling by car. This was the most painful and aggravating activity that I did when I was in crisis. It was agony, particularly when I was getting myself into and out off the car. If you do have to travel in a car, obviously get somebody else to drive. Use the strength of your hands and arms to get you in and out of the car. Activate your core before entering or leaving by contracting your abdominal muscles to take some of the load off the lumbar spine. To get into the car, open the door, face away from the car, and gently lower yourself onto the seat, then move both legs at the same time into the car. To get out of the car, repeat this in the opposite order, moving your legs from the seat to facing outside of the vehicle then slowly lift yourself, while the core is activated. Use the car and any props for support. Receiving help from somebody at this time can actually increase the pain because the person does not know when and what positions are aggravating your pain. For many people, the car is one of the first obstacles faced after spending time at home resting, usually to go to the doctor or hospital. Prepare yourself for the trip. Put ice on the affected area first and walk at least 10 minutes to loosen the tight muscles and joints which have been immobile during this time of recovery. Do not drive! You may be able to enter the car in a position to drive, but even a slight movement or position change could cause tremendous pain, increasing the risk of exacerbating the tissue damage. If there is nobody to take you where you need to go, call a cab and follow the rules detailed above!
9. When resting, always lie in the position that gives the most relief, or makes you as comfortable as possible. If on your back, bend your legs and put a pillow under your knees. If you feel more comfortable on your side,

put a pillow between your knees. This will remove a bit of the load on your lumbar spine. For neck problems, a brace may help in severe cases, especially when moving the neck causes pain. This is one of the only times that I recommend the use of a brace, as the neck needs to move, even in crisis, and the brace impedes this from happening. Use a brace when you have pain or tingling down your arm or arms and get an MRI taken as soon as possible to study the state of the discs and nerve roots.

10. Walk as soon as you can. When I was in crisis, I spent three days lying, only getting up to go to the bathroom or to eat, but on the third day, I walked for 40 minutes. In the beginning, it hurt like crazy and I questioned whether this rationale was sensible or not. I found however that the intense pain slowly subsided as I walked. When walking on the street, make sure that you clearly look where you are putting your feet. Any irregular surface that causes you to recruit sore muscles from your back will cause more pain. Step with one foot first and then shift your weight onto it, whilst moving the other foot forward. You must think about each step if you want to avoid that electrical shock-type pain that an incorrect step or irregular surface will cause. When crossing the street to the footpath, lift one foot first, transfer your weight to it and then lift the other. Do not place excessive weight on one foot. Take small steps to distribute the weight evenly and allow both feet to take similar loads.
11. Avoid going to events such as meetings, parties, etc., if you are not sure whether you will need to be standing for long periods. If for some reason you do find yourself in such a situation, walk slowly and shift your weight from one foot to another whilst standing.

Following this routine will help you to deal with your moment in crisis better. Lie down for 20 minutes on the floor or in a resting position for the neck (when the problem is in the neck), ice the area for 20 minutes, and walk for 20 minutes (in the case of the neck, follow the video on simple neck exercises in the following chapter). Repeat this procedure all day if you have to. Your spine is inflamed and needs to be rested so that it can recover. Do not lose faith! Do not panic, stay strong and determined. Follow the rules and you'll get out of this crisis. Remember that your body is in crisis to protect you.

When the crisis begins to pass, do not get carried away! Do not forget that more than likely the original problem is still present. Go slowly, do not push yourself, avoid sudden movements, and, if you have not yet investigated the cause, do it now!

The fall that caused my crisis was due to carelessness and resulted in a fracture of the L3 (lumbar) transverse process. It is a fracture that is painful but luckily without serious consequences after the 6 weeks of healing has occurred.

The fall also damaged other areas of my spine; however, the lower back problems were more serious. In these cases the brain often highlights the most serious problem via pain etc. while leaving other areas often asymptomatic until the original, more serious problem has started to heal. I only became aware of the other problems when I started to become more mobile. Moral of the story: after a trauma or accident, don't forget that just because you don't feel pain at the time of the accident, it doesn't mean that nothing happened, especially when other areas have been injured.

The bitter-sweet irony of my fall was that it allowed me to test firsthand much of what I had learned from my patients in over two decades of work with them. We learn so much when we are in crisis. The idea is that we remember the lessons as they are often warning signs of a future that may be waiting with more intense and more frequent pain. A future that impedes us from enjoying our life to the fullest.

Painful neck crises are scary. Pain can be intense and can radiate down the arm to the fingers and can be aggravated by even the slightest of movements in the neck. You must remember that this is a warning sign from your brain that there is a real risk of damage to the delicate nervous system, principally the spinal cord or nerve roots that exit between each vertebra. Something that you have done once or repeated/maintained many times has inflamed these nerve roots and as a result, your brain has put your neck into lockdown. Literally. There are many things that you must do at this moment.

1. Don't aggravate it more by continuing with the activity that caused it. Such activities commonly include poor posture such as lying down on the couch using the armrest as a pillow, sleeping on your belly, looking down at a smartphone or laptop for extended periods of time, or working in this same posture (think hairdressers and dentists). Identify what caused the problem ASAP and avoid it at all costs.
2. Taking an anti-inflammatory can be vital as it removes the inflammation from the nerve root. If you feel relief, please don't think that your problem has been solved. It hasn't. You must now get your neck examined and have its function restored by a spinal health specialist that you trust. One that focuses on the restoration of bio-mechanical function as opposed to one that will simply focus on pain relief.
3. Rotate between ICE, REST, and very minimal movements. Some of the exercises detailed in the exercise section will be beneficial. Make sure that they do not exacerbate your pain when you do them.

4. Use a neck brace *only* if you cannot otherwise avoid aggravating the pain and if you have sharp radicular pain down your arm or shoulder. Using a brace for too long will weaken the muscles of your neck and make it harder for you when you want to stop using one, as these muscles will not be capable of supporting your neck the way they were before using the brace.

Stay persistent with these rules, introduce movement a little more every day, find a good professional who focuses on the restoration of function and on what actually caused the crisis, and good luck!

HOT OR COLD?

When a biological tissue is overloaded or damaged enough to impair its normal function, our body triggers an unconscious reflex. This process is called inflammation and occurs to aid the healing of damaged tissues. Local blood flow increases to bring nutrients to the muscles and other tissues, and remove any toxins that may impede healing.

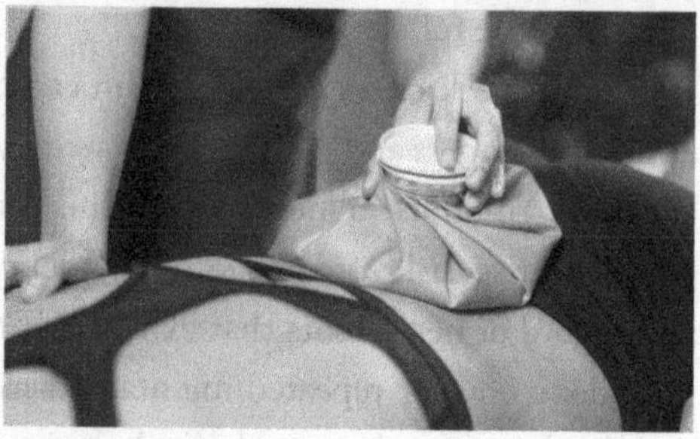

The increase in blood flow gives a heightened red colour to the area. This area is also warmer since there is more blood and blood is warm. Other symptoms include pain, heightened sensitivity, numbness, or tingling (paresthesia). Remember that inflammation is a positive response to tissue damage and is a normal part of the healing process, especially when it is acute (a recent injury).

Applying heat at this time, via a hot shower or a hot water bottle, an ointment, or infra-red heat lamps can actually worsen the inflammation and increase the level of discomfort. This strategy is successful when a problem has become chronic as heat is more effective at relaxing tight muscles and relieving achy joints.

ICE

Ice should always be applied in these situations because it is an anti-inflammatory and natural analgesic, i.e., it helps reduce swelling and reduces blood flow, reducing inflammation and helping to relieve the pain.

The application of ice should occur as follows:

- 20 minutes with ice;

- 20 minutes without ice;
- 20 minutes with ice;
- 1 hour without ice;
- 20 minutes every hour after that.

Be careful not to leave the ice applied for longer than 20 minutes, as this will cause vasodilation and a subsequent increase in inflammation.

The ice can be placed inside a slightly damp cloth or gauze or it can be used as a gel compress. Don't use frozen veggies as they will thaw fast and be ineffective.

The initial feeling, just after applying ice, is unpleasant. It can even feel like it is burning. It isn't. You simply aren't used to the sensation and, if wrapped in a wet towel, it will not burn you. Don't let this feeling discourage you.

Do not forget that this strategy serves only to lower the inflammation and to reduce the pain momentarily, and the cause must always be detected as soon as possible. The activity that aggravates the condition should also be avoided while the problem is being rectified.

In the spine, regions that tend to inflame and require ice are: the neck (especially when it is referring pain or pins and needles down the arms to the hands and fingers), dorsal spine (especially when a rib is subluxated, sometimes causing severe pain radiating to the chest, arms or shoulders) and lumbar spine, sacroiliac and piriformis muscle in the buttocks (which often radiates sciatic pain to the leg). If the episode is traumatic, an appointment with your chosen spinal practitioner should be made as soon as possible to restore normal function to the joint.

Heat should never be applied while the lesion is in its acute phase, i.e., the first day of inflammation and up to six weeks after, depending on the region of the body affected.

When the lesion enters a semi chronic or chronic phase, the application of heat can be helpful. At this time, you can alternate between ice and heat. If you are not sure what stage the trauma is in, do not use heat until it is advised by a health professional.

HEAT

The effect of heat on blood vessels is converse to that of cold. It stimulates the dilation of blood vessels, allowing more blood to enter, increasing blood flow, and allowing the region to be nourished.

In the case of chronically contracted muscle, blood flow decreases, and, consequently, nutrients and biological factors that are required to relax the

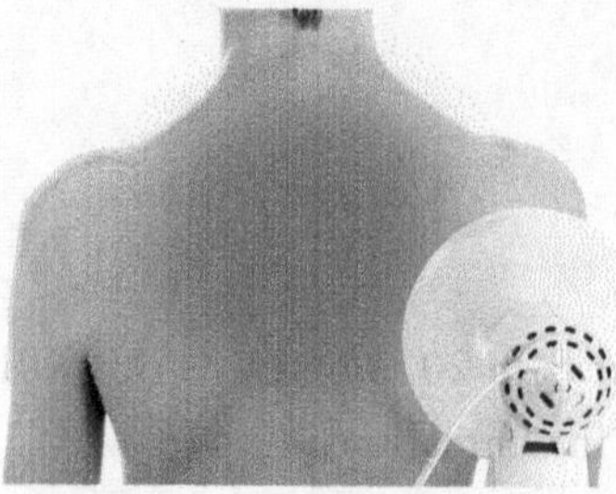

contracture cannot reach the affected muscle. A vicious circle begins and this can result in a muscle being dysfunctional for many years.

The use of heat in this case quickly helps, relaxing the spasm and greatly reducing the pain. However, just as ice is not the solution by itself, neither is the use of heat. It should be used as a way to facilitate healing and act as an adjunct to any corrective treatment that you are doing to rectify the primary problem, the one that caused the contracture in the first place.

You can apply heat in the following ways:

- A heating pad that is heated in a microwave – A sports gel or liniment
- An infra-red lamp

WHEN SHOULD YOU SEEK URGENT MEDICAL ATTENTION?

Back pain and other spinal-related symptoms are warnings signs of problems that usually do not represent an immediate danger. They can, however, occasionally be warning signs that something more serious is occurring. This includes processes such as tumours, infections, or diseases in other regions of the body. Please seek urgent medical attention if one or more of these signs is present:

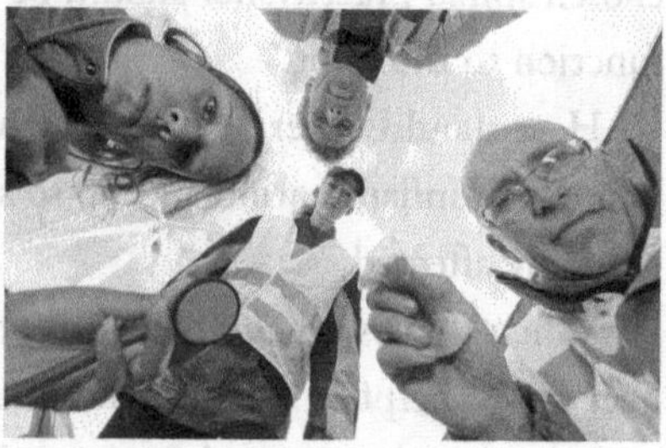

- Fever
- Sudden and severe pain that appears for no obvious reason
- Pain that awakens you in the night
- Pain coinciding with notable, unexplainable weight loss
- Severe headache accompanied by sudden severe neck pain when flexing the neck (looking down)
- Unexplained loss of consciousness
- Loss of control of bladder, bowel, or sexual function.

Once again, your symptoms are more than likely not serious. That said, it is always best to be on the safe side, investigate what is happening and why, before devising a sensible strategy for restoring function and health to your body.

CONCLUSION

We usually don't wait until it's too late to start taking care of our car, bicycle or anything else in our lives that is of value to us. Sadly however, our spine commonly is not one of the assets that receives this type of attention before it gives painful signals that there is something wrong. I have worked with spinal problems and associated symptoms for nearly 30 years. I feel a tremendous sadness every time I see an elderly patient for the first time and discover advanced degeneration in their spine. The degeneration that could have easily have been avoided if they were aware of how to care for their spine appropriately. I have seen no particular economic class, gender, nationality or occupation that suffered more than any other. People often report doing heavy physical work on farms, sitting at desks, lifting up heavy loads and a myriad of other actions that compromise spinal function. Many of these people passed years and decades with these asymptomatic problems only to realise, when their spine eventually advised them that there was a problem, that their level of comfort and/or mobility would never be the same again. Pain and symptoms are such important signals that should never be ignored. If only they received an instruction manual on how to use their spine before spinal dysfunction occurred. As pain is the parameter for most of us, we understandably only think about a problem when the warning light is flashing. While putting oil or fuel into a car's engine is enough to turn its warning light off, unfortunately for many people the pain will be permanent as the underlying problem has reached the stage of degeneration that cannot be reversed. Even if they do turn to painkillers to help relieve them of the pain, they are soon reminded of the underlying problem as soon as the painkillers wear off.

From my personal experience, do all you can to avoid spinal problems in the future and the debilitating symptoms that come with it. Please learn how to use your spine and care for it in the same way that you care for anything else in your life that is important. Quite likely your spine is much more important to you than what you realise. Stop to think of all of the important things in your life. Your relationship with spouse and family, your friends, the exercise that you practice and maybe even your work. Now think how each of these important aspects would be if you lived with permanent back pain. Without feeling pain it is understandably easy to overlook the importance of spinal care.

But I guarantee you there are factors in your life that are compromising the correct function of your spine. If you know that your posture is incorrect, the technique that you use to lift a box is wrong or even the fact that you sleep face down, is detrimental and that one-day will cause you grief, why wait until then to do something about it? There are no lack of people in the world with chronic problems to tell you firsthand that they wish they had done something about their problem earlier. This also applies to our diet, the food we eat, the liquids we drink, the thoughts we have, our quality of sleep and so many other factors. Use your pain and other symptoms as an alert guiding you towards an underlying cause. And a cause that when rectified will help you avoid a decrease in the quality of life that you enjoy today. If you do suffer back pain have the confidence that by following the basic little rules outlined in his book and by being empowered by the knowledge on how to use your spine correctly, that you can revert your situation. You cannot only live a pain-free life you can also be more mobile, active and emotionally fulfilled than ever. In the course of my 30 year career I have seen countless people turn their lives around to have lives that allow them to do things that they never dreamt were possible. And what is even more encouraging is to know that the modifications involved to turn their lives around were usually simple. They implemented basic principles. Principles that we should all learn, especially when we recognise just how important our spine is to our happiness and our health.

Good luck on your journey and know that when it comes to spinal care, knowledge is paramount.

> *"There where the pain resides is what can save you."*
> FREIDRICH HÖLDERLIN